B. M. Czarnetzki · Urticaria

Beate M. Czarnetzki

Urticaria

With 40 Color
and 21 Black-and-White Figures

Springer-Verlag
Berlin Heidelberg New York Tokyo

Professor B. M. Czarnetzki, M. D.
Department of Dermatology School of Medicine
University of Münster
Von-Esmarch-Str. 56
D-4400 Münster

ISBN-13: 978-3-642-70315-7 e-ISBN-13: 978-3-642-70313-3
DOI: 10.1007/978-3-642-70313-3

Library of Congress Cataloging in Publication Data
Czarnetzki, Beate M.: Urticaria / B. M. Czarnetzki. –
Berlin; Heidelberg; New York; Tokyo: Springer, 1986.

Softcover reprint of the hardcover 1st edition 1986

Product Liability: The publisher can give no guarantee for information about drug dosage and application thereof contained in this book. In every individual case the respective user must check its accuracy by consulting other pharmaceutical literature.

Typesetting, printing and binding: K. Triltsch, Würzburg
2329/3321-543210

Table of Contents

Abbreviations

Ab	antibody
ACTH	adrenocorticotrophic hormone
ADCC	antibody dependent cellular cytotoxicity
Ag	antigen
AGEPC	acetyl glyceryl ether phosphorylcholine
ANA	antinuclear antibody
Aqu. U.	aquagenic urticaria
ATP	adenosine triphosphate
BHA	butylated hydroxyanisole
BHT	butyrylhydroxytoluol
BK	bradykinin
BSP	bromosulfophthalein
C	complement
Ca	calcium
cAMP	cyclic adenosine 3′,5′-phosphoric acid
CG	cysteinyl-glycinase
cGMP	cyclic guanosine 3′,5′-phosphoric acid
chol u	cholinergic urticaria
chr u	chronic urticaria
CNS	central nervous system
co	cyclooxygenase
Con A	concanavalin A
CT	connective tissue
CU	cold urticaria
d	dalton
DMSO	dimethyl sulfoxide
DS	dextran sulfate
DSCG	disodiumcromoglycate
DU	dermographic urticaria
$EAC1\bar{s}$	a complex of erythrocytes, antibodies against erythrocytes and $C1\bar{s}$
EACA	epsilon-aminocaproic acid
ECF(A)	eosinophil chemotactic factor (of anaphylaxis)
ESR	erythrocyte sedimentation rate
GGTP	γ-glutamyl transpeptidase
GI	gastrointestinal
h	hour
HETE	hydroxyeicosatetraenoic acid
HF	Hageman-factor
HHT	hydroxyheptadecatrienoic acid
H MW	high molecular weight
HPETE	hydroperoxyeicosatetraenoic acid
5-HT	5-hydroxytryptamine
HU	heat urticaria
IC	immune complex
IFA	inflammatory factor of anaphylaxis
Ig	immunoglobulin
kd	kilodalton
LIF	leukocyte migration inhibiting factor
L/M	lymphocyte/macrophage
LO	lipoxygenase
LPS	lipopolysaccharide
LT	leukotriene
lys enzyme	lysosomal enzyme
MC	mast cell
MIF	migration inhibiting factor
MLC	mixed lymphocyte culture
min	minute(s)
neg	negative
NK	natural killer (assay)
NSAID	nonsteroidal antiinflammatory drugs
NT	neurotransmitter
OPT	oral provocation test
P	properdin
PAF	platelet activating factor
PG	prostaglandin
PLA_2	phospholipase A_2
pos	positive
PTA	plasma thrombin activator
PU	pressure urticaria
PUPPP	pruritic urticarial papules and plaques of pregnancy
PUVA	psoralen-UVA combination therapy
RA	rheumatoid arthritis factor
RAST	radioallergosorbens test
RBC	red blood cells
RIST	radioimmunosorbens test

s	second
SLE	systemic lupus erythematosus
SRS	slow reacting substance(s)
ST	skin test
TX	thromboxane
UV	ultraviolet light
zy	zymosan

Preface

Urticaria is a vexing problem, to the patient who suffers from the annoying pruritus and the fear of life-threatening reactions, to the physician who faces the challenge to find the cause of the eruption and to control the symptomatology, and to the scientist who is asked to explain the process that elicits tissue swelling at the cellular and molecular levels.

The last thorough treatise on urticaria was the superb monograph by R.P. Warin and R.H. Champion, published more than a decade ago. Since then, there have been major advances in the field. This holds particularly for the clinical aspects of anaphylactoid reactions, the urticarial vasculitis syndrome, and the understanding of the pathogenesis of all major types of urticaria. Progress has become possible through new insights into the biology of mast cells and basophils and through the study of mediators of acute allergic reactions of which one type, the leukotrienes, have only very recently been discovered.

This book is meant to provide an in-depth review of all major basic and clinical aspects of urticaria. It is intended to serve as a reference for clinicians who are confronted with diagnostic and therapeutic problems and as a source of information for scientists about the state of our current understanding of the pathogenesis of urticaria. Hopefully on this basis, researchers can progress in their endeavor to unravel the many unknown factors in the pathogenesis of the broad spectrum of diseases with urticarial reactions.

Seneca once said that a long way is made short and efficient through guidance and example. The list of teachers who have stimulated my interest and helped me to understand the basic and clinical aspects of mast cell-related problems is long. I would like to specifically mention J.N. Fink during medical school training in Milwaukee, J.R. Pomeranz and R.W. Belcher during dermatology residency in Cleveland, L.M. Lichtenstein and P. Norman during a research fellowship at the Department of Clinical Immunology and Allergy at Johns Hopkins University in Baltimore, and E. Macher at the University Clinics in Münster where much of what I have learned in the past could be broadened through further basic research and clinical experience.

My thanks go also to all the following friends and colleagues who have critically reviewed parts of this book: P.J. Frosch, Heidelberg; G. Goerz, Düsseldorf; H. Kästner, J. Knop and E. Macher, Münster; E. Kownatzki, Freiburg; M. Loos, Mainz; H. Merck, Cologne; W. Opferkuch, Bochum; J. Ring, Munich; H. Schadewaldt, Düsseldorf; W. Sterry, Kiel; G. Stingl, Vienna; V. Voigtländer, Mannheim; R.P. Warin, Bristol; H.H. Wolff, Lübeck.

The book could never have been finished without the untiring, enthusiastic help of Ms M. v. Lovenberg and Ms K. Staigis who did the typing even during their free time, and of Ms J. Bückmann and Mr. P. Wissel who did the photographic work. Finally, a word of appreciation should go to those closest to me who patiently and generously shared with me many trying months of reading and writing.

Münster, February 1985

1 History of Urticaria

1.1 Indroduction

The history of urticaria represents a fascinating account of man's gradually increasing understanding of medicine as such, and of the unique clinical features of the pathomechanisms of urticaria in particular. Over many centuries, the prevailing view of medical thinking on the cause of diseases has led to the evolution of theories that were to explain also the causes of urticaria and its possible treatment. The following pages give a very brief account of these theories and developments, since they form the background on which our current knowledge and our search for a better understanding of urticaria is based.

1.2 Nomenclature

Many different names have been applied to urticaria during the past centuries. They are well worth reviewing since they mirror the thinking of each particular period on the most prominent clinical and pathogenetic aspects of the disease (Table 1.1).

The School of Hippocrates (4th century B.C.) associated urticaria with *nettles* and insect bites. The name nettles appears frequently thereafter in several languages, up until the middle of the last century. At that time, Alibert introduced the name "knidosis" which was in use until the beginning of the 20th century.

Table 1.1. Different names applied to the urticarial eruption in the course of time.

Names	Source
Uredo	Plinius, 1st cent.
Essera (Arabic: elevation)	Hali Ben Abbas, 10th cent.
Nesselsucht (German: nettle-rash)	Valentini, 1690
Nettle rash	Hartford, 1740
Urticatio (*urere*, Latin: to burn)	Zedler, 1740
Randados (Spanish: nettles)	Cleghorn, 1751
Morbus porcinus (pig's disease)	Astruc, 1759
Morbus porcellaneus (porcelain disease)	Astruc, 1759
Scarlatina urticaria	Sauvages, 1763
Urticaria	Frank, 1792
Knidosis (*knide:* Greek: nettle)	Alibert, 1833

The sensation of burning at sites of wheals received special attention in the writing of the Roman school, and Plinius first applied the name *uredo* to the disease. The burning sensation (*urere* = burning) became again the focus of attention when Zedler called the disease *urticatio* in the 18th century. At the end of the same century, Frank referred to the disease as *urticaria*, a name which has remained valid until today (Schadewaldt 1981a).

A few additional names have been in use for the disease (Table 1.1). Hali Ben Abbas, in the 10th century, coined the name *essera*, meaning mountain or elevation (Schadewaldt 1981a), in allusion to the slightly raised nature of the wheal above skin level. This name persisted in the medical literature until the end of the last century. The name *Morbus porcellaneus* alluded to the porcelain-white color of the central wheal, while the name *Morbus porcinus* is in no way related to the symptomatology, but may have come into the medical literature through a misspelling of the word porcelaine by a transcriber of books (Schadewaldt 1981a).

1.3 Pathogenetic Theories (Table 1.2)

From the time that Hippocrates noted an association between urticaria, nettles, and insect bites, it took many centuries until the concept arose that food (strawberries, shellfish, etc.) might also cause urticaria (16th century). At about the same time, Libavius was the first author to clearly identify the major clinical aspects of urticaria: (1) sudden onset, (2) elevation (tumor), (3) redness (rubor), (4) itching (pruritus), and

Table 1.2. Theories on the etiology of urticaria.

Theory	Source
Idiosyncratic theory	Behrens, 1700
Humoral theory	Chemniz, 1703
Theory of sympathies	2nd half, 18th cent.
Toxin theory	Chalmers, 1776
Nervous theory	Eulenburg, 1867
Meteorological theory	Frank, 1823
Menstrual theory	Mosler, 1864
Microthrombosis theory	Philipson, 1899
Theory of inflammation	Török, 1903
Allergic theory	Joltrain, 1930

(5) evanescence (cessante per aliquot dies) (Schadewaldt 1981 a). The description of these features formed the basis for a number of theories on the cause of the disease. The importance of this clinical description is all the more apparent since Sydenham (1624–1689) still considered nettle fever a part of erysipelas.

In the 18th century, Behrens (who suffered himself from allergy to seafood), argued rightly that an *idiosyncracy* of the patient was responsible for the urticarial reactions since not everyone who ingested the same food reacted to it with urtication. Chemniz (1703) proposed his *humoral theory* at about the same time, explaining the waxing and waning of the wheals as part of the local inhibition of the flow of the fluids or humors (*stasis theory*). The *theory of sympathies* was fashionable during the course of the 18th century since it offered an explanation for the association between the stomach (ingestion of strawberries) and the skin (urticae).

At about the same time, Chalmers proposed the *toxin theory* which was still discussed by the American dermatologist Gilchrist in 1908. Toxins were considered to be present within the food, such as in shells, or the food was thought to be transformed by the body into a toxic agent. The toxins would induce *local stasis* and urtication.

Eulenburg, a protagonist of the *nervous theory*, suggested that certain substances in food affect the nervous system in predisposed persons. Thus, his theory also incorporated the idiosyncratic theory.

At the turn of the present century, the *angioneurotic theory* which had been part of the nervous theory of Eulenburg (1867), was expanded by Neisser (1901) who considered urticaria a *secretory neurosis with vasodilatation*.

Three other theories of the last century are worth mentioning, mostly for the sake of curiosity:

1) The *metereological theory* of Frank (1823) suggests that allergy is determined by the constellation under which a person is born. In a recent international allergy meeting, this theory was reconsidered in so far as the incidence of allergic rhinitis seems to be higher in persons who are born in certain months of the year.

2) The *menstrual theory* (1864) was based on an observation which holds even today, that some female urticaria patients suffer from a hypersensitivity to their own endogenous hormones (see Chapter 3, p. 42).

3) *The microthrombosis* theory by Philipson (1899) represents a fascinating attempt to explain the migrating nature of the wheals through microthromboses. Philipson rejected the angioneurotic theory by showing that urticae can develop in denervated regions of the body (for details see Schadewaldt 1981 a).

At the start of the 20th century, *the theory of inflammation*, as proposed by Török (1928) and Gilchrist (1908), coexisted for a while with the angioneurotic theory. In 1907, Windaus and Vogt synthesized histamine, and Dale and Laidlaw (1910) demonstrated its pharmacological effects on smooth muscles and vessels. Soon thereafter Eppinger (1913) showed that cutaneous whealing, erythema, and pain developed at sites of local injections of histamine. It gradually became apparent that histamine (*histos*, Greek: tissue) was present in many tissues and that it could explain anaphylaxis and the broad clinical spectrum of acute allergic reactions. In 1927, Lewis further detailed the effect of histamine on the skin by describing the triple response named after him: (1) a local vasodilatation followed by (2) an arteriolar dilatation of the surrounding tissues due to an axon reflex, and (3) an increased permeability of the capillaries. The picture was rounded off when it was shown that the main source of histamine in the skin was the mast cell (Riley 1953).

More recently, other mediators of inflammation beside histamine, in particular kinins, leukotrienes, and acetylcholine, have been demonstrated at sites of urticarial reactions. They have been implicated as causes for the persistence of therapeutic unresponsiveness in certain types of wheals. Nevertheless, histamine remains the single most important mediator of urticarial reactions (see also Chapter 2, p. 5).

Almost in parallel with the theory of inflammation, the view arose that urticaria has an *allergic basis*. Since urticae were frequently seen in association with serum sickness, a protein hypersensitivity reaction was considered to be the basis of the underlying problem. In their classic experiments, Prausnitz and Küstner (1921) transferred serum from an allergic individual into the skin of a normal subject and then provoked local whealing by letting the test subject eat the allergen. They provided thus convincing evidence that a humoral factor as well as the allergen are necessary for the production of the cutaneous wheal. The humoral factor or "reaginic antibody" in allergic patients was shown to belong to a separate class of immunoglobulins, the immunoglobulin E (IgE) (Ishizaka et al. 1966, Johnsson and Bennich 1967). The link to cutaneous mast cells as the primary effector cells in allergic reactions was made with the demonstration that mast cells bind IgE via high affinity receptors to their cell surface. The combination of an allergen with allergen-specific IgE on the mast cell membrane results in the release of potent mediators such as histamine into the surrounding tissue which then leads to urtication of the skin (see Chapter 2, p. 5).

In more recent years, thinking has shifted away from the view that urticaria is primarily an allergic event. This came about after it was noted that an allergic cause can be identified in at most 20% of patients with chronic urticaria. Other frequent eliciting factors of chronic urticaria are physical forces or certain chemicals in foods and drugs. The mechanisms for histamine liberation from mast cells in these entities are only poorly understood (see Chapters 5, p. 57 and 7, p. 104). Since IgE is not involved in the reactions to many chemicals despite the presence of all the symptoms of anaphylactic reactions, the terms anaphylactoid or *pseudoallergic reactions* have been coined in recent years (Dukor et al. 1980). As in allergic urticaria and hereditary angioedema, genetic factors can play a role in these types of reactions (see also Chapter 7, p. 106).

1.4 The Physical Urticarias

(see also Chapter 5)

Contact urticaria was the first type of physical urticaria to be described in association with the provocation of wheals on contact with nettles (Hippocrates) (Table 1.3). *Urticaria factitia* was recognized in the Middle Ages, when, according to Török (1928), patients with this affliction were beheaded or burnt alive because of their proven association with the devil. In the medical literature, urticaria factitia was first described by Heberden in 1767. Gull coined the term "factitious urticaria" (1853), and Köbner mentioned the German word "Inscriptionsmethode" (1864). The condition became much publicized when a "femme autographique" was presented at a medical meeting in Paris by Dujardin-Beaumet in 1880 (Schadewaldt 1981c).

Table 1.3. First descriptions of the different types of urticaria (see Schadewaldt 1981 and the respective later chapters for references).

Types	Source
Contact urticaria	School of Hippocrates (4th cent. B.C.)
Angioedema	Donato, 1586
Solar urticaria	Borsch, 1719
Urticaria factitia	Heberden, 1767
Cold urticaria	Frank, 1792
Urticaria pigmentosa	Nettleship, 1869
Heat contact urticaria	Frank, 1921
Cholinergic urticaria	Duke, 1924
Pressure urticaria	Urbach and Fasal, 1929
Familial cold urticaria	Kile and Rush, 1940
Aquagenic urticaria	Shelley and Rawnsley, 1964
Vibratory angioedema	Patterson, 1972

Solar urticaria was first recognized by Borsch (1719), but it took more than a century before Veiel (1887) demonstrated in an ingenious way that only solar rays and not heat from a stove or light from a candle were responsible for this affliction. Apart from *cold urticaria* which was first noted in the 18th century, all remaining types of the physical urticarias have been described in the 20th century (Table 1.3). Except for *cholinergic urticaria*, the incidence of these more recently recognized physical urticarias is relatively low (Schadewaldt 1981c).

1.5 Urticaria pigmentosa

(see also Chapter 9)

Nettleship, while a resident physician at the Black Friars Hospital in 1869, described the first case of what he called "chronic urticaria leaving brown stains." The basic underlying cutaneous pathology, namely the local proliferation of mast cells, was subsequently identified by Unna (1887), after Paul Ehrlich had discovered mast cells by means of a special staining method (1879). Once the disease had been accurately described, numerous case reports appeared in the literature. Sangster (1887) was the first to name the disease urticaria pigmentosa, and Sézary (1936) expressed his preference for the name mastocytosis, stressing the frequent systemic involvement and the potentially fatal outcome of the disease (reviewed in Sagher and Even-Paz 1967).

While the latter term is in most frequent usage, various other names have been applied to the disease. They underline the variable clinical picture of the condition: xanthelasmoidea (T. Fox 1875), papular erythema (Morrow 1899), xanthomoidea (Duhring 1898), urticaria perstans hemorrhagica (Pick 1881), urticaria neviformis (Klotz 1907), nevus pigmentosus urticans (Török 1928), teleangiectasia macularis eruptiva perstans (Weber and Hellenschmied 1930), mast cell reticulosis (Sézary 1952), solitary mast cell nevus (Drennan and Beare 1954) (reviewed in Sagher and Even-Paz 1967).

1.6 Angio(neurotic)edema

(see also Chapter 4)

The first case report of a typical angioedema in association with urticaria was published by Marcello Donati (1586). He described a young count who was allergic to eggs (Schadewaldt 1981b). Quincke published his famous treatise on acute circumscript edema of the skin in 1882, but his doctoral student Eugen Dinkelacker, in his treatise which appeared in the same year, discussed 14 other cases which he had published earlier. Quincke was well aware of detailed descriptions of the disease which had appeared in Britain, Scandinavia, Germany, and the United States (Rook 1974). Sir W. Osler described the first fatal cases of angioedema due to asphyxiation in 1888, and he was also the first one to note the occurrence of angioedema in families. A clear distinction between angioedema that is associated with urticaria and hereditary angioedema became possible in 1963 when Donaldson and Evans reported that patients with hereditary angioedema have a defect of the inhibitor of the first complement component. The most important recent progress in the understanding and the treatment of the disease was initiated by the observation of Spaulding (1960) that androgens can inhibit attacks and, as was proven many years later, increase the inhibitor levels in these patients (see Chapter 4, p. 47).

1.7 Treatment

(see also Chapter 11)

Already in the second half of the 19th century, physicians stressed that any treatment of urticaria must be based on the recognition of its causes. Fox stated in 1883 that the number of remedies in use for urticaria were directly proportional to the ignorance of physicians regarding the pathogenesis of the disease.

For acute urticaria due to ingested food, the administration of emetics such as rhubarb, magnesia, or castor oil was recommended. Pruritus was treated topically with cologne, vinegar, benzoic acid, or chloroform. Prescriptions for oral intake of sodium bicarbonate, colchicine, bismuth, and diluted fluoric acid or a dyspeptic diet were found to be at times helpful. Quinine derivatives were noted to cure and also cause urticaria. The same was known even at that time for sodium salicylate. Arsenic, strychnine, ergot, and even nettle tea were other remedies in common use (Fox 1883).

With the discovery of sympathomimetic amines at the turn of this century, a valuable tool became available to combat life-threatening anaphylactic reactions. Systemic administration of calcium and of the patient's own blood were in vogue in the late twenties of this century. But even at that time, more sophisticated therapeutic approaches such as desensibilization with the putative allergen, were already practiced (Török 1928). The discovery of antihistamines in 1937 by Bovet and Staub ushered in a new era of systemic treatment of urticaria. The corticosteroids (Swingle and Pfiffner 1930) provided another powerful tool for the treatment of acute urticaria. However, use of the latter in chronic urticaria was rapidly discredited because of the potential dangers of long-term use.

The battery of tools available for the symptomatic treatment of urticaria is not entirely satisfying even today since certain rare forms of urticaria are unresponsive to them and no treatment is without potential dangers and side effects. As in the last century, the aim of treatment remains therefore the identification of the causative agent, its elimination, and, only if this approach is unsuccessful, modern drug therapy may be instituted as a symptomatic measure.

2 Basic Mechanisms

2.1 The Wheal

Urticaria is defined by its primary lesion which is named wheal, urtica, or hive. This lesion is characterized by three major features:

1) a transient edema of the dermal tissue,
2) a surrounding reflex erythema (Fig. 2.1), and
3) intense pruritus or itch at the same site.

Except for the itch, such a cutaneous reaction can be readily reproduced in any type of skin by intradermal injection of histamine, certain other vasoactive mediators, or agents that cause the release of vasoactive mediators from mast cells in tissue (Table 2.1). Whealing is produced by a local increase in capillary and venular permeability, with the exsudation of plasma fluid into the surrounding tissue. The flare reaction is mediated by an axon reflex, is blocked by local anesthetics, and does not develop at all in denervated regions (Umemoto et al. 1976). Local pruritus is also mediated via nerve fibers, but the mechanisms by which it is produced are only poorly understood.

Plants and stinging animals cause wheals as a means of repelling other animals. The resulting increased vascular permeability and blood flow might serve to improve the absorption of toxins.

The normal role of the wheal in host defense is not readily evident. Conceivably, the associated increased capillary permeability serves to improve the influx of antibodies or other serum components into tissue and to counteract the invasion of foreign noxious substances. The pruritus or pain during urtication is, however, perceived as a nuisance by the host in most instances. This reaction seems therefore rather disadvantageous. Like the IgE-dependent immune system, the whealing reaction can thus be viewed as an evolutionary derailment of the mammalian host defense system rather than as a means to improve survival.

In recent years, much has been learned about the mechanisms causing the production of wheals. In particular, the mediators which induce them have been thoroughly studied. On the other hand, little is known about the way in which the wheal is resorbed and how the skin returns to its basic physiological condition.

Two types of wheals can be differentiated by the kinetics of their development and resorption: an immediate, transient wheal, and a wheal that occurs several hours later as part of the late phase cutaneous reaction. Both types can develop during IgE-dependent or nonspecific mast cell releasing mechanisms (Gleich 1982, Kaliner 1984). The immediate wheal is

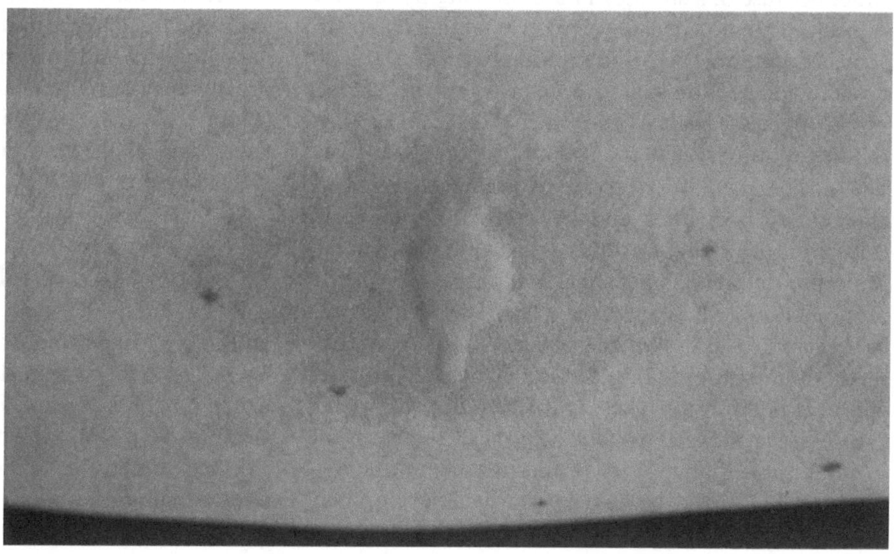

Fig. 2.1. Wheal and flare reaction after intracutaneous injection of compound 48/80 (0.1 %).

Table 2.1. Agents causing histamine release via three major mechanisms (Stanworth 1980, Lagunoff et al. 1983).

Cytotoxic Stimuli	Noncytotoxic Reactants		Anaphylatoxin Generators
Terminal complement components	*Immunological stimuli*	*Enzymes*	dextran
Surfactants	antigen – specific IgE	phospholipase A_2	starch
Detergents	aggregated immunoglobulins	chymotrypsin	endotoxin
Polycations	*Basic polypeptides*	peroxidase + H_2O_2	radiocontrast material
Hypotonicity	bradykinin	xanthine oxidase	aspirin
Lysolecithin	polistes kinin	*Therapeutic agents*	
Phospholipid reactants	mellitin	morphine	
Mellitin	compound 48/80	codeine	
Chlorpromazine	mast cell degranulating peptide	tubocurarine	
	substance P	ketotifen	
	polylysine	ionophore A 23187	
	polyornithine	*Other*	
	polyarginine	dextran	
	protamine	mannitol	
	polymyxin B	protein A	
	C3a, C4a, C5a	concanavalin A	
	Phagocytizable particles	ATP	
	(mast cell granules, zymosan)	lymphokines	
	Hormones	formylmethionyl polypeptides	
	ACTH	neurotensin	
	parathyroid hormone	acetylcholine	
	somatostatin		

transient, persists for only 1 or 2 h, is not associated with a cellular infiltrate, and depends on rapidly released mediators such as histamine. Such mediators are also eliminated again rapidly from the tissue site through digestion by enzymes such as histaminases, or through further oxidation or binding to tissue proteins. In addition, the target tissue may become rapidly refractory to the action of the mediator, and the wheal resolves.

The late wheal, or the late phase cutaneous reaction, arises from 4–8 h after the resolution of the immediate wheal, at times without an intermediary lag phase. It develops at sites of very intense immediate reactions, either because of a strong stimulus or a highly reactive subject (Umemoto et al. 1976). Histamine, platelet-activating factor (PAF) and several products of arachidonic acid metabolism have been found in suction blisters over the lesions (Dorsch et al. 1985). Possibly, the coagulation system is also involved (deShazo et al. 1979). The mediators in late phase reactions have chemotactic properties, and they recruit inflammatory cells from the blood into the tissue. Initially, neutrophils predominate, but after 24 h there are mostly mononuclear cells (Lemanske et al. 1983). These cells can secrete additional chemotactic and vasoactive mediators to amplify the reaction. When the primary stimulus is no longer present to maintain the wheal, the lesion resolves, usually after 48 h, due to the normal anti-inflammatory properties of the tissue.

Figure 2.2 shows the kinetics of wheal development and resorption in a normal person after injection of normal saline, histamine, concanavalin A (Con A), and compound 48/80. The NaCl wheal resolved very rapidly, followed 6 h later by the histamine and 24 h later by the 48/80 wheals. The mitogen-induced wheal persisted for more than 24 h. Intense infiltrates of neutrophils, eosinophils, and mononuclear cells were present at the sites of the 48/80 and Con A injections 7 h later (Fig. 2.3, see also James et al. 1982), but not at sites of histamine or normal saline injections. This suggests that mediators other than histamine, particularly chemotactic factors, caused the persistence of the lesions with compound 48/80 and Con A.

The pattern of wheal formation and resorption is the same for allergic and non-allergic individuals and depends only on the mediators. Patients with delayed pressure urticaria and angioedema are an exception (Dolovich et al. 1983) since the pressure of injection itself can elicit delayed wheals, even with NaCl (Czarnetzki et al. 1984a).

2.2 The Mast Cell

In the clinical setting, formation of wheals is almost exclusively mast cell dependent. There are a few exceptions, for example in hereditary angioedema (see Chapter 4, p. 47), or when vasoactive mediators are injected directly into the skin, as occurs on contact with stinging plants or insects (see Chapter 6, p. 91).

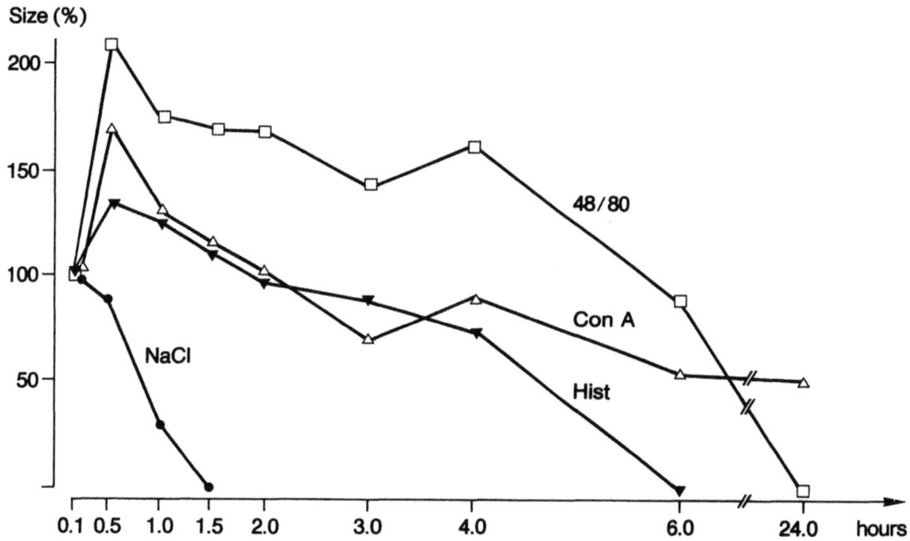

Fig. 2.2. Kinetics of whealing in a volunteer in response to normal saline (*NaCl*), 0.1% histamine (*Hist*), 0.01% concanavalin A (*Con A*), and 0.1% compound *48/80*. The size of the wheal is expressed as percent of the 5 min wheal which is set at 100% (see also Pokropp and Czarnetzki 1983).

An understanding of the morphological and functional aspects of mast cells provides therefore an important clue to the pathological processes that are involved in urticaria.

2.2.1 Morphological Aspects

Mast cells are large, mononuclear, resident tissue cells which are unique in that they contain high affinity receptors for IgE on their cell membrane and large, electron-dense, intracytoplasmic granules which store preformed mediators of inflammation (Fig. 2.4).

2.2.2 Mast Cell Heterogeneity

Currently, three different types of mast cells are differentiated: the connective tissue mast cell, the mucosal mast cell, and the peripheral blood basophil. Connective tissue mast cells are independent of T-lymphocytes, and they are present in large quantities in T cell-deficient animals and humans (Mayrhofer and Bazin 1981). During in vitro culture, mononuclear phagocytes can be transformed into mast cells by very specific stimuli (Czarnetzki 1984b). The exact precursor of the other types of mast cells is not known, although all three are derived from the bone marrow (Kitamura et al. 1977).

Mucosal mast cells have been identified primarily in the gut. They resemble basophils in that they are about half the size (~ 10 μm diameter) of connective tissue mast cells. They have only relatively few electron-dense cytoplasmic granules which contain less histamine, no heparin, and instead only lowly sulfated glycosaminoglycans, such as chondroitin sulfate and heparan sulfate. Furthermore, while they respond to IgE-dependent stimuli, they are unresponsive to compound 48/80 or bee venom peptide 401, and their secretory activity cannot be suppressed by chromone-like drugs (Bienenstock et al. 1982). Whereas mucosal mast cells depend in part on T-cell factors for their growth (Tertian et al. 1981), this does not hold for connective tissue mast cells (Czarnetzki et al. 1984b). All three types of mast cells increase at sites of immediate and delayed type reactions, also in chronic urticaria (Natbony et al. 1983), but whether this is due to local proliferation or immigration of the cells, is unclear.

Connective tissue mast cells are long-lived cells (Padawer 1974), and they are located chiefly in the loose connective tissue surrounding blood vessels (Fig. 2.5), hair follicles, sebaceous and sweat glands of the skin, along the bronchial airway tissue and the peripheral alveolar spaces in the lungs, and in the subserosa and submucosa of the intestine. Mast cells are scarce within the parenchyma of organs. They are located predominantly in the serous and synovial membranes of internal organs. The skin has a very high density of mast cells (7225/mm^3; Eady et al. 1979), and this holds also for the thymus, other lymphoid organs and the lung. This tissue distribution reflects the main effector function of mast cells.

2.2.3 Mast Cell Receptors

Mast cells and basophils are unique in that they carry high affinity receptors for IgE on their membranes (Ishizaka et al. 1970). IgE has been isolated and identified as a 180 kdal glycoprotein, having all the properties formerly assigned to the so-called reaginic or cytophilic antibody (Ishizaka and Ishizaka 1967). The receptor for IgE on mast cells is a 50 kd, two-

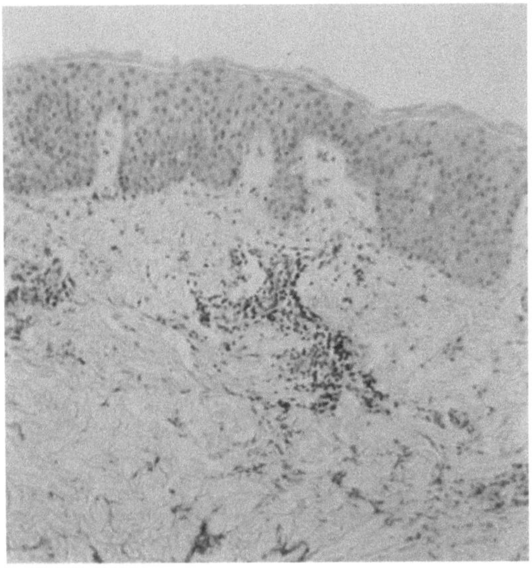

Fig. 2.3. Histological section of human skin 7 h after injection of 0.1% compound 48/80. Note the intense perivascular dermal infiltrate which consisted of mononuclear cells and variable numbers of neutrophils and eosinophils. Toluidine blue, orig. magn. 100 ×.

chain glycoprotein (Metzger et al. 1982) which studs the membrane at a density of 3×10^5 to 1×10^6 molecules and has an association constant of 10^{10} to 10^{11}. In normal persons, only about 10% of these receptors are occupied in vivo, and the number of total receptors and receptors occupied by IgE is higher in subjects with high serum levels of IgE and in atopics (Feltkamp-Vroom 1977; MacGlashan et al. 1983). IgE receptors with low binding affinity have recently also been identified on human lymphocytes (Parker et al. 1983), monocytes (Melewicz and Spiegelberg 1980), and eosinophils (Hübscher 1975). However, eosinophils have a secretory response only on contact with aggregates of IgE. In humans, a homocytotropic

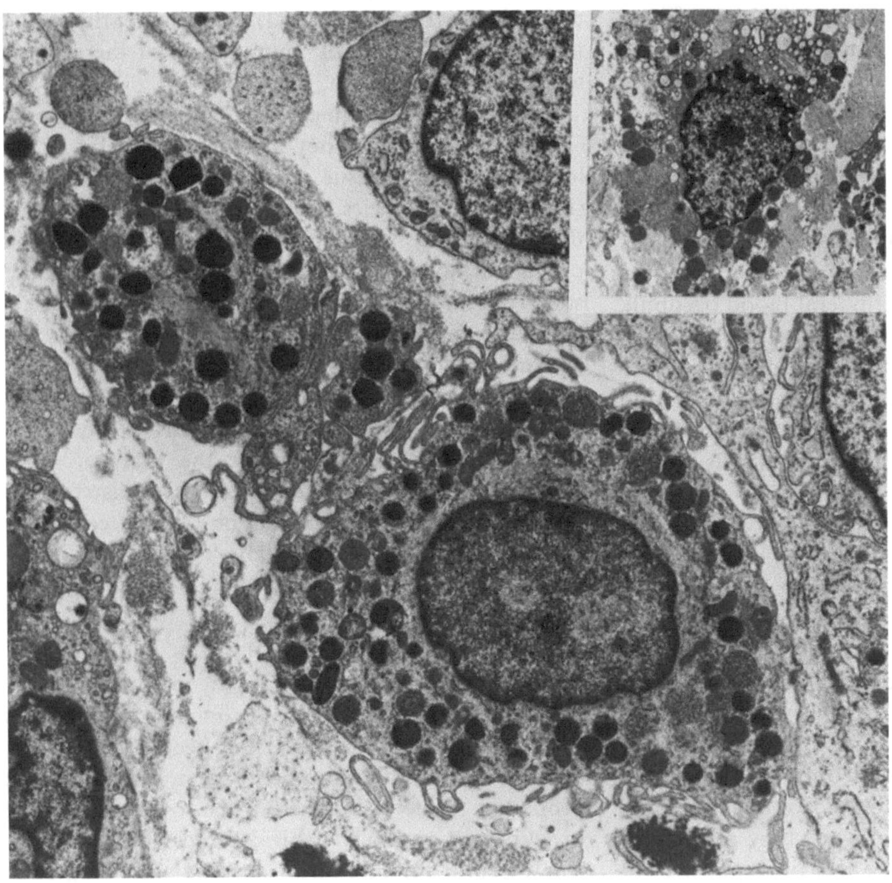

Fig. 2.4. Electron micrograph of cutaneous mast cells from the lesions of a patient with pressure urticaria (× 6300). Note the varying degree of electron density of the intracytoplasmic granules. The granules have become strikingly electron-lucent in the degranulated cell shown in the *inset* (orig. magn. 2800 ×). Note also individual granules in the interstitial tissue (produced in cooperation with Dr. G. Kolde, Münster).

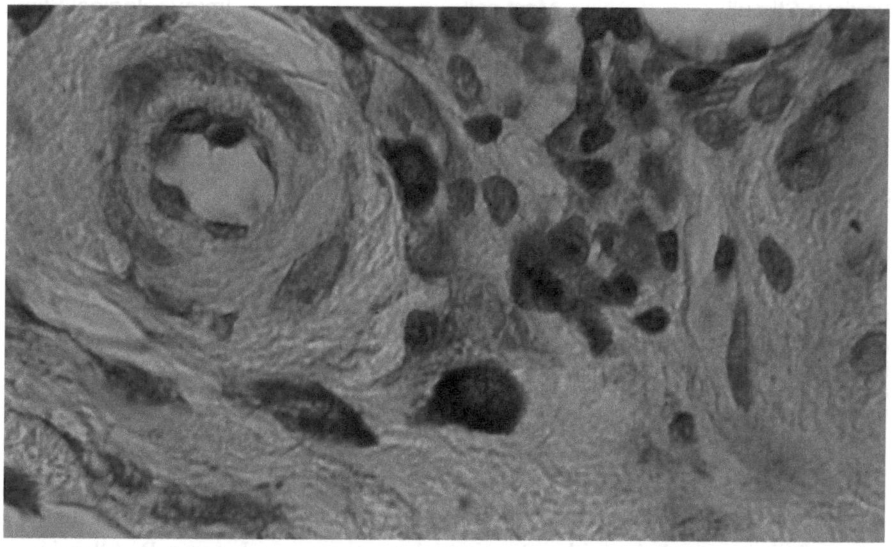

Fig. 2.5. Histological section of dermal tissue, showing a blood vessel and four mast cells in close proximity. The metachromatic staining characteristics of the mast cell granules, as recognized by the bluish-purple cytoplasmic staining, help to differentiate mast cells from other mononuclear cells. Toluidine blue, orig. magn. 400 ×.

antibody of the IgG class has also been found (IgG_4). It seems to be functionally important for it can be used to passively sensitize monkey and human skin to specific antigen. Its ability to induce in vitro histamine release from human basophils is however still controversial. This antibody functions as a blocking antibody when it is present in high concentrations, such as in bee keepers (reviewed by Perelmutter 1984).

Certain recognition units on mast cell and basophil membranes are also found on other cell types. They include receptors for IgG (Ishizaka et al. 1979) and, at least on the rat mast cell, receptors for C3b (Sher et al. 1979) and for products of the K and D regions of the major histocompatibility complex (Daëron and Voisin 1979) (Fig. 2.6). Murine mast cells lack Ia antigens, and this holds also for cultured human cells (Mossmann et al. 1979, Czarnetzki et al. 1984b). Human mast cells often have fibronectin on their surface which may aid in their attachment to surfaces within the connective tissue (Forni et al. 1983).

2.2.4 Mast Cell Triggering

In Fig. 2.7, the most important stimuli that can induce urticaria are shown, grouped into immunological and noxious agents. There is good evidence for a pathogenetic role of the immunological stimuli only for IgE-dependent mechanisms and the anaphylatoxins. A possible involvement of lymphokines is discussed with delayed pressure urticaria (see Chapter 5, p. 55).

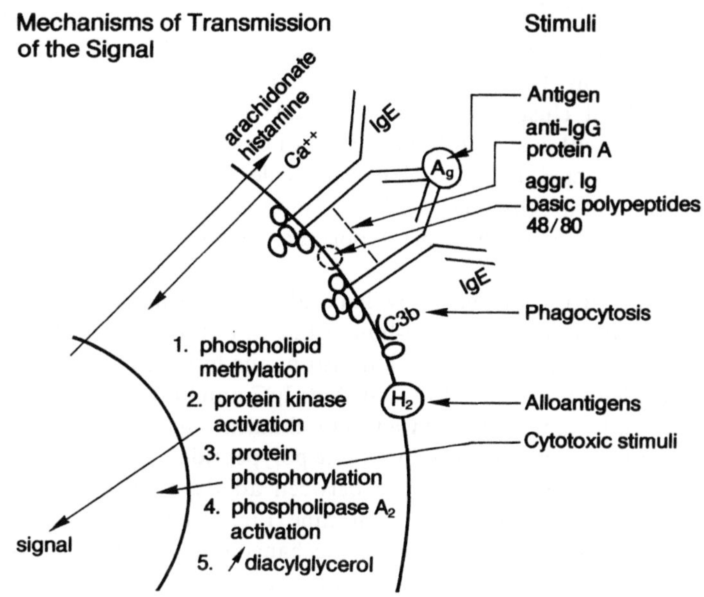

Fig. 2.6. Mechanisms of mast cell activation. Besides stimulation by binding of antigen (*AG*) to free Fab arms of two adjacent IgE molecules, stimulation via IgE or its membrane receptor occurs by two additional mechanisms (Stanworth 1980). A cascade of enzymes is activated within the membrane after stimulation. Ca^{++} flows into the cell, and histamine and arachidonic acid are secreted into the cell exterior.

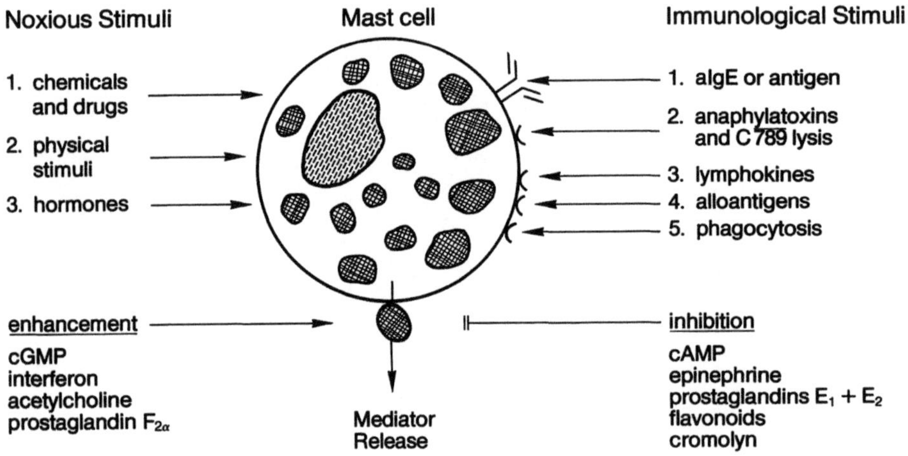

Fig. 2.7. Major types of stimuli which cause mast cell mediator release and also induce or maintain the urticarial reaction. The possible modulating role on this process by certain agents is indicated in the lower part of the scheme.

There is no doubt that noxious stimuli are the major cause of all the anaphylactoid and urticarial reactions which are seen clinically. Their mechanism of action is, however, only poorly understood.

IgE-mediated induction of mast cell mediator release is the most thoroughly studied mechanism of mast cell stimulation. A series of investigations have provided evidence that binding of antigen to a single IgE molecule does not suffice to trigger the cells, but that at least two adjacent IgE molecules must be tied together or bridged at their free Fab arms for this event to take place (Fig. 2.6). Larger aggregates of IgE are not much more effective.

Antigen-IgE-receptor coupling induces the following major intramembraneous events:

1) phospholipid methylation,
2) Ca^{++} influx,
3) arachidonic acid release, and
4) histamine release.

A brief, transient rise of cAMP precedes phospholipid methylation (Ishizaka 1982, Siraganian et al. 1982). Glycolipid clustering occurs (Curtain et al. 1981), together with a several-fold increase of diacylglycerol (Kennerly et al. 1979). The latter molecule can serve as source of arachidonic acid and monoacylglycerol triglyceride and thus of important mediators of inflammation.

Stanworth (1980) has provided evidence that stimulation of mast cells via cell-bound IgE can occur not only by the free Fab arms, but also by the linking of two adjacent Fc arms (Fig. 2.6). Anti-IgG and protein A cause histamine release via this mechanism, whereas aggregated immunoglobulins, basic polypeptides, and compound 48/80 form a tie between adjacent IgE receptors at the level of the membrane (Fig. 2.6). Basic polypeptides which act via this mechanism include a long list of important mediators of inflammation (see Table 2.1), such as the anaphylatoxins, kinins, and substance P. Allergic sensitization is not required for this type of release.

There is recent evidence that histamine release by dextran and mannitol is also IgE-dependent (Findlay et al. 1984, Hanahoe 1984). These investigators observed that after removal of IgE, compound 48/80-induced degranulation remained unaltered, while dextran- and anti IgE-mediated release was inhibited. It is thus possible that IgE-dependent release occurs by additional mechanisms than those proposed by Stanworth (1980).

There are three other basic ways by which mast cells can be stimulated for mediator release. Morphologists have repeatedly reported on the ability of connective tissue mast cells to phagocytize small and large particles. This fits well with the ontogenetic relationship of the cells to mononuclear phagocytes. Mast cells take up diverse microorganisms, ranging from viruses to fungi, metals, colloids, and antigens. C3b receptors augment particle uptake and histamine release during phagocytosis of mast cells (Sher et al. 1979, Czarnetzki 1982). This phagocytic uptake of particles is inefficient and its role in disease is unclear.

There are also special receptors for H2 antigen-mediated release of histamine (Daëron and Voisin 1978). Opiates release mast cell mediators in vivo and in vitro by both receptor-mediated and receptor-independent mechanisms (Grosman 1982, Casale et al. 1984). A final release mechanism which results in cell death operates through the influence of cytotoxic agents on mast cells (Fig. 2.7, Table 2.1). The terminal complement components, surfactants, and detergents are important examples. The intense inflammatory reaction that follows the action of some of these substances causes far more tissue damage than would be expected to underly a fleeting wheal. On topical application of cytotoxic agents, contact urticaria may nevertheless be the predominant lesion (see Chapter 6, p. 91).

For many of the agents which cause noncytotoxic histamine release (see Table 2.1), the release mechanisms are not known. Most of these substances are discussed in the reviews by Stanworth (1980) and Lagunoff et al. (1983). More recent observations of interest are the reports of mast cell or basophil release due to neurotensins (Kurose and Saeki 1981, Krüger et al. 1982), parathyroid hormone (Kraeuterkops et al. 1982), substance P (Renner et al. 1982), the enzyme myeloperoxidase (Stendahl et al. 1983), chymotrypsin (Nials et al. 1983), and phospholipase A2 (Chi et al. 1982). The latter observation underlines the importance of arachidonic acid metabolism in the release process (Fig. 2.6).

Other biological agents which may play a role in non-IgE dependent and also in non-urticarial disease are lymphokines and analogues of chemotactic products from bacteria, the N-formyl-methionyl-peptides, which also cause mast cell release (Siraganian and Hook 1977, Thueson et al. 1979; Sedgwick et al. 1981).

A final group of agents (Table 2.1) is able to activate the complement system and can potentially cause mast cell release via the anaphylatoxins which are generated in this process (see 2.3.7, p. 19). Complement activation by these substances occurs, however, equally well in normal persons as in patients with urticaria and would therefore not be an explanation for clinically observed reactions in a small subgroup of patients (see Chapter 7, p. 106).

2.2.5 Modulation of Mast Cell Release (Fig. 2.7)

The inhibition of mediator release from mast cells is a basic goal in the treatment of urticaria, and enhancement of that same process may explain the exacerbation of the disease in certain settings. Urticaria can be modulated at the level of the released mediators or the responding target tissue by blocking or eliminating the mediators, or by changing the cutaneous vascular response. The latter explains, for example, the exacerbating effect of alcohol in patients with urticaria, due to the increased peripheral vasodilatation caused by this chemical. Enzyme defects could also allow for uninhibited production of anaphylatoxins and would be an example of modulation at the mediator levels.

Cyclic AMP/GMP

It is a frequent clinical observation that stress, emotion, premenstrual tension, and exercise aggravate urticaria. With the recognition of the regulating role of the cyclic AMP system on basophil histamine release, Lichtenstein and Margolis (1968) provided a first plausible explanation for the effect of the sympathetic and parasympathetic nervous system on this process. The findings of these authors were later substantiated by in vitro studies of human skin and of isolated rat and human tissue mast cells (Yamamoto et al. 1973, Winslow and Austen 1982, MacGlashan et al. 1983).

The data showing an inhibitory role of β-adrenergic agonists were generally confirmed in all these cell systems, but marked species and cell type variations were observed with regard to the response of the cellular cyclic AMP/GMP system to antigen stimulation. In addition, a direct correlation between the modulation of histamine release and the changes in the cyclic AMP/GMP system could not always be established. For example, antigen stimulation of rat mast cells causes a bimodal rise of intracellular cAMP and cGMP levels which does not occur in human basophils or mast cells. In human basophils, addition of β-adrenergic agonists (epinephrine, isoproterenol), of prostaglandins (PG) E_1 and E_2, of phosphodiesterase inhibitors (caffeine, theophylline), of high concentrations of histamine and of adenosine cause a sustained increase of intracellular cAMP levels and a concurrent inhibition of basophil histamine. In this same system, prostaglandin D_2, which should act similarly on the intracellular cAMP, enhances release. In human mast cells, β-adrenergic agonists and prostaglandin E_2 also decrease histamine release, but histamine and prostaglandin D_2 are ineffective although they raise cyclic AMP levels, in case of histamine via the H2 receptor. In the rat mast cell, adenosine and prostaglandin D_2 also cause a rise of intracellular cyclic AMP, but adenosine potentiates histamine release (Marquardt et al. 1978), whereas prostaglandin D_2 has no modulating effect on this process.

The cyclic GMP system was initially thought to always cause the opposite effect of the cAMP. Increased intracellular levels, as occur with cholinergic stimulation or on incubation with prostaglandin $F_{2\alpha}$, also facilitate mediator release. Other factors which potentiate mast cell secretion were however later found to operate not necessarily via the cGMP system, and the importance originally attributed to the regulatory role of the cAMP/cGMP system can no longer be sustained.

Interferon

Chronic urticaria and extrinsic asthma are frequently exacerbated during viral infections. Ida et al. (1977)

and Busse et al. (1983) gave a possible explanation for this phenomenon: They showed that several types of viruses enhance basophil mediator release, and that interferon is responsible for this effect. In lymphokine preparations, Ida et al. (1980) identified interferon and an additional enhancing factor. Skurkovich et al. (1983) showed that interferons α, β, and γ enhance the binding of IgE to basophils which might explain the observations that interferon enhances histamine release. Beside this effect of interferon, Skurkovich et al. (1983) discussed another potentially modulating function of interferon in allergic disease: Allergen can induce interferon production from lymphocytes, macrophages, basophils and mast cells, and interferon is in turn able to cause a decrease of T-suppressor cells. It would thus be possible that interferon plays a pivotal role in the induction of the allergic state.

Arachidonate metabolism

In addition to the modulatory role of different prostaglandins, products of the lipoxygenase pathway of arachidonate metabolism can also modulate mediator release. Elevated levels of 5-hydroperoxyeicosatetraenoic acid and 5-hydroxyeicosatetraenoic acid enhance basophil release, but have no effect on human mast cells (Peters et al. 1981, MacGlashan et al. 1983). When basophils are stimulated with lymphokines rather than with antigen, arachidonate metabolites have, on the other hand, no modulating effect on mediator release at all (Ezeamuzie and Assem 1984). There is also good in vivo evidence that corticosteroids, which block the entire arachidonate metabolism at the level of the phospholipase A_2 (Fig. 2.11), have no effect on antigen-induced mediator release from cutaneous mast cells (Slott and Zweiman 1974), whereas they are effective inhibitors of the leukocyte-dependent late cutaneous response (Poothullil et al. 1976).

Cromoglycate and flavonoids

Cromoglycate is a powerful inhibitor of mast cell histamine release but has no effect on human basophils or mucosal mast cells. Its mechanism of action is still puzzling, and an effect on the central nervous system may explain its therapeutic benefit in extrinsic asthma. Local injections of the drug into the skin do not modulate IgE-dependent release (Ting et al. 1983).

Flavonoids are naturally occurring, widely distributed compounds in plants which are responsible for the coloring of some flowers. They have a basic 2-phenyl-4-chromone structure and resemble thus cromoglycate which is a bischromone. Several of the flavonoids, for example quercetin, are more powerful inhibitors than cromolyn. Some flavonoids also affect gut mast cells and basophils. These compounds are thought to act at the level of the membrane Ca^{++} ATPase or on phospholipid metabolism (reviewed by Foreman 1984).

In vivo modulation of mediator release

Kern and Lichtenstein (1976) observed a defective histamine release from basophils in patients with chronic urticaria. This observation could be extended to the release of eosinophil chemotactic factor (ECF) from basophils (Czarnetzki et al. 1976), but its relevance for the pathophysiology of chronic urticaria is unclear, since the main changes in this condition are localized to the skin where mast cells rather than basophils are the main effector cells.

2.2.6 Mast Cell Granules

The granules within mast cells and basophils are modified lysosomes which contain hydrolases and which develop by fusion of progranules that derive from the Golgi zone (Chi et al. 1978). On electron microscopy (Fig. 2.4), the granules consist of a crystalline lattice core. In human mast cells, they contain additional inclusions which are constituted of small stacks of lipid membranes, the so-called whorls or scrolls. The granule matrix is made up of a dense complex of acid glycosaminoglycans which are attached to a protein core. Numerous enzymes, biogenic amines, and zinc are bound to the acid mucopolysaccharide matrix by ionic forces (Murphy et al. 1974), and immunoglobulins, C1q, and a factor VIII-like substance are present as well (Simson et al. 1977, Igarashi et al. 1982, Kindblom 1982). In the human mast cell, the acid glycosaminoglycans consists mostly of highly sulfated heparin, although hyaluronic acid has also been demonstrated in dermal mast cell granules (Sasai and Ichihashi 1975). In the basophil, there is no heparin, and only glycosaminoglycans with lower sulfatation, such as chondroitin, heparan or dermatan sulfate (Orenstein et al. 1978), are found instead. This explains the water solubility of basophil granules and their lack of staining with metachromatic dyes in formalin-fixed, routine histological sections.

In the rat, heparin comprises one-third of the total dry mass of the mast cell (Mellblom and Enerbäck 1979). It has a molecular weight of 150–750 kd, with many sites for ionic binding to other, oppositely charged molecules. This explains its low molar ratio in the granule, compared to smaller molecules [heparin :

chymase : serotonin : histamine = 1 : 45 : 42 : 1352, Schwartz and Austen (1980)]. Heparin makes the granule function as a place of storage of several important mediators of inflammation (Fig. 2.8).

There is good morphological evidence that the granules are interconnected with each other like sausage links and that their matrix acts as an ion exchange resin (Padawer 1979). When common mineral cations such as Na^+, K^+, Ca^{++} or Mg^{++} enter the granules, they replace positively charged molecules such as histamine, and these can then diffuse, via the intergranular channels, to the cell exterior. This process explains why early after stimulation of mast cells with antigen, one sees only a swelling and a loss of electron density of the granules of skin mast cells in parallel to early histamine secretion. Within 5 to 10 min, when histamine release is maximal, granules themselves are released into the cell surrounding. The granules that remain within the mast cells often contain only a fribrillar residue, or empty vacuoles take their place (Ting et al. 1980) (see also Fig. 2.4).

Mast cell granules release some of their contents only in an environment of very high ionic strength. Examples of such tightly bound substances are trypsin in human mast cells and an "inflammatory factor of anaphylaxis" (IFA) described by Oertel and Kaliner (1981). IFA has a molecular weight of 1400 d and consists of 12 amino acid peptides; it causes a transient vasodilatation during the first 30 min and a leukocyte accumulation within 2–8 h after injection into rat skin. This factor may play a role in the development of late cutaneous reactions.

The fate of mast cell granules after release of their contents is not known. They may be digested by their own enzymes, by enzymes in the interstitial tissue, or by enzymes within other phagocytes after being taken up into these cells. Murine mast cells (Ginsburg et al. 1978) and guinea pig basophils (Dvorak et al. 1982) can regranulate in vitro and resynthesize histamine for several days after noncytotoxic degranulation; this has not been observed in human cells (Drobis and Siraganian 1976).

2.3 Mediators

In recent years, it has become apparent that mast cells are the potential source of a host of mediators and that their complex interplay provides a possible explanation for the diverse clinical aspects of urticaria. Mast cells release three major groups of mediators:

1) muscle-contracting and vasoactive agents such as histamine, serotonin, slow-reacting substances (SRS), kinins, and prostaglandins,
2) chemotactic agents such as eosinophil chemotactic factor (ECF, leukotriene B_4), platelet activating factor (PAF), or neutrophil chemotactic peptides, and
3) heparin and enzymes which modulate or stimulate mediator production and activity.

Mast cell mediators exist either preformed within the specific mast cell granules, or they are generated de novo on stimulation of the cells from phospholipids within the membrane (see Fig. 2.8). In addition, plasma-derived mediators, such as peptide fragments of the complement and kinin systems, may also participate in the inflammatory events occurring in urticaria.

2.3.1 Histamine

Of all the mediators known to date, histamine has been studied most thoroughly, both with regard to its

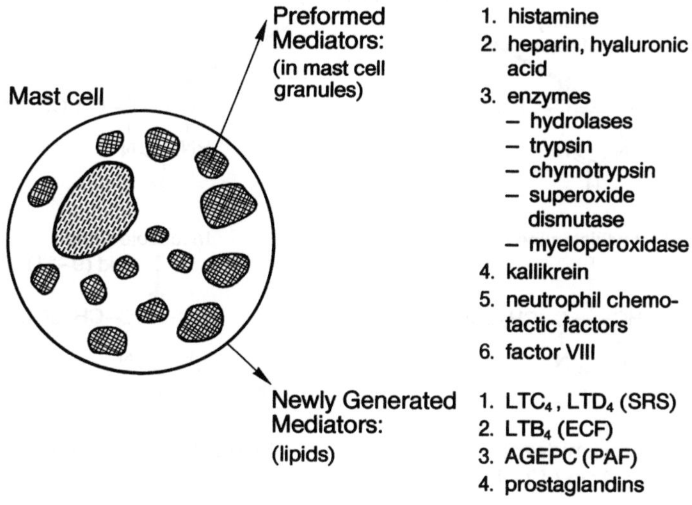

Fig. 2.8. The major preformed mediators within mast cell granules and of the lipid mediators that are newly generated on stimulation of mast cells. *LTC_4*, leukotriene C_4; *LTD_4*, leukotriene D_4; *SRS*, slow-reacting substance; *LTB_4*, leukotriene B_4; *ECF*, eosinophil chemotactic factor, *AGEPC*, acetyl glyceryl ether phosphorylcholine; *PAF*, platelet-activating factor.

chemistry and its biological effects. Its role in urticaria is unquestioned for two reasons. On injection into the skin, histamine produces the hallmarks of urticaria:

1) an initial red macule at the injection site,
2) a surrounding reflex erythema, and
3) a central edema (the wheal) within 1–2 min afterward.

This so-called triple response of Lewis (1927) is accompanied by burning pain or a sensation of itching.

Intravenous injections of histamine cause bronchoconstriction, cutaneous erythema (flush), headache, tachycardia, edema, and hypotension (Kaliner et al. 1982). All these symptoms can be observed in association with urticaria, and the entire symptomatology of urticaria is thus mimicked by histamine alone. Additional proof for a role of histamine in urticaria is given by the demonstration of elevated levels of this mediator in lesions of chronic urticaria and of most physical urticarias in the venous effluent of involved skin (Kaplan et al. 1978; see Table 5.4, p. 58 for the physical urticarias).

Histamine is a β-imidazolethylamine (molecular weight of 111 d) (Fig. 2.9) and is formed by the enzymatic decarboxylation of L-histidine, with pyridoxal-5-phosphate as cofactor. In humans, its breakdown is catalyzed either by a diamine oxidase, resulting in imidazole acetic acid, or by a methyl transferase, with N (3)-methyl-histamine as the product. Histamine, and more so its metabolites, can be measured in the urine (see Fig. 2.9).

Histamine is universally distributed in the plant and animal kingdoms. In humans, it is located primarily in tissue mast cells and peripheral blood basophils (1–5 $\mu g/10^6$ cells), but it also exists at high concentrations in non-mast cell locations within the stomach and in the central and peripheral nervous system (Levy 1974). Normal serum levels in humans are 0.2–0.4 pg/ml (Dyer et al. 1982).

The diverse effects of histamine on different cells and organ systems are listed in Fig. 2.10. Cells have special receptors for histamine, and the molecule attaches to them via either its amino terminal end (H1 receptor) or its imidazole ring (H2-receptor) (Fig. 2.9). Some tissues and cells carry both types of receptors, and their stimulation may have opposing effects (Fig. 2.10).

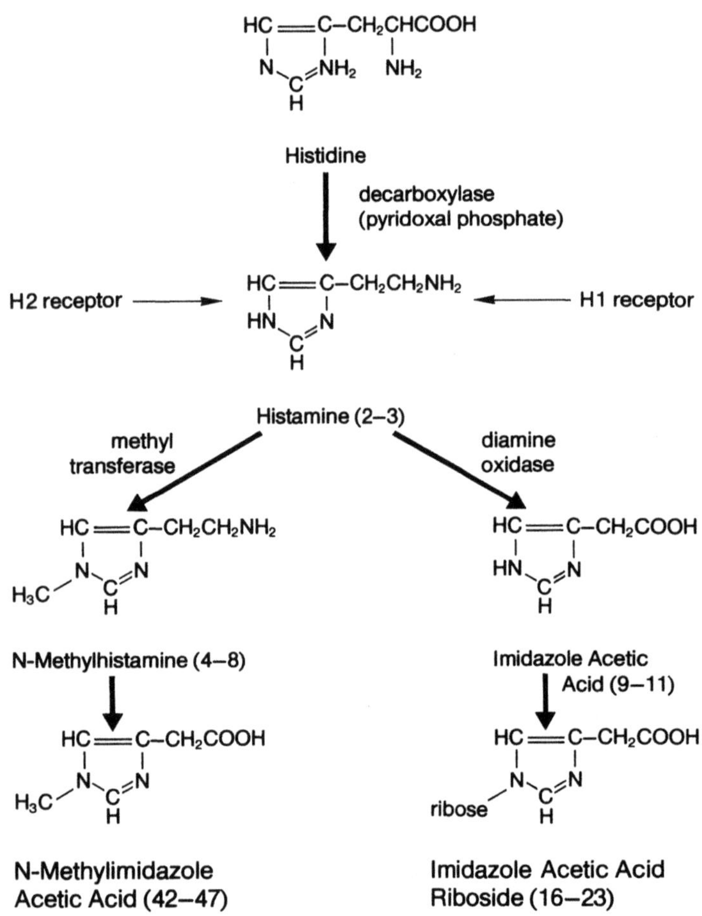

Fig. 2.9. Generation and metabolic degradation of histamine. Note also the site of the histamine molecule that attaches to either the H1- or the H2-receptor sites on target tissue. The numbers in parentheses indicate the % of catabolites recovered in the urine.

Histamine

Target Tissue	Effect	Receptor
vessels 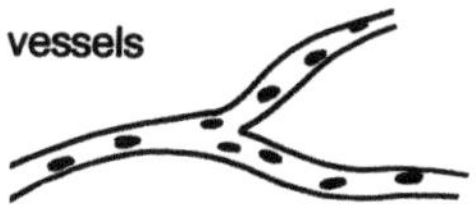	1. endothelial cell contraction of postcapillary venules (increased permeability)	H1
	2. dilatation, terminal arterioles	H1 + H2
	3. stimulation, prostaglandin secretion	H1
smooth muscle 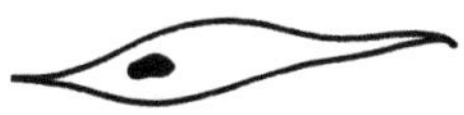	4. contraction (bronchoconstriction)	H1
	5. relaxation	H2
nervous system 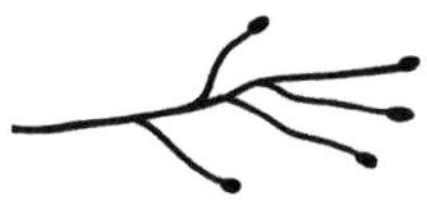	6. pruritus	H1
	7. decreased AV conduction, heart	H1
	8. increased sinus node frequency, heart	H2
	9. thermoregulation (CNS)	H1 + H2
neutrophil, basophil 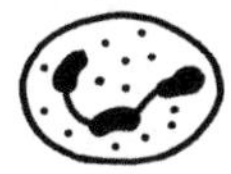	10. inhibition of secretion and chemotaxis	H2
	11. enhancement of secretion and chemotaxis	H1
eosinophil 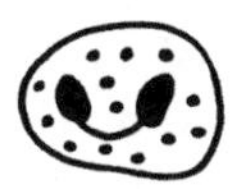	12. inhibition of chemotaxis	H2
lymphocyte 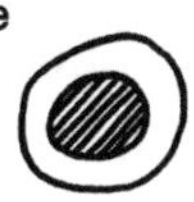	13. stimulation of LIF production	H1
	14. stimulation of chemotactic lymphokine production	H2
	15. decreased MIF production, decreased NK, ADCC + MLC activity	H2
stomach 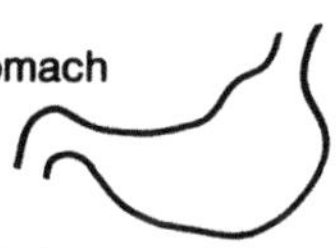	16. increased gastric acid secretion	H2
glands 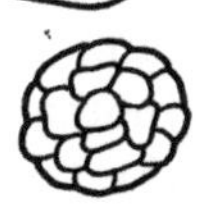	17. increased secretion of mucus, saliva	–
keratinocytes 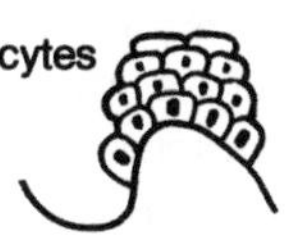	18. inhibition of mitoses	H1 + H2

Fig. 2.10. Biological effects of histamine on diverse cell types via either its H1 or H2 receptor on the target tissue. *LIF*, lymphocyte inhibitory factor; *MIF*, migration inhibiting factor; *NK*, natural killer cell; *ADCC*, antibody dependent cellular cytotoxicity; *MLC*, mixed lymphocyte culture.

Histamine-induced edema is thought by some to develop as a result of endothelial cell contraction. It depends both on the increased hydrostatic pressure within the capillaries and on the decreased colloid osmotic pressure gradient (Haddy 1960). Dilatation of the terminal arterioles accounts for flush and decreased central blood pressure during massive in vivo histamine release. Histamine causes also the secretion of PGE, PGI_2, $PGF_{2\alpha}$, and PGD_2 from peripheral vessels and might thus modulate its own effect on this organ system (Juan and Sametz 1980). Smooth muscle cells respond to histamine with either a contraction or a relaxation. There are marked variations in this response, depending on the different species. In the lung, part of the action of histamine is mediated via the vagus nerve. Little is known about the response of human cardiac muscle to histamine (Douglas 1980), but here too, the molecule acts on the electrical conduction system, causing an increased sinus node frequency and a decreased AV conduction of the heart.

Histamine also acts on the peripheral nervous

Table 2.2. Action spectrum of vasoactive and bronchospastic mediators.

Biological Effect	Mediators					
	histamine	serotonin	kinins	LTC_4/D_4 (SRS)	PAF	prostaglandins
Vasodilatation	+	−	+	−	−	+ (PGE_2, I_2, D_2)
Vasoconstriction	−	+	−	+	+	+ ($PGF_{2\alpha}$, TXA_2)
Increased vascular permeability	+	+	+	+	+	+ (PGE_2, I_2, D_2)
Smooth muscle contraction	+	+	+	+	+	+ (PGG_2, H_2, $F_{2\alpha}$, D_2, TXA_2)
Pain-pruritus	+	+	+	−	+	+ (PGE_2, D_2)

LT, leukotriene; PG, prostaglandin; PAF, platelet-activating factor; TX, thromboxane; SRS, slow reacting substance.

system to produce pruritus (Hagermark and Strandberg 1977) which is thought to be mediated via the afferent pain fibers. This explains why agents causing pain on injection are also implicated as mediators of pruritus (Table 2.2). Itching cannot be reproduced consistently by injection of histamine or histamine-liberators into human skin (Pokropp and Czarnetzki 1983), and other inflammatory mediators or central factors may be responsible for or modulate the expression of pruritus.

Histamine does not readily cross the blood-brain barrier, but it is present within the brain at high concentrations, particularly in the hypothalamus. Neurons have both H1 and H2 receptors, and histamine functions as a neurotransmitter. Histamine is also present within mast cells of the brain and exerts a control on the vasculature and the immune response within the central nervous system. Injections of histamine into the ventricle result in increased blood pressure and heart rate, emesis, hypothermia, and increased adrenocorticotrophin and prolactin secretion. Little is known about the effect of histamine on cortical function since none of these studies were done with humans (Lomax and Green 1981).

Histamine regulates granulocyte and lymphocyte functions. At high concentrations ($10^{-2}-10^{-4}$ M), it inhibits the migration of neutrophils and eosinophils (Rivkin and Becker 1972, Clark et al. 1975, Czarnetzki et al. 1975) and the secretion of lysosomal enzymes from neutrophils and of histamine from basophils (Lichtenstein and Gillespie 1973, Sosman and Busse 1976). At lower concentrations (10^{-6} M), histamine enhances migration and secretion of neutrophils (Sosman and Busse 1976). In contrast to the findings of Clark et al. (1975), works from several laboratories could not demonstrate a chemotactic effect of histamine on neutrophils or eosinophils (Czarnetzki et al. 1975, Ting et al. 1980).

Subsets of T-lymphocytes with H1 receptors produce a leukocyte migration inhibiting factor (LIF), while H2 receptor-bearing lymphocytes secrete a lymphocyte chemotactic factor (Center et al. 1983). The latter cells also respond to histamine with decreased production of migration inhibiting factor (MIF) (Rocklin et al. 1980) and a decreased response in natural killer assays, antibody-dependent cytotoxicity, and mixed lymphocyte cultures (Nair and Schwartz 1983). These functions of histamine are probably not important in the pathogenesis of urticaria because of the fleeting nature of the disease and the rapid degradation of histamine. Similarly, the effect of histamine on gastric acid secretion, on bronchial mucus secretion, and on keratinocyte proliferation (Fig. 2.10) has little clinical significance for the cutaneous whealing response.

2.3.2 5-Hydroxytryptamine (Serotonin)

Like histamine, serotonin can induce smooth muscle contraction and enhanced vascular permeability, but unlike histamine, it causes increased vasoconstriction (Table 2.2). The compound is formed by hydroxylation and deamination of tryptophan. In humans, 90% is present in the enterochromaffin cells of the gastrointestinal mucosa, and the rest is found in platelets and the central nervous system, particularly in the hypothalamus (Levy 1974, Plaut and Lichtenstein 1978). Human mast cells and basophils do not synthesize serotonin, but they might take it up passively, as do murine mast cells, since serotonin has been measured in human mastocytomas (Morishima 1970). Platelet activating factor (PAF), which is secreted by basophils and mast cells (Fig. 2.8), can also secondarily induce secretion of serotonin from platelets (Levy 1974, Plaut and Lichtenstein 1978). Serotonin plays probably no significant role in urticaria, although elevated serum levels have been measured in one patient with cholinergic urticaria after exercise challenge (Kaplan et al. 1975; see Chapter 5, p. 78).

2.3.3 Kinins

The third group of potent vasoactive and bronchoconstrictive agents, the kinins, consists of bradykinin

(BK) (H-Arg-Pro-Pro-Gly-Phe-Ser-Pro-Phe-Arg-OH), lyso-BK (kallidin), and methionyllysyl-BK. These compounds are generated in mammalian plasma from inactive high and low molecular weight precursor molecules, the kininogens, by the action of kininogenases (kallikreins). Proteases such as trypsin, plasmin, and leukocyte-derived enzymes can act as kallikreins, and their action is inhibited by α_2-macroglobulin, α_1-antitrypsin, antithrombin III, and by the C1-esterase inhibitor. Kinins are rapidly destroyed in plasma and tissue through the action of inactivating enzymes, the kininases.

Kinins are as potent or even more potent than histamine in their ability to cause bronchoconstriction and increased vascular permeability. Cutaneous edema is maximal 10–30 min after injection and disappears rapidly thereafter. There is also local vasodilatation, and a drop in blood pressure occurs on intravenous injection. In animals, elevated serum levels, together with histamine, have been measured during anaphylactic shock. Intense pain but no pruritus develops at the cutaneous injection sites. Kinins have no significant in vitro leukotactic activity on their own (Ward 1971), and leukocytes accumulate in tissue instead due to complement activation of the kinin.

The kinin system is related to the coagulation and the fibrinolytic system in that

1) high molecular weight kininogen augments the activation of factor XI by Hageman factor, and
2) kallikreins can function as plasminogen activators, causing conversion of plasminogen to plasmin, a fibrinolytic enzyme.

The inhibitory role of the C1-esterase inhibitor has been mentioned before, and its absence explains the activation of kinins and complement in hereditary angioedema (see Chapter 4, p. 47). Kinins have been measured in wheals, particularly in physical urticaria (see Chapter 5, p. 55). A special role for basophils in kinin generation is likely, since these cells contain a kinin-generating principle. Also, epinephrine which causes kinin generation, depends for this activity on the presence of mast cells in the rat (reviewed in Garcia Leme 1978, Yecies and Kaplan 1980).

2.3.4 Slow-Reacting Substances (Leukotrienes C_4, D_4, E_4)

These mediators, the slow-reacting substance(s) (SRS), were originally identified by their ability to cause a slowly increasing, prolonged contraction of smooth muscles (Feldberg and Kellaway 1938) which was not inhibited by antihistamines. SRS was shown to be released by immunological challenge of diverse tissues, but cells other than mast cells, such as neutrophils and monocytes, seemed to contribute significantly to its production.

Recently, SRS has been found to belong to the leukotrienes (LT), a group of arachidonate metabolites which derive their name from their leukocyte source, the conjugated trienes, and the four (subscript 4) double bonds in their chemical structure (see Fig. 2.11; Samuelsson et al. 1979). After production of the unstable intermediates 5-hydroperoxyeicosatetraenoic acid (5-HPETE) and LTA_4 through the action of a lipoxygenase on arachidonic acid, the addition of a glutathione results in the production of LTC_4. Removal of the glutamyl group results in LTD_4, and with further enzymatic splitting off of the glycine, the relatively inactive LTE_4 is formed (Fig. 2.11). LTC_4 is the main product of murine mastocytoma cells (Murphy et al. 1979) and rat basophilic leukemia cells, whereas purified human mast cells produce mainly LTD_4 (Parker et al. 1979, Orning et al. 1980, MacGlashan et al. 1983). SRS-LTs are also produced by human neutrophils, eosinophils, and macrophages (Borgeat and Samuelsson 1979, Du et al. 1983, Weller et al. 1983).

LTC_4 and LTD_4 constrict small and large bronchi, peripheral airway tissue, and smooth muscles of ileum and blood vessels (Parker 1982). They also cause intense constriction of arterioles which is however short-lived and is rapidly followed by a markedly increased permeability of postcapillary venules and by a drop in blood pressure (Dahlen et al. 1981).

The relative potencies of LTC_4 and LTD_4 vary somewhat, depending on which tissues they influence. In all their biological activities, they are more potent than histamine by one to several log molar concentrations. Until now, they have not been demonstrated in urticarial tissue, but they cause erythema, wheals, and increased blood flow when injected into human skin (Bisgaard et al. 1982, Camp et al. 1983, Soter et al. 1983). The pain on injection does not exceed that induced by saline alone (Camp et al. 1983). LTD_4 and E_4 are also potent inhibitors of in vitro lymphocyte transformation and antibody formation (Webb et al. 1982), and LTC_4 induces generation of PGI_2 and TXA_2 in guinea pigs in vivo (Omini et al. 1981).

2.3.5 Platelet Activating Factor

PAF, a soluble mediator from rabbit basophils with platelet activating properties, has recently been identified as an ether phospholipid that derives from mast cells, basophils, neutrophils, macrophages, and plate-

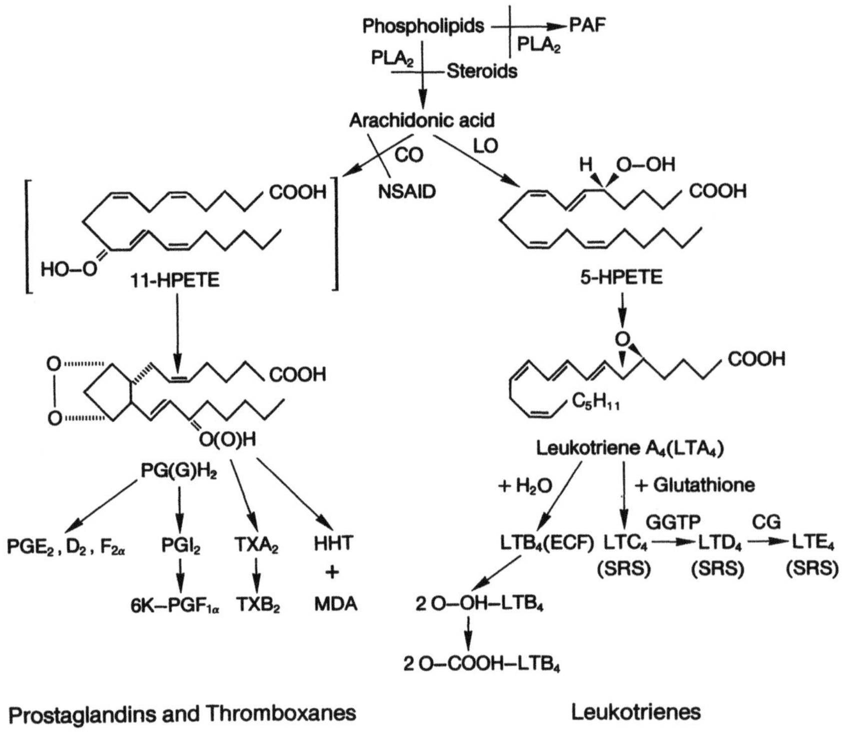

Fig. 2.11. Pathways for the production of platelet-activating factor (*PAF*), prostaglandins (*PG*), thromboxanes (*TX*), leukotrienes (*LT*) B_4 (eosinophil chemotactic factor, *ECF*), LTC_4, D_4 and E_4 (*SRS*). PLA_2, phospholipase A_2; *CO*, cyclooxygenase; *LO*, lipoxygenase; *GGTP*, γ-glutamyl transpeptidase; *CG*, cysteinylglycinase; *HPETE*, hydroperoxyeicosatetraenoic acid; *NSAID*, nonsteroidal anti-inflammatory drugs.

lets (Pinckard et al. 1982, Benveniste and Vargaftig 1983, MacGlashan et al. 1983). Production of PAF from phospholipids is thought to proceed via a lyso-PAF through the action of phospholipase A_2 and via a subsequent acetylation of this hydrolysis product by an acetyl transferase. As with prostaglandins and leukotrienes, the production of PAF can thus be blocked by corticosteroids (Fig. 2.11).

PAF has no direct bronchoconstrictive and hypotensive properties of its own in animals, but mediates this activity through platelet aggregation (Vargaftig et al. 1981). Secondarily released histamine and serotonin have been implicated as the mediators of these biological effects. PAF causes also coronary artery spasms, cardiac dysrythmia, bradycardia, and myocardial depression (reviewed by Wasserman 1983).

Studies in human skin have shown that injection of PAF results in a transient blanching, indicating acute vasoconstriction, and a burning pain. Within 5 min, erythema and edema develop at injection sites, with maximal reactions by 10 min which subside within 60 min. Histamine was 100 × less potent than PAF in these studies (Pinckard et al. 1982) (Table 2.2). Archer et al. (1984) also observed an area of erythema but no whealing at the injection sites in 54% of their subjects. The reactions appeared 3–6 h after injection and subsided within 1–2 h. A platelet-mediated secondary effect can therefore not be excluded in this delayed reaction. The combination of prostaglandin E_2 and PAF caused a synergistic enhancement of whealing.

Neutrophils may also contribute to these cutaneous changes of PAF, particularly to the late-phase erythema. They accumulate at sites of cutaneous injections of PAF within 25 min, are maximal at 3–6 h, and disappear by 24 h (Pinckard et al. 1982). This corresponds to the in vitro ability of PAF to cause neutrophil and monocyte aggregation and chemotaxis (Czarnetzki and Benveniste 1981, Pinckard et al. 1982, Czarnetzki 1983). PAF also enhances the secretory response of these cells (Pinckard et al. 1982, Czarnetzki 1982), although the chemotactic response to PAF is 100 × weaker than that to LTB_4.

2.3.6 Prostaglandins

All nucleated cells are capable of generating prostaglandins (PG), but the type produced varies, depending on the cell type, tissue, and stimulus. The production of these potent mediators of inflammation from arachidonic acid through a cyclooxygenase is inhibited by aspirin, other nonsteroidal anti-inflammatory drugs, and by dapsone (Fig. 2.11). Anaphylactic challenge of guinea pig or human lung results in the release of $PGF_{2\alpha}$, E_2, I_2, D_2, G_2, H_2, B_2, thromboxane (TX) A_2 and hydroxyheptadecatrienoic acid (HHT). Histamine, SRS, and a prostaglandin-releasing factor that is generated during anaphylactic challenge can also induce the production of some of these compounds from the same organs (Metcalfe et al. 1981). Purified human mast cells release PGD_2, $F_{2\alpha}$, E, I_2, and TXB_2, and purified basophils PGD_2 and TXB_2 (MacGlashan et al. 1983).

Prostaglandins have a great diversity of biological effects which oppose each other in part. PGI_2, D_2, and E_2 raise intracellular cAMP and inhibit secretion of mediators such as histamine and LTB_4 (Ham et al. 1983), while PGG_2 and $F_{2\alpha}$ raise cGMP levels and facilitate the same activities.

Injections of PGE_2 and D_2 into the skin cause vasodilatation, whealing, itching, and pain (Crunkhorn and Willis 1971, Sondergaard and Greaves 1971, Soter et al. 1983) (Table 2.2). $PGF_{2\alpha}$ and TXA_2 are vasoconstrictors; PGG_2, H_2, $F_{2\alpha}$, D_2, and TXA_2 have smooth muscle contracting properties, while PGE_2 and I_2 are muscle relaxants. Other activities of prostaglandins which are potentially important in allergic disease are the modulation of mucus secretion (PGE_2 is inhibitory, other PGs are enhancing), the stimulation of platelet aggregation (TXA_2), and the chemotactic activity of HHT for eosinophils and neutrophils (reviewed in Marom and Casale 1983).

PGE_2 causes hyperalgesia, and PGI_2 is even more potent in this respect although its effect is more short-lived. PGE_2 potentiates the pain or the itch produced by histamine or bradykinin (Hagermark and Strandberg 1977, Higgs and Moncada 1983), and the vascular leakage, induration, and tenderness caused by PGE_2 and D_2 in the skin is augmented by LTB_4 or histamine (Soter et al. 1983).

The role of prostaglandins in urticaria is nevertheless unclear, nor have they been sought in wheals. Many cell types, including mast cells and diverse leukocytes, can produce them, and they mimick or potentiate the actions of several mediators of anaphylaxis. It is possible that certain types of prostaglandins, such as PGD_2 which causes flushing and hypotension in patients with mastocytosis, and which is elevated in patients' urine (see Chapter 9, p. 120), play a more specific role in mast-cell related diseases.

2.3.7 Complement

The complement system is comprised of a cascade of factors and enzymes which function primarily as cell activators but can also lead, through the late components, to cell lysis and death. More than 20 components of the complement system have been isolated by now (Fig. 2.12). Factors C1–C9 constitute the classical pathway of activation; factors B, D, and P are the main constituents of the alternative pathway; and four distinct inhibitor molecules function as regulator molecules in both systems. The classical complement pathway is activated by immune complexes that contain IgG_{1-3} or IgM; the alternate pathway is activated by complex polysaccharides or lipopolysaccharides, as may be found in snake venom or pollen antigens, by immune complexes that contain IgA, and by C3b, a split product of C3 which provides an amplification mechanism and a way of involving the alternate pathway secondarily when activation occurs through mechanisms I or III (Fig. 2.12). A third

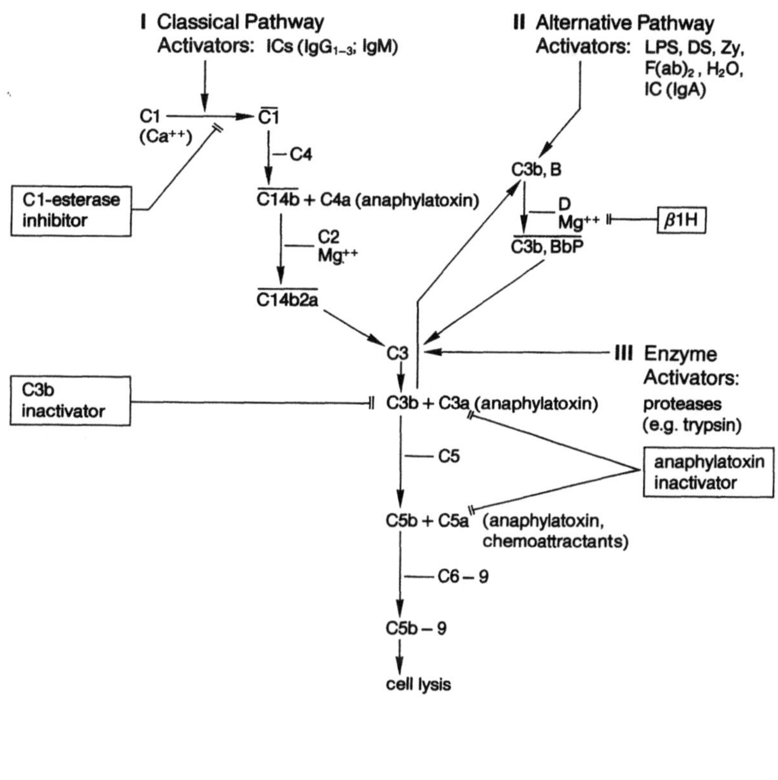

Fig. 2.12. Complement activation (I, II, III), resulting in the generation of biologically active peptides or in cell lysis. Inactivators of the system (in *squares*) are shown, with their points of attack. *IC*, immune complex; *LPS*, lipopolysaccharide; *DS*, dextran sulfate; *Zy*, zymosan; *P*, properdin.

possibility of complement activation is through direct action of proteases on C3, resulting in the biologically active peptide component of this factor.

The complement molecules are distributed throughout the mammalian organism and are found in plasma, lymph, interstitial tissue, and cerebrospinal fluid. Since they can be activated constantly, even by minor trauma, the mechanisms which control their activation are very important. This control occurs through the rapid decay of the activated enzymes and through the lability of the membrane-binding sites of C4b, C3b, and C5b. In addition, there are four distinct inhibitors of the system (Fig. 2.12).

The C1 inhibitor is an α-globulin that binds the C1s and inhibits irreversibly its capacity to cleave C4 and C2. It also blocks C1r activation of C1s and affects other proinflammatory systems by inhibiting active Hageman factor and the kinin-generating activities of kallikrein (Nicholson et al. 1978). The anaphylatoxin inactivator is an α_2-macroglobulin which cleaves enzymatically the C-terminal arginine from C3a, C5a, and bradykinin and destroys thus the histamine-liberating and spasmogenic properties of these mediators. Beta1H is a β-glycoprotein that binds to fluid phase C3b and displaces factor B, interrupting in this fashion the alternate pathway complement activation. Finally, C3b inactivator, a β-glycoprotein, cleaves the α-chain of C3b and inhibits thus the amplification of the alternate pathway.

Like PAF, components of the complement system function as spasmogens, edema-producing agents, cell activators, and chemoattractants. The spasmogenic and edema-generating activity is not only primary, but it also mediated through liberation of histamine from mast cells and basophils, and through stimulation of the secretion of serotonin from platelets (Hadding 1981) and of leukotrienes from diverse leukocytes (Regal and Pickering 1981).

All these activities are due to the C-terminal arginine of the so-called anaphylatoxin peptides, primarily to C5a (which is also inactivated more slowly by the anaphylatoxin inactivator than C3a) and the recently described, biologically less active C4a (Gorski et al. 1979). The anaphylatoxins also stimulate the non-cytotoxic secretion of lysosomal enzymes from neutrophils which provides an additional way of amplifying the inflammatory process.

Of all the complement components, only the C5 split products are capable of inducing cell migration. This occurs through the action of the methionine in position 70 of the amino acid sequence of the molecule. The anaphylactically inactive $C5a_{des\text{-}arg}$ can also cause the directed migration of cells in the presence of a cochemotaxin in normal serum (Perez and Goldstein 1981). C5a is the most potent chemoattractant known, with the broadest spectrum of action (Table 2.3). It attracts neutrophils, eosinophils, basophils, monocytes, macrophages, lymphocytes, fibroblasts and tumor cells by binding to specific receptor units on these cells, and it may well play a role in the migration of cells into urticarial lesions.

Other functions of the complement system which have probably no major impact in the development of urticaria, are the enhancement of phagocytosis of cells through membrane-bound C3b, the lysis of cells, also of mast cells, through the terminal complement components, the binding of cells to each other which may be important in lymphocyte activation, and the induction of the respiratory burst and the liberation of PGE and lysosomal enzymes from macrophages (Sandberg 1981, Hadding 1981 for review).

There is good evidence that the complement cascade plays a role in the pathobiology of urticaria. Activation through immune complexes, altered tissue antigens, and exogenous antigens (e.g., pollen, grain extracts) may be involved. In anaphylactoid reactions, complement activation has been implicated as the primary eliciting event, but activation also occurs in normal persons; therefore, additional factors must be responsible (see Chapter 7, p. 106). Undoubtedly, complement consumption plays an important role in the urticarial vasculitis syndrome (see Chapter 8, p. 109), but activation of the system has also been shown in some patients with chronic urticaria. Laurell et al. (1977) measured abnormal levels of C1q and C1s in 30% of their 150 patients with chronic urticaria and angioedema. These patients had no genetic defects of the complement system. Marder et al. (1976) reported on one patient with selective C1q deficiency,

Table 2.3. Comparative data on the potency and target-cell specificity of the four best characterized chemotactic factors which may be important in urticaria.

Target Cells	Chemotactic Factors			
	C5a	LTB_4 (ECF)	PAF	Lymphokines
Neutrophils	++	++	+	+
Eosinophils	++	++	−	+
Monocytes/ macrophages	++	+	+	+
Lymphocytes	++	−	−	+
Basophils	++	−	−	+
Fibroblasts	++	+	−	+

++ = very potent, in macromolar concentrations; + = potent, in micromolar concentrations; − = inactive or not studied. PAF, platelet activating factor; LTB_4 = leukotriene B_4; ECF = eosinophil chemotactic factor.

urticaria, and vasculitis. Mathison et al. (1977) observed alterations in 10 of 72 patients with chronic urticaria with involvement of classical or alternate pathway components or both. In contrast, Lieberman et al. (1977) and Oehling et al. (1979) found no changes at all. Deficiency of the C1-inhibitor will be discussed separately in the chapter on angioedema (Chapter 4, p. 47).

Table 2.4. Biological activities of LTB_4.

Leukocyte chemotaxis (see also Table 2.3)
Leukocyte chemokinesis
Leukocyte aggregation
Enhanced leukocyte secretion
Augmentation of PGE_2- and PGD_2-induced vascular permeability
Induction of T-suppressor and cytotoxic cells
Enhancement of γ-interferon production

2.3.8 Chemotactic Factors

The chemotactic properties of C5a and PAF have been discussed in the preceding sections. Another important group of chemoattractants are derived through lipoxygenation from arachidonic acid (Fig. 2.11), and a final group comprises cell-derived proteins and peptides of varying sizes and target-cell specificities, of which the lymphocyte- and mast cell-derived factors are the most thoroughly studied of this latter group.

Table 2.3 summarizes the cell-specificity and potency of these factors. C5a is the most potent chemoattractant with the broadest spectrum of activities. PAF is active only at concentrations of $\geq 10^{-6}$ M, has no significant effect on eosinophils, and attracts human monocytes only in patients with widespread inflammatory diseases (Czarnetzki 1983, Czarnetzki and Grabbe 1983). LTB_4 is the most powerful chemoattractant among the arachidonate metabolites (Fig. 2.11). It is as potent as C5a on a molar basis, has a selective action on eosinophils, and resembles in these and all other properties the low molecular weight eosinophil chemotactic factor (ECF) that is released from mast cells, basophils, neutrophils, and monocytes (Czarnetzki and Grabbe 1983).

A metabolite of LTB_4, 20-OH-LTB_4, is about 100 times less active than the parent compound during in vitro or in vivo chemotaxis (Czarnetzki and Rosenbach 1984), while the 20-COOH-LTB_4 is practically inactive. LTB_4 is also chemotactic for monocytes of patients with inflammatory dermatoses such as erythrodermic or atopic eczema (Czarnetzki 1983) and attracts human fibroblasts (Mensing and Czarnetzki 1984). It causes enhanced, nondirected migration (chemokinesis), aggregation, and enhanced secretion of cells (Goetzl 1980) and has recently been observed to modulate suppressor cell induction and γ-interferon production (Rola-Pleszczynski et al. 1982, 1983) (Table 2.4). Vasoactive properties of the molecule are mediated through the release of products from immigrated inflammatory cells or through a combined action of LTB_4 with prostaglandin E_2 (Goetzl 1980). Elevated levels of LTB_4-like activity have been identified in skin of patients with urticaria pigmentosa (Czarnetzki et al. 1985), pressure urticaria (Czarnetzki et al. 1984a), and a variety of non-urticarial inflammatory disorders, ranging from rheumatoid arthritis (Klickstein et al. 1980) and psoriasis (Grabbe et al. 1982) to atopic eczema (Ruzicka et al. 1984). While LTB_4 may thus play a potentially important role in the induction of the leukocyte infiltrates in more persistent wheals, it is not specific for urticaria.

Other chemotactic arachidonate metabolites are the cyclooxygenase product 12 L-hydroxy-5,8,14-heptadecatrienoic (HHT) acid and several lipoxygenase-dependent monohydroxy-5,8,10,10-eicosatetraenoic acids (HETEs) (Goetzl 1980). They are less potent than LTB_4 and have no action on eosinophils in our experience (Czarnetzki and Grabbe 1983). LTB_5, which is formed from eicosapentaenoic acid, is 30 times less active in its biological activities than LTB_4 (Terano et al. 1984). With the rapid burst of new information of biologically active lipid mediators, many more chemotactic lipids will certainly be detected in the near future. Studies on their respective role in the pathogenesis of urticaria or asthma may help to better understand the diverse clinical aspects of urticaria and aid in the therapy for allergic diseases.

Several oligopeptides with eosinophil and neutrophil chemotactic activity have been isolated from rat mast cells (Boswell et al. 1978). These high molecular weight (> 750 kdal) neutrophil chemotactic proteins have also been detected in the serum of patients with various types of physical urticaria (reviewed by Wasserman 1983) and of asthma (Atkins et al. 1977). In contrast to the chemotactic lipids, these factors are preformed within mast cell granules. The synthetic tetrapeptides, which were originally reported to represent the ECF-A (eosinophil chemotactic factor of anaphylaxis) (Goetzl and Austen 1975), have been found subsequently to be biologically inactive during in vitro chemotaxis assays in several laboratories (Czarnetzki and Grabbe 1983). The inflammatory factor of anaphylaxis (IFA) in mast cell granules consists of several peptides (molecular weight, 1400–4000 d) which cause neutrophil influx soon (1–3 h) and mononuclear leukocyte infiltration later (2–24 h) after intracutaneous injection (Oertel and Kaliner 1981). It is unclear whether this factor causes cell migration by itself or through secondary mechanisms. This should not, however, distract from its ability to mimic the temporal sequence of events and the cell types that are observed in the infiltrates of chronic and of physical urticarias.

Finally, a group of lymphocyte-derived chemotactic factors should be mentioned that attract neutrophils, eosinophils, and lymphocytes (Cohen and Ward 1971, Colley 1973, Center 1983). In addition, infiltration of basophils has been shown to be lymphocyte-dependent (Dvorak and Hammond 1978). Lymphokines are also able to induce eosinophil proliferation in the bone marrow; this does not occur with any of the several potent eosinophil chemotactic factors, like C5a or LTB_4 (Czarnetzki and Pawelzik 1983). This fact, together with the dependency of eosinophilia on genetic factors (Vadas 1982), provides a plausible reason why eosinophils are only variably present in the infiltrates of urticarial lesions and why urticaria is not associated with a significant eosinophilia.

2.3.9 Heparin

The characteristic metachromatic shift from blue to red on exposure of toluidine blue to mast cell granules is due to the action of sulfated glycosaminoglycans in mast cells and basophils. Human lung mast cells contain 2.4–7.8 µg heparin/10^6 mast cells. In mucosal mast cells and basophils, more lowly sulfated glycosaminoglycans, such as chondroitin sulfate, are stored instead. Although the latter compounds share a number of biological activities with heparin, heparin is more potent and has the broadest spectrum of action.

The major constituent of heparin is a hexasaccharide, consisting of 2 × [(2,6 disulfoglucosamine-2-sulfonic acid) – (2,6 disulfoglucosamine-glucuronic acid)] (Jacques 1979). Macromolecular heparin (molecular weight 60–1000 kd), which is released together with histamine on stimulation of mast cells, contains a 20 kd molecular weight protein core to which the glycosaminoglycans side chains are attached (Stevens and Austen 1981).

The fate of heparin, once it is secreted into the tissue, is not well understood. It is very resistant to the action of proteolytic enzymes like trypsin, or chymotrypsin, but binds rapidly to cells. Neutrophils, eosinophils, macrophages, and fibroblasts can phagocytize mast cell granules, and heparin is broken down within these cells, probably through progressive desulfatation of the molecule (Atkins and Metcalfe 1983). Heparin within mast cells has only 10% of the anticoagulant activity of commercial heparin which is an extract from beef lung or porcine intestinal mucosa.

The biological activity of heparin is mediated mostly through its highly negative charge, due to the multiple acid groups forming stable complexes with many substances. Heparin binds inorganic ions, plasma proteins, biogenic amines, drugs, basic proteins, alkylamines, and alkaloids. It modulates the biological activity of some 50 different enzymes, either by activation of proenzymes, formation of adducts, stabilization of the molecules, inhibition of the latter, or activation of their inhibitors and release of enzymes from cells (Jacques 1979).

Some important functions of heparin are listed in Table 2.5. The anticoagulant activity of the molecule

Table 2.5. Major aspects of the effect of heparin on various defense systems.

Target System	Effect
Coagulation	1. binds antithrombin 2. inhibits factors XII, XIa, Xa, IXa, kallikrein, plasmin, and antithrombin II
Complement	1. interferes with C1q binding to immune complexes 2. interferes with interaction of $C1\bar{s}$ with C4 and C2 3. inhibits activation of C3 by cobra venom (alternative pathway)
Inflammatory system	1. interferes with the action of many enzymes and inactivates them (e.g., histaminase, lysosomal enzymes) 2. binds histamine, MIF, lymphocyte-derived chemotactic factor, and ECF 3. binds eosinophil major basic protein 4. potentiates binding of fibronectin to collagen 5. binds to fibronectin 6. stimulates release of lipoprotein lipase and plasminogen activator from endothelium 7. stimulates release of phospholipase A from liver membranes 8. inhibits formation of PGE_2 and TXA_2 9. binds platelet factor 4
Immune system	1. increases positive sensitization of basophils 2. modulates the priming activity of protein antigen 3. inhibits mitogen-induced lymphocyte blastogenesis

MIF, migration inhibiting factor; ECF, eosinophil chemotactic factor; TXA_2, thromboxane A_2; PGE_2, prostaglandin E_2.

Table 2.6. Major enzymes in human mast cells and their potential functions.

Enzymes	Function
Neutral proteases	mast cell degranulation (chymotrypsin)
trypsin (tryptase)	cleavage of C3 to C3a and C3b (trypsin)
chymotrypsin (chymase)	cleavage of high molecular weight (kininogen)
	cleavage of proteoglycans and protein core of cartilage
	inactivation of lipoprotein lipase
	digestion of collagen and bradykinins
	activation of Hageman factor
Lysosomal hydrolases	
β-glucuronidase	cleavage of terminal glucuronide } e.g. attack of heparin
β-hexosaminidase	hexosamine and sulfate esters } e.g. attack of heparin
arylsulfatases	cleavage of sulfuric acid ester bond } e.g. attack of heparin
acid phosphatase	
Peroxidase	inactivation of leukotrienes and peroxides

which resides in only a few side chains, is abolished by binding to eosinophil major basic protein or to platelet factor 4. The activities of heparin extend from a modulation of the kinin, fibrinolysis, and complement systems to binding and inactivation of potent mediators of inflammation (Czarnetzki et al. 1980) and to alterations of the lymphocyte-dependent immune response (Atkins and Metcalfe 1983; reviewed in Jacques 1979, Metcalfe et al. 1981, Metcalfe 1983).

2.3.10 Enzymes and Enzyme Inhibitors (Table 2.6)

During IgE-dependent reactions, mast cells release neutral proteases and acid hydrolases into their surroundings (Schwartz et al. 1981, Wilhelms and Roesch 1981). One must therefore assume that these enzymes modulate mast cell-dependent reactions. Mast cell enzymes have been studied for many years by cytochemical methods; their biology and biochemistry have been examined more recently.

Practically all the enzymes which have been demonstrated in mast cells are also present in other cell types. Enzymes from these latter sources also contribute to an amplification of the inflammatory response that is initiated by mast cells. Studies in cytochemistry have shown that paraffin-embedded human and rat mast cells contain abundant chloroacetate esterase (also found in neutrophils but not in macrophages) which helps to differentiate mast cells better than the pH-dependent toluidine blue reaction. Alpha-naphthyl-acetate-esterases give minor, diffuse reactions in mast cells and also in macrophages. Beta-glucuronidase and diaminopeptidase IV are additional enzymes that give positive reactions in human skin mast cells. Acid phosphatases and peroxidases cannot be demonstrated cytochemically (reviewed by Sterry 1984).

Biochemical analysis has revealed that the major protease in human mast cells is a trypsin. Only minute amounts of a chymotrypsin can be measured, although these enzymes are present in large quantities in rat mast cell granules. Human mast cells contain 6–19 μg trypsin/10^6 cells, and the enzymes make up 50–40% of the total granule protein (reviewed by Wasserman 1983). The enzyme is tightly bound to the granule matrix, is released from there only at high ionic strength, and is not inhibited by plasma antiproteases. It may be identical to the cytochemically demonstrated chloroacetate esterase.

A chymotrypsin-like enzyme which constitutes 15% of the total protein in rat mast cell granules remains complexed to heparin after degranulation of rat mast cells in vivo and can cleave only smaller molecules in this situation.

Both the trypsin and chymotrypsin are potentially important in urticaria (see Table 2.6). They are released from mast cells and basophils on antigen challenge, together with histamine (Wilhelms and Roesch 1981; personal communication). Arthur and Shelley (1955) observed that they caused pruritus when injected into the skin. Lagunoff et al. (1983) see Table 2.1) showed that chymotrypsin causes histamine release from rat mast cells. The enzymes cleave C3 into C3b and the anaphylatoxin C3a (Fig. 2.12), digest collagen, attack the proteoglycans and the protein core of cartilage, and inactivate lipoprotein lipases. A trypsin-like enzyme has also been described which activates Hageman factor (Metcalfe et al. 1981, Wasserman 1983).

Acid hydrolases which are generally found in primary lysosomes of cells, are also present in mast cells. Beta-hexosaminidase is the most active enzyme in human mast cells (Schwartz et al. 1981), making up 1% of the total granule protein in the rat. It is released together with histamine, β-glucuronidase, arylsulfatase, and trypsin. The lysosomal hydrolases cleave glucuronides, hexosamines, and sulfate esters, as implied by their name. They can therefore also attack glycosaminoglycans chains, for example, in heparin. Acid phosphatase is not released during degranulation and has been demonstrated on electron microscopy in pinocytozing mast cell granules only (Komiyama and Spicer 1975) (Table 2.6). Mast cell granules can take up peroxidase from other cells such as eosinophils, and the peroxidase found in their granules by some workers may derive from that source. Peroxidases can inactivate leukotrienes such as SRS and superoxides which may prove otherwise toxic to the cells (Henderson and Kaliner 1979).

Inhibitors of proteases have already been discussed in conjunction with the kinin and complement systems. They oppose the action of mast cell enzymes once released from the cells. Inhibitors of trypsin and chymotrypsin are α_1-antitrypsin, β_2-macroglobulin, and serum trypsin and chymotrypsin inhibiting capacity. Juhlin and Michaelsson (1969) have postulated that a deficiency of these inhibitors might allow for the uncontrolled production of mediators in some types of chronic urticaria. Such a possibility was made more likely by the discovery of a deficiency of the C1-esterase inhibitor in hereditary angioedema (see Chapter 4, p. 47).

Doeglas and Bleumink (1975) have thoroughly studied this hypothesis in 92 patients with chronic urticaria. They found decreased levels of α_1-antitrypsin and total antitrypsin activity in patients with acquired cold urticaria. In patients with acquired angioedema, they also found decreased α_1-antitrypsin levels, but also lowered antichymotrypsin, antitrypsin, and antikallikrein activities. The remaining patient groups with chronic idiopathic urticaria and other physical urticarias, however, had normal levels. Thus, other pathogenetic mechanisms must be sought in these diseases.

2.4 Overview of Pathogenetic Aspects

The recent rapid advances in the understanding of mast cell and mediator function and of the mechanisms that control their activity should foster hope that the basic aspects of urticaria are now well elucidated. Current science is far from claiming this. A few facts are however generally accepted, namely that mast cells and their analogues are the central effector cells in almost all types of urticaria and that vasoactive mediators are responsible for the typical, fleeting cutaneous edema.

Figure 2.13 depicts in a simplified fashion the sequence of events that leads to the inhibition, amplification, and termination of urticaria. The primary stimulus which acts on mast cells is well known in cases of allergic urticaria, but these represent only a minor fraction of all cases of urticaria. To what extent other stimuli (see Fig. 2.6, Fig. 2.7 and Table 2.1) play a role in specific types of urticaria is greatly undetermined and will be discussed in later chapters. In angioedema, there is good evidence that mast cell activation and mediator release are not the primary pathogenetic events (Chapter 4, p. 47). In urticarial vasculitis (Chapter 8, p. 109), mast cells may be only secondarily involved through complement activation.

The variety of mediators released from mast cells (Fig. 2.8) have several major effects (Fig. 2.13):

1. They contract smooth muscle, causing bronchoconstriction and vasodilatation or constriction and leakage of vessels (Table 2.2), resulting in tissue edema, hypotension, and asthma. Histamine, kinins, serotonin, prostaglandins, and SRS type leukotrienes can each cause these effects alone or in combination. PAF and anaphylatoxins can induce the generation of the smooth muscle-active mediators in target tissue.

2. Certain mast cell constituents can activate plasma to generate potent mediators such as the complement-derived anaphylatoxins and kinins. Mast cell enzymes belong to this group. The complement and kinin-type mediators can act on muscles and nerves on their own. They can also stimulate, together with other mast cell-derived mediators, the additional production of mediators from mast cells or other tissue.

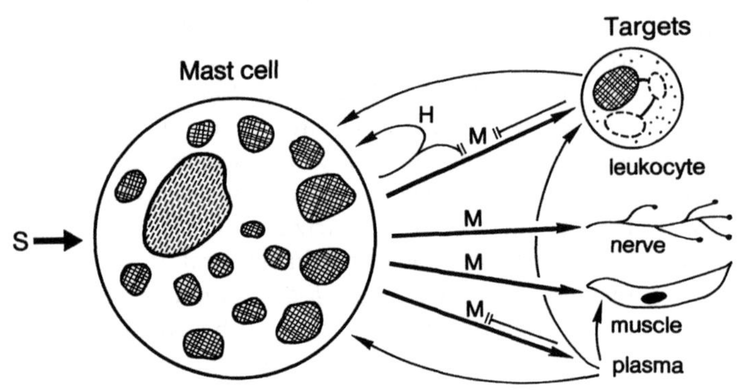

Fig. 2.13. Model of potential events initiated by mast cell secretion of mediators (*M*). The effect of mediators may be amplified by recruitment of further mediator-secreting cells or by synergism of the different mediators with each other. The reaction is downregulated through inactivation of mediators and their biological effects (*S*, stimulus; *H*, histamine).

3. Finally, mast cell mediators can aid in the recruitment of other leukocytes to the site. Chemotactic factors which are potentially involved in this activity, are protein- and peptide-type preformed chemotactic factors in mast cells, newly generated chemoattractants that derive from arachidonic acid and phospholipids (see Table 2.3 and Fig. 2.11), and the complement fragments C5a and $C5a_{des\,arg}$. Chemotactic factors play a role in more persistent urticarial reactions secondary to intense mast cell stimulation.

4. The pruritus which is typically observed in urticaria may be due to the action of several of the vasoactive mediators (Table 2.2) or to enzymes.

It is striking that most mediators have several possible modes of action within the tissue. They even develop additional activities when acting in concert with other mediators. An example of this is provided by LTB_4 which has vasoactive properties only in the presence of PGE_2 or PGD_2. The activities of vasoactive or leukotactic mediators is also synergistically amplified when they are combined in individually low amounts (Czarnetzki and Grabbe 1983). These and the enhanced secretory activity of mast cells and other leukocytes cause the rapid and efficient, potent inflammatory reactions that characterize urticaria and anaphylactic processes.

Normally this inflammatory system has so many inhibitory barriers that it cannot develop its full picture unless the stimulus is overpowerful or the inhibitory system is defect. The down-modulating mechanisms (Fig. 2.13) are also responsible for the rapid disappearance of urticarial reactions. Practically every mediator has its inactivator, whether in form of inactivating enzymes, hydroxyl radicals (Henderson and Klebanoff 1983), or binding proteins. Some of these inhibitory principles are present within the cells and are released by mast cells and other leukocytes. Examples are heparin or leukocyte enzymes. Other inhibitors are present in plasma and tissue fluid. The protease inhibitors comprise the most powerful system in this compartment. In fact, the increased vascular leakage during urticarial reactions is an efficient way of allowing the protease inhibitors to become available in larger quantities and to help the involved tissue to return to its original state of integrity.

3 Acute and Chronic Urticaria

3.1 Definition

Urticaria is defined by the appearance of wheals (hives or individual urticae) of any size and configuration on any part of the skin. The wheals consist of a circumscribed, slightly elevated, erythematous, usually pruritic, edematous swelling of the upper dermal tissue which disappears within minutes to hours, leaving a basically unaltered, normal appearing skin (restauratio ad integrum). Similarly transient, erythematous swellings of the deeper cutaneous and the subcutaneous tissue are called angioedema and appear in about 50% of patients in association with ordinary urticaria (see Chapter 4, p. 47).

3.2 Classification

Most urticarial eruptions appear suddenly because of exposure of the organism to some specific, noxious agent, and the crops of lesions gradually decrease in severity after the cause is eliminated. This type of urticaria is called acute urticaria and is defined by most authors as a tendency for whealing that persists or reappears intermittently for not longer than six weeks.

Illig and Paul (1978) (Table 3.1) further differentiate acute intermittent from ordinary acute urticaria.

Table 3.1. Classification of urticaria on the basis of its time course (after Illig and Paul 1978).

Type	Course	Duration
I. Acute urticaria	appears only once	a few days, up to 6 weeks
II. Acute intermittent urticaria	short episodes, with long intervals inbetween (weeks or months)	> 6 weeks, up to many years
III. Chronic recurrent urticaria	free intervals of a few or many days	> 6 weeks, up to many years
IV. Chronic continuous urticaria	new wheals daily	> 6 weeks, up to many years

Acute urticaria occurs usually only once or twice in a lifetime, whereas acute intermittent urticaria tends to reappear in bouts of intense whealing episodes, possibly with angioedema, shock, malaise, and fever. Weeks and months of symptom-free intervals may lie inbetween.

The same authors further subdivide chronic urticaria into chronic recurrent urticaria, with symptom-free intervals of only a few days, and chronic continuous urticaria, with whealing on a daily basis. This classification of the urticarias is useful in that it helps to better delineate the clinical course of the disease.

Urticaria develops in the context of a wide spectrum of circumstances and diseases, and the clinical picture varies considerably depending on these factors. A classification of urticaria on the basis of its patho-

Table 3.2. Classification of urticaria, based on possible pathogenetic mechanisms.

I. Immunoglobulin-dependent urticaria (mostly IgE)
  1. Atopic diasthesis
  2. Specific antigen sensitivity (drugs, pollens, foods, contactants, insect venoms)
  3. Physical urticaria
    1. Dermographic urticaria
    2. Cold urticaria
    3. Solar urticaria
    4. Cholinergic urticaria

II. Complement-mediated urticaria
  1. Hereditary angioedema
  2. Acquired angioedema
  3. Necrotizing vasculitis
  4. Heat urticaria
  5. Serum sickness
  6. Reactions to blood products or substitutes

III. Non-immunologic urticaria
  A. Direct mast cell-releasing agents
    1. Opiates
    2. Antibiotics
    3. Curare
    4. Radiocontrast media
    5. Chemical contactants
  B. Intolerance reactions
    1. Aspirin and nonsteroidal anti-inflammatory agents
    2. Azodyes and benzoates

IV. Mastocytosis, urticaria pigmentosa

V. Idiopathic urticaria

genesis which is useful for both the diagnosis of the underlying cause and for treatment, is presented in Table 3.2. It should, however, be remembered that the underlying pathomechanisms causing the different types of urticaria, are far from being exactly understood, and in some of them, even more than one mechanism may be involved.

The individual disease categories, as listed in Table 3.2, are described in more detail in this or one of the several subsequent chapters dealing with the specific subtypes of urticaria.

3.3 Epidemiology

3.3.1 Incidence

The incidence of urticaria varies greatly, depending on the age and the geographic location of the population studied. Swinny (1941) reported that 23.6% of Virginians had urticaria at some time in their life, whereas Hellgren and Hersle (1964) observed an incidence of only 1.85% in their survey of five geographic areas in Sweden. The prevalence figures at any one time for the same population of 36,575 persons were 0.11% for males and 0.14% for females (Hellgren 1983).

McKee (1966) reported that 11.8% of patients attending a general medical outpatient department had suffered from urticaria at some time in their life, whereas only 1.4% of the patients seen at a Dutch dermatology outpatient department in a university referral center sought help because of urticaria (Doeglas 1975).

3.3.2 Age

Urticaria may occur at any age, but it develops most frequently during the third and fourth decades of life. Its first appearance after the age of sixty is extremely rare which may be due to a decreased ability of the immune system to recognize and react to neoantigens. The incidence among newborns in India has been reported to be as high as 23.5% (Singh et al. 1980), compared to 3.4% among infants and children in Western civilizations (Warin and Champion 1974). Among college students, 15.7% had been affected with urticaria at one time in their life (Sheldon et al. 1954).

3.3.3 Sex

In almost all patient series, females are reported to have urticaria slightly more frequently than males. Since this sex predilection is not observed among children (Halpern 1965), it may simply be due to a greater tendency of females to seek medical attention. The increased incidence of mechanogenic urticarias (see chapter on physical urticarias) among male patients may similarly be based on the greater nuisance that this condition causes among men during heavy manual labor.

3.3.4 Types of Urticaria

Acute urticaria accounts for 33% or more of all urticarias (Hellgren 1983), and it occurs more frequently among young adult males and females. A cause can be identified in only about one-half of the cases (Wüthrich and Häcki-Herrmann 1980).

About 10% of patients with acute urticaria proceed to have chronic urticaria which lasts by definition for more than 6 weeks. In these patients, a cause is even more difficult to elucidate. Older series report an identifiable cause in only about 20% (Champion et al. 1969), but with a better characterization and more recent awareness of the physical urticarias and the intolerance reactions, this figure has much improved (Table 3.3). In other reports, this same trend to better diagnosis is apparent, with a cause being identified in 31% (Mathison et al. 1977) and 28% (Wüthrich and Häcki-Herrmann 1980) of patients with chronic urticaria. In contrast, Harris et al. (1982) found a cause in only 8% of children with urticaria (7% cold urticaria, 1% food allergy).

Table 3.3. Percent incidence of different types of chronic urticaria in different patient series.

Underlying cause	Incidence		
	Champion et al. (1969)	Doeglas (1975)	Illig and Paul (1978)
Idiopathic	79.0	45.0	60–70
Allergic	3.1	?	3– 8
Physical	17.0	55.0	12–17
Intolerance	–	?	15–26
Other	0.9	–	–

3.3.5 Atopy

Most authors agree that acute urticaria occurs more frequently in atopics, with symptoms lasting for only a few days, and the cause being in general an allergen to which the patient is known to be allergic (Warin and Champion 1974). Singh et al. (1980) reported that newborns with urticaria have an increased family history of atopy and a twofold higher risk of developing allergic disorders during infancy. Harris et al. (1982) obtained a family history of urticaria in 33%

and of atopy in 54% of their pediatric patients with urticaria. In 30% a history of atopy was found.

In contrast, patients with chronic urticaria and their relatives have no increased incidence of atopy (Champion et al. 1969). Doeglas (1975) agrees with this, but when he took the increased reactivity to skin tests against multiple allergens as a criterion for atopy, he found more atopics among patients with chronic idiopathic and dermographic urticaria. Such an approach must however be viewed with caution since, as Wüthrich and Häcki-Herrmann (1980) have pointed out, the clinical relevance of positive skin tests is very unclear in patients with urticaria. In contrast to asthma, rhinitis, and atopic eczema, urticaria should therefore not be viewed as part of the atopic syndrome. This is underlined by the fact that the majority of the urticarias are not based on an IgE-mediated allergic reaction.

3.4 Clinical Aspects

3.4.1 Cutaneous Lesions

The individual wheal starts as a pinkish erythema that is rapidly transformed into a slightly elevated, edematous papule or plaque (Fig. 2.1). After a brief time, the redness often becomes more accentuated at the margin of the lesion, with the center assuming a yellowish-white hue, due to the pressure of the edema and the constriction of larger arterioles. This color is even more apparent when the skin is stretched. The lesion may be surrounded by a brightly red reflex erythema. On squeezing the erythematous skin between two fingers, the typical orange peel appearance of the lesion becomes apparent (see Fig. 5.6, p. 65).

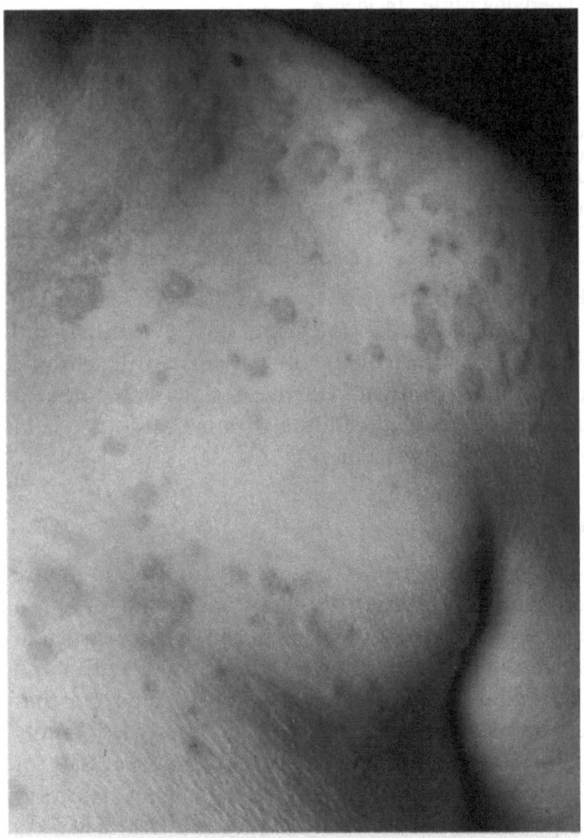

Apart from this basic aspect of the appearance of the wheal, the clinical picture of urticaria can be extremely diverse. Wheals may be small (Fig. 3.1), even pinpoint-sized, as in cholinergic urticaria (Figs. 5.9 and 5.10, p. 76), or they can attain the size of a palm. Their shape may be annular (Fig. 3.2), and gyrations may develop due to union of several patches (Fig. 3.3). In this way, large, confluent areas of the skin can become involved.

Due to intense edema, vesiculation or bulla-formation may develop on top of the wheal. This rare occurrence is seen more frequently on top of insect bites and on lesions of infants with urticaria pigmentosa (see Fig. 9.2, p. 118). Some lesions maintain a more papular appearance after the urticarial component has faded. This is seen more often in wheals due to insect bites and in chronic urticaria, particularly when there is an underlying vasculitis. In the older literature, papular urticaria is called strophulus (Török 1928). On the basis of histological findings, the condition represents a cutaneous vasculitis, with immunoglobulin and complement deposits in the vessel walls (Heng et al. 1984).

Rarely, more intense lesions can become hemorrhagic. Hyperpigmentation is not a feature of ordinary urticaria, but is seen at sites of cutaneous mast cell proliferation in urticaria pigmentosa. Whether this increased melanization is due to mast cell-derived mediators or to the stimulus that causes mast cell proliferation, is unknown. The hallmark of urticaria is otherwise its lack of epidermal involvement.

The typical urticae develop within seconds to minutes on any part of the skin or the mucosa, and they are generally gone from the involved site by 3–4 h, at most 48 h after they have been initiated. This ephemeral character of the lesions may be due to an exhaustion of local mast cell histamine stores. Other lesions arise adjacent to old sites or in totally different locations. The fleeting, migratory nature of the wheal

Fig. 3.1. Relatively small urticarial lesions in an elderly midwife with chronic idiopathic urticaria of more than 10 years duration.

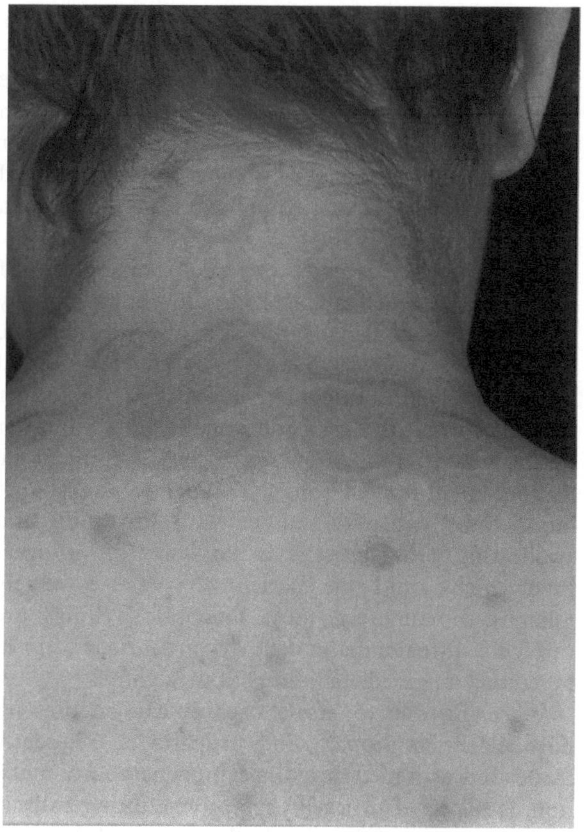

Fig. 3.2. Annular wheals with surrounding erythema in a patient with acute urticaria due to penicillin.

can often be best appreciated by marking the edge of the lesions with a pen and checking its progression several hours later. The reason for this varying and unpredictable distribution of lesions is unclear. It may be due to changes in local blood flow and the transport of the eliciting stimulus to mast cells. More likely, the activity of local factors which regulate the firing threshold of mast cells, or an intrinsic "releasability" of the mast cells, is involved.

Some types of urticaria have special configurations and sites of predilection, particularly the physical and contact urticarias. The time course of the wheal may vary from very fleeting lesions as in most physical urticarias, to more persistent lesions, as is typical of urticarial vasculitis. The tissue edema may also extend to the deeper cutaneous and subcutaneous tissue, as in angioedema or in delayed pressure urticaria (see the respective chapters).

Wheals are almost invariably pruritic, and in contrast to the itching that is associated with eczema, urticarial lesions tend to be rubbed or pressed by the patient. This explains why their surface is practically never excoriated. Some patients report stinging, burning, tingling, pricking, or crawling sensations in the lesions. Itching is felt more readily in regions where the skin is tight, such as on the scalp, the palms, the soles, and over bony prominences. Deep swellings may be painful.

In chronic urticaria, lesions tend to develop during the night, and patients suffer much more from pruritus while sleeping or during periods of nervous tension. This may be due to changes in adrenal and autonomic nervous function, particularly to low cortisol levels at night.

3.4.2 Noncutaneous Symptomatology

The restriction of much of the symptoms of urticaria to the skin is surprising in view of the fact that the

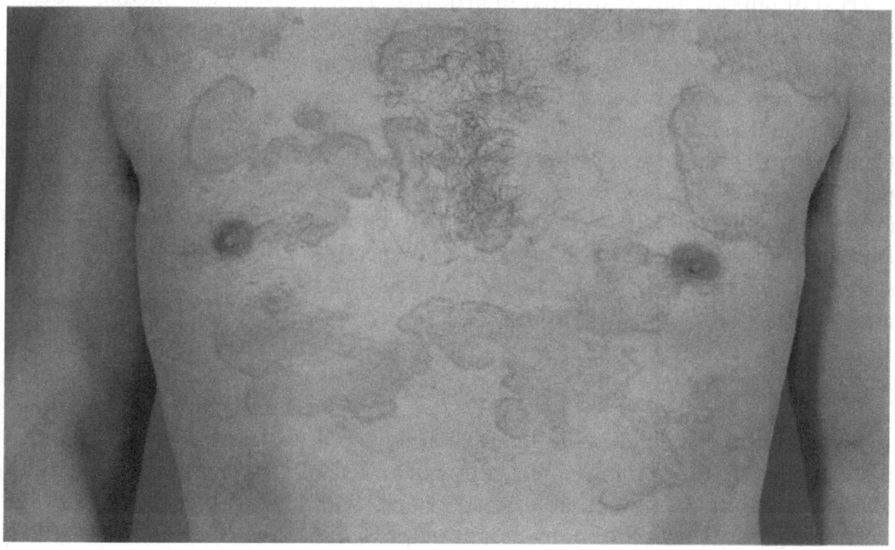

Fig. 3.3. Large, gyrating, erythematous wheals in a patient with chronic idiopathic urticaria.

route of access of antigens, if known, is mostly systemic. Nevertheless, internal organs can be involved, particularly during very severe and acute reactions. The reason may either be due to a reaction of local mast cells to the antigen or noxious agent, or alternately, to a response of other organs to mast cell mediators which are carried to them from the skin via the blood stream.

Some patients experience a prodromal phase of their urticaria which can last from a few hours to a day or two and is associated with loss of appetite, malaise, headache, and fever. The most frequent internal organs involved during acute urticaria are the upper respiratory and the gastrointestinal tracts, the latter particularly after ingestion of antigens. Swelling of the mucous membranes of tongue, soft palate, pharynx, or larynx may cause difficulties with breathing and swallowing. Hoarseness is an early sign of laryngeal involvement, and the patient may be extremely anxious. Fortunately, these mucosal swellings are rarely life-threatening in ordinary urticaria, except in hereditary angioedema and cold urticaria.

Wheezing due to bronchospasm can be present, particularly in atopics, and urticaria is frequently associated with allergic asthma. In general, not much note is taken of urticarial symptoms during asthma attacks because of the more bothersome and threatening pulmonary symptomatology.

Involvement of the gastrointestinal tract causes crampy abdominal pain, vomiting and diarrhea, particularly after ingestion of foods that cause release of mediators from intestinal mast cells. In chronic urticaria, increased acidity may lead to chronic gastric ulceration and bleeding.

Arthritic complaints are part of the urticarial vasculitis syndrome and of serum sickness. Other internal organs are rarely involved in urticaria. There are isolated reports of renal, hepatic, and pancreatic symptomatology and of central nervous system complications, such as cerebral edema, mental confusion, coma, hemiparesis, or convulsions (Warin and Champion 1974). Cardiac involvement such as chest pain and EKG changes due to transient ischemia (Warin and Champion 1974, Bork et al. 1980) are also extremely rare and were not observed in a prospective study of 98 patients with acute urticaria and angioedema (Siegel and Bergeron 1954).

3.4.3 Anaphylaxis

In highly sensitive individuals, systemic anaphylaxis is a potentially life-threatening manifestation of an acute allergic reaction. Non-immunologic reactions, with the same clinical manifestations as an anaphylactic reaction, are called "anaphylactoid". Symptoms occur mostly after intravenous or intramuscular injections, but in highly sensitive persons, the eliciting agent can also penetrate via the oral, gastrointestinal, respiratory, cutaneous, and even the epicutaneous route.

The reaction develops rapidly and reaches its peak after 5–30 min. At the onset, patients may notice itching of the palms and soles, the genital area, or the external auditory meatus. Tingling of the soft palate, nausea, vomiting, substernal pressure, or shortness of breath are other early symptoms. Hypotension, pruritus, bronchospasm, urticaria, angioedema, diffuse erythema, pruritus, laryngeal edema, cardiac arrythmias, and hyperperistalsis may be present alone or in various combinations. This diversity of possible clinical manifestations stands in contrast to observations in animals where the shock organ is always very predictable: the lungs in the guinea pig, the intestine in the dog.

Patients who have reacted with urticaria at several previous incidents may experience shock at subsequent exposures to the antigen or noxious agent. A severe urticarial reaction, if left untreated, may also proceed to hypotension and anaphylaxis. If the patient survives an anaphylactic reaction, hives may develop over the subsequent hours.

Anaphylaxis is mediated by IgE antibodies, possibly also by the IgG_4 subtype which has a high affinity for mast cells and basophils. Bee and wasp stings and reactions to penicillin are probably the most frequent causes of fatal systemic anaphylaxis. Atopic individuals are more endangered (Rajka and Skog 1965).

Other drugs that may cause anaphylaxis are organic mercurials, opiates, organic iodides in radiopaque contrast media, local anesthetics, streptomycin, bromosulfophthalein (BSP), dehydrocholate sodium (Decholin), fluorescein, Congo red, dextran, aspirin, heparin, vitamin B_{12}, tetracycline (especially demethyltetracycline), and cephalosporins. Foreign antisera, allergen extracts, and hormones can also cause anaphylaxis. The specific mechanisms involved, whether IgE-mediated or anaphylactoid, are not always clear (Parker 1975) (see also Chapter 7, p. 96).

3.4.4 Serum Sickness

When antigens persist for prolonged periods of time in the circulation, allowing for antibody and subsequently for immune complex formation, serum sickness may result. A maculopapular, and less frequently an urticarial reaction, may first be present at the injection site and thereafter in a generalized distribution. Fever, lymphadenopathy, arthritis, nephritis, angioedema, neuritis, or severe gastrointestinal symptoms are other features of the disease. There is usually a leukocytosis, an elevated ESR, and a moderate eosinophilia.

In former times, the most frequent causes of serum sickness were injections with foreign sera. Drugs such as penicillin, sulfonamides, thiouracils, radiocontrast media, diphenylhydantoin, aminosalicylic acid, and streptomycin are more common causes nowadays. After initial exposure, a latency period of 4–6 days is necessary before sufficient quantity of antibody is secreted by the immune system for the formation of circulating immune complexes. Reactions occur faster on repeated exposure to the antigen and for up to 3 weeks after administration of long-acting penicillins or sulfonamides. Symptoms persist for a few days to a week, lasting longer when drugs with depot release are involved. In cases of accelerated reactions due to repeated exposure to the eliciting drugs, cardiovascular shock, convulsions, asthma, and diarrhea can lead in rapid succession to coma and death.

3.4.5 Course and Prognosis

In about 90% of patients with acute urticaria, whealing subsides in 2–3 weeks and never recurs again. In the remaining group with chronic urticaria, symptoms will subside if the causative factor is found and meticulously avoided. Most of the patients with idiopathic urticaria lose their tendency to wheal within 5 years. Even the IgE-dependent reactivity, such as a penicillin allergy, has been observed to become less severe with time, and the skin test reactivity is lost after 5–10 years in up to 90% of the patients if no reexposure occurs (Finke et al. 1965). For the individual patient, the duration of the urticaria is, however, unpredictable and may range from a few months to many decades.

3.5 Histopathology

The usual, fleeting urticarial lesions show very few distinctive pathological features on light microscopic examination of skin biopsies. Edema of the papillary and reticular dermis may be so intense as to cause a separation of the epidermis from the dermis (Fig. 3.4). The small venules of the upper dermis are dilated, but the capillaries of the subpapillary plexus may be narrowed due to pressure of the intense dermal edema. A cellular infiltrate is absent in early lesions. Electron microscopy shows mast cell degranulation (Fig. 2.4, p. 8) or only swollen, more electron-lucent, intracellular mast cell-specific granules. Epidermal cells, endothelial cells, and neurons may contain vacuoles (Majno et al. 1969, Cauna et al. 1970).

In chronic urticaria, lesions of the fleeting type contain a sparse, perivascular infiltrate of lymphocytes and possibly also eosinophils (Monroe et al. 1981). The infiltrate is more intense in lesions that persist beyond 24 h. Features of a leukocytoclastic vasculitis, with all the typical histopathological features of that syndrome, may also be present in these older lesions (see Fig. 3.4 and Section 8.4, p. 110).

In lesions with a predominantly mononuclear infiltrate, the lymphocytes are mainly T-cells with the helper phenotype, and they coexpress Ia (HLA-Dr) antigens. This suggests that delayed type hypersensitivity reactions also play a role in chronic urticaria (Mekori et al. 1983).

Mast cell numbers may also be increased in the wheals, compared to normal patient skin (Natbony et al. 1983 and Chapter 5.3.3), but such changes are known to occur also in other diverse inflammatory reactions (Asboe-Hansen 1950, Walton and DeSouza 1983).

3.6 Laboratory Findings

In accordance with the ephemeral character of the clinical and histopathological findings, there are no striking changes in laboratory values during acute urticaria, unless an underlying disease is present.

In chronic idiopathic urticaria, several larger patient series have been studied with an equally meager result. Thus, laboratory examinations offer little diagnostic help in acute or chronic urticaria (see Chapter 10.3, p. 124). Specific laboratory changes that are typically found in certain subtypes of urticaria are discussed in the respective chapters (see Chapters 4, p. 53, 5, p. 55 and 8.6, p. 112). A few data of special interest will however be presented in the subsequent paragraphs.

3.6.1 Leukocytes

In 17% of patients, neutrophil counts can be elevated in chronic urticaria (Brown et al. 1974), but a leukopenia has also been reported in 8% of children (Harris et al. 1982). These changes can be associated with an elevated ESR in up to 21% of patients (Green et al. 1965). An eosinophilia ($> 5\%$) is not found at all (Stemmler and Lischka 1979) or at most in 15% of patients (Green et al. 1965). Even though its presence may indicate an allergic or parasitic cause, a specific search for it is not warranted. A basopenia has been

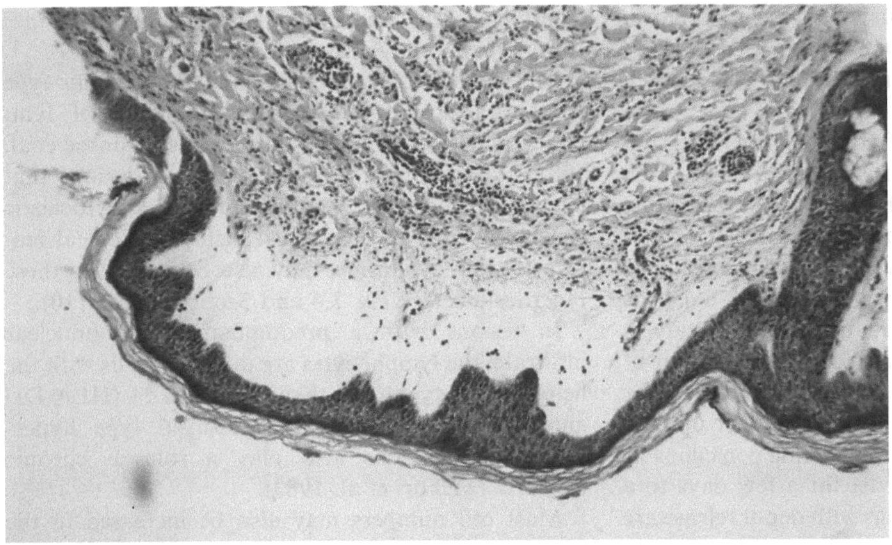

Fig. 3.4. Histopathology of bullous lesions in a patient with urticarial vasculitis. A massive papillary edema and a moderate mononuclear cell infiltrate are present, particularly around the small vessels, orig. magn. 100 ×.

reported in several older studies (Warin and Champion 1974), but has received no further attention in recent years.

3.6.2 Immunoglobulins

Routine screening for pathological serum values is fruitless (Stemmler and Lischka 1979). Total serum IgE is normal (Juhlin et al. 1969, Greaves et al. 1974, Wüthrich and Kopper 1974), or it is elevated in a small percentage of patients (13% according to Harris et al. 1982 and Small et al. 1982). Such elevations are mostly seen in patients with parasitoses or insect sting allergies. Serum IgG and IgA levels are generally normal, whereas IgM may be increased in up to 42% of patients for no obvious reasons (Brown et al. 1974).

3.6.3 Complement and Protease Inhibitors

Complement levels are generally normal, and the decrease in a small percentage (10%) of patients with urticaria may be related to increased serum immune complexes which can be demonstrated in 38% of the patient sera (Small et al. 1982). Similar abnormalities are frequently observed among the subgroup of patients with vasculitis (Chapter 8.6, p. 112; discussed in detail).

Transient elevations of serum albumin and total protein have been observed in > 50% of patients. No attempt has been made to explain this phenomenon (Warin and Champion 1974).

Because of a possible pathogenetic relationship between whealing and the kallikrein system, serum protease inhibitor profiles have been examined and have been found to be normal for trypsin-, chymotrypsin-, kallikrein- and C1-esterase inhibitory capacities (Doeglas and Bleumink 1975; Crovato and Rebora 1977). Abnormal changes in these parameters are however present in hereditary angioedema and in cold urticaria (see respective chapters).

3.7 Specific Causes of Reactions

3.7.1 General Aspects of Drug Reactions

In adults, the leading causes of urticarial reactions are drugs, whereas in children, the major responsible factors are foods and infections (Halpern 1965).

Drug reactions can have a bewildering array of clinical appearances. Cutaneous manifestations are most frequent, mostly in the form of maculopapular eruptions. Urticaria, angioedema, and anaphylaxis occur at almost the same frequency (14% Haneke et al. 1980; 25% Tay 1974). Other cutaneous manifestations are photosensitivity reactions, erythema multiforme, exfoliative dermatitis, purpura, and fixed drug eruptions. Specific drugs tend to cause one type of skin lesions more than another, and several reaction types may also overlap.

All major immunological and non-immunological pathomechanisms may be involved in drug reactions, alone or in combination, although cytotoxic and tuberculin-type reactions can be excluded as causes of urticaria and anaphylaxis.

Most drugs are small molecules and cannot be allergenic by themselves. They are generally degraded into activated derivatives which bind through firm, covalent bonds to endogenous macromolecules. especially proteins, but also to polysaccharides and polynucleotides. This requires a high degree of chemical reactivity of the drug or its metabolic product. The carrier molecule and its hapten is then processed by macrophages and lymphocytes to initiate the immune response, and B-cells are stimulated subsequently to produce hapten-specific antibodies. A complex set of regulating factors, derived from T-cells and B-cells, and finally also the genetic makeup to the individual, will determine whether the major class of antibodies that is produced will be of the IgG or the IgE type.

Other factors that modulate this system relate to the chemical nature of the hapten or adjuvans, the route of administration, the dosage and frequency of administration, and a possible underlying disease that predisposes to the drug reaction (Parker 1975). Thus, anaphylaxis to drugs is observed far less frequently after oral than after parenteral administration, and atopics are more prone to produce IgE antibodies, whereas maculopapular rashes to ampicillin occur more readily in patients with infectious mononucleosis, lymphatic leukemia, or hyperuricemia. High doses of drugs, administered at frequent intervals, have been used to induce a switch from IgG to IgE production during rapid hyposensitization. But this does not imply that anaphylactic sensitization can be prevented by treating nonallergic individuals with high doses of the drugs they need. Also, in contrast to certain allergic reactions, such as hemolytic anemia which becomes more likely with increased duration of therapy and dosage, anaphylactic reactions can occur already upon first administration of drugs, or any time thereafter, due to an unrecognized previous sensitization by trace contaminants of the drug in foods.

Finally, the chemical nature of the antigen will also determine which type of immunological reaction will take place. For mast cell or basophil release, the antigen must have several combining sites on its molecule to allow for interaction with two adjacent IgE molecules on the cell surface. The number of binding sites will also play a role in the type and size of antigen-antibody complexes that are formed. These in turn, together with the type of antibody and antigen that may be involved, will determine whether the complement cascade will be activated or not.

3.7.2 Penicillin

Antibiotics, including penicillin and related compounds, are the most frequent causes of drug reactions and of urticaria (Idsoe et al. 1968, Tay 1974, see Table 3.4). Up to 10% of all patients who are treated with penicillin, become sensitized, and 14–25% of them will have urticaria, angioedema, and anaphylaxis (Tay 1974, Haneke et al. 1980). Fortunately, anaphylaxis occurs in only a small minority (0.14%) of patients who are treated with penicillin, and only one death has been reported in a survey of 94,655 patients (Warin and Champion 1974).

Table 3.4. Causes of various drug reactions among 171 hospitalized patients in the Far East (Tay 1974) and among 300 hospitalized patients in North America (Speer et al. 1978).

Cause	Percentage	
	Tay	Speer et al.
Antibiotics	49.1	83
Antipyretics and analgesics	12.8	12
Sedatives, hypnotics	7.6	5
Diuretics	5.8	–
Antihistamines	4.1	–
Miscellaneous	20.6	–

Antigens

The major amount (95%) of the injected benzylpenicillin reacts with its carrier molecule in the circulation in the form of a benzylpenicilloyl. Minor antigenic determinants, such as penicilloates, peniloates, penicillamine, and penaldate (Levine 1966), are contaminants that are carried over from the fermentation processes during the production of penicillin and derive therefore from microorganisms and from the special culture media. Major and minor determinants can cause anaphylactic reactions.

Recently, high molecular weight impurities have been identified by radioimmunoassay in both biosynthetic and semisynthetic penicillin preparations (Ahlstedt et al. 1980a). The authors suggest that these contaminants can be easily eliminated, thus further reducing the general risk of penicillin reactions.

Special aspects

The high incidence of allergy to penicillin in humans is surprising, and a number of possible reasons have been offered to explain this phenomenon. Cross-reactions with any of the semisynthetic penicillins due to the common 6-amino-penicillenic acid nucleus may be one reason. This does not hold for ampicillin since its common morbilliform rash is due to toxic and not to allergic mechanisms. True allergy, with positive skin tests, occurs only among the few patients who react to ampicillin with urticarial reactions (Bierman et al. 1972). Treatment with cephalosporin or penicillamines, and even a tinea infection, have been thought to induce sensitization to penicillin (Blum and DeWeck 1966, Thoburn et al. 1966, Parker 1975).

Penicillin allergy presents a specific problem since

the penicillin molecule cannot be destroyed by boiling or steam sterilization. Traces may remain therefore on syringes or on dental instruments. Pasteurization will not remove the material from milk or other dairy products, and it may even be present in vaccines prepared from serum of animals treated with the drug. Recently, an anaphylactic reaction of a patient with known penicillin allergy was traced to penicillin-like contaminants in a soft drink (Wicher and Reisman 1980). Chicken or pork are also possible sources of trace amounts of penicillin which can maintain an urticaria in highly sensitive individuals.

Penicillin treatment is often followed by dermographic urticaria (see Chapter 5, p. 62) or by an exacerbation of chronic urticaria. These observations as well as the beneficial effect of penicillin in cold urticaria (see Chapter 1.1.4, p. 145) remain unexplained. Similarly puzzling is the finding that some patients with chronic urticaria have positive skin tests to penicillin without any apparent causal relationship between penicillin and their disease (Haneke et al. 1980, Boonk and Van Ketel 1981).

Clinical aspects

Urticaria or anaphylactic reactions to penicillin differ clinically in no way from reactions caused by other drugs. Levine (1966) has divided allergic reactions to penicillin into three major types. *Immediate reactions* occur within 2–20 min, are rare, IgE-dependent, and associated with urticaria, hypotension, shock, and less commonly wheezing, rhinitis, and laryngeal edema. *Accelerated reactions* develop between 2–40 h after administration of penicillin, are also IgE-dependent, and are almost always urticarial, rarely with laryngeal edema. *Late reactions* are of the serum sickness type, occur 7–10 days after administration, and are associated with various skin rashes, arthritis, fever, hemolytic anemia, thrombocytopenia, and proteinuria. The simultaneous presence of IgE antibodies may enhance this reaction, possibly by improving immune complex deposition due to the action of histamine.

Immunological aspects

Levine (1966) made the intriguing observation that practically all patients who are treated with penicillin will develop hemagglutinating antibodies, even if no drug reaction is evident. Ahlstedt et al. (1980b), in a comparative study of azidocillin, ampicillin, and benzylpenicillin, found that the induction and the specificity of the IgE response are influenced by the nature of the carrier, the number of epitopes, and the different acyl side chains. According to Fellner and Baer (1967), the IgE antibodies persist over many years, whereas the IgG antibody levels drop. Other authors have also noticed a decline in skin test reactivity with time (Finke et al. 1965).

Table 3.5. Test procedures for penicillin allergy, depending on previous clinical reactions (after Bäurle and Haneke 1980; Parker 1975).

Type of reaction	Test procedure
1. Anaphylactic shock	in vitro techniques only (RAST, in vitro histamine release)
2. Urticaria, angioedema	epicutaneous, then scratch test: 1. penicilloyl, 10^{-5} M (higher doses, if tolerated) 2. penicillin G, 50–200 units (higher doses, if tolerated) if both 1 + 2 are negative: prick test and increasing concentrations of both reagents
3. Serum sickness	as under 2; fewer precautions are necessary

Diagnosis

Allergy to penicillin can be diagnosed by several means (see Table 3.5 and Chapter 10, p. 122). In patients with a history of anaphylactic reactions, it is advisable to perform only RAST tests on the serum. Skin tests must be done with great caution, and minimal quantities should be applied if a high degree of sensitization is suspected. This can be accomplished by high dilutions of the antigen and by applying the test substance only topically. If reactions are negative, intradermal tests and higher doses can be applied at 10 min intervals. Despite a positive history, tests may be positive in only 44% of patients (Haneke et al. 1980), but positive reactions might occur on further testing by oral provocation (Stemmler and Lischka 1979). Emergency drugs and equipment should be readily available at all times during these procedures. The test reagents should be (1) benzylpenicilloyl-polylysine for the major determinants and (2) benzylpenicillin or a mixture of major and minor determinants.

Other tests such as the in vitro basophil degranulation, histamine release, or lymphocyte transformation tests are currently of little practical importance or of scientific interest only.

3.7.3 Sulfonamides and Antibiotics Other Than Penicillin

Next to penicillin, other antibiotics, and in particular sulfonamides and tetracyclines, are leading causes of urticaria (Table 3.4). The list of antibiotics includes chloramphenicol, streptomycin, p-aminosalicylic acid, griseofulvin, nystatin, polymyxin, and vaginally applied nifuroxime. As with most drugs, the pathomechanisms are only poorly understood, and reaginic (IgE) antibodies, other immunoglobulins, immunoglobulin- or antigen-antibody aggregates, complement, and a direct release of histamine by the drugs or their metabolites from mast cells may be involved. Quinine, morphine, codeine, and curare are direct histamine liberators and are particularly dangerous for patients with mast cell proliferative disease since they can precipitate acute shock and death due to massive histamine release (Sutter et al. 1962).

3.7.4 Various Other Drugs

The list of drugs that cause urticaria is long; only a few drugs cause no reactions at all (Wintroub et al. 1979). Mention should be made of hypersensitivity to lidocaine hydrochloride (four cases in 10 years) (Chin and Fellner 1980). Procaine, prilocaine, and mepivacaine cause no cross-sensitivity and can be used as alternatives to lidocaine. Antipyretics and aspirin-like analgesics have recently been recognized as causes of urticaria and anaphylaxis via non-immunological mechanisms. They will be discussed separately, together with food additives, in Chapter 7, p. 96, because of their special significance as a frequent cause of chronic urticaria.

3.7.5 Implants

Surgical implants should be considered in the search for causes of urticaria. In a patient with a 10-month history of urticaria after implantation of tantalum staples, the immediate skin test to tantalum was positive; the disease improved with desulfiram therapy and after surgical removal of the staples (Werman and Rietschel 1981). Orthodontic bands are another potential source of allergens (Tinkelman and Tinkelman 1979). Platinum can cause urticaria through very small groups of ionic complexes containing reactive halogen ligands (Cleare et al. 1976).

3.7.6 Vaccines

Vaccines can cause anaphylactic or anaphylactoid reactions because of the allergens contained in them in the form of foreign sera, constituents of eggs on which the viruses are grown, microbial products, antibiotics, and contaminants. They were a far more frequent cause of urticaria before the antibiotic era. Tetanus toxoid, perhaps the most widely used vaccine in the Western world, can cause reactions of any kind in up to 5.3% of patients, 2.7% of them being at the site of injection, and 2.5% in generalized forms of serum sickness. Urticaria may persist in rare instances for several weeks. Anaphylactic shock is extremely rare: 2/7,589 treatments (Moynihan 1955). Serum sickness and more recently anaphylaxis are also seen with vaccination against rabies, snake bites, gas gangrene, and with antilymphocyte serum.

3.7.7 Blood Products and Substitutes

Transfusion of blood and blood products often causes minor skin rashes, with urticaria occurring in only 1–3%. The reaction may be truly allergic, due to specific antigens (penicillin, food), IgE antibodies, or basic constituents in the transfused plasma (Routledge et al. 1976). IgE-dependent mechanisms, complement activation, or direct histamine release may be involved.

Urticaria and anaphylactic shock also occur upon infusion of volume substitutes such as gelatin, hydroxyethyl starch, dextran, mannitol, and plasma proteins. Reactions are most frequent with gelatin (0.1%) and least common with plasma proteins (0.01%). Clinical details and mechanisms involved in these reactions are discussed in Chapter 7, p. 96.

3.7.8 Seminal Plasma

About 20 patients are on record who developed symptoms ranging from minor pruritus to severe anaphylaxis after intercourse (Kroon 1980). The antigen is common to seminal plasma in all men, has a molecular weight of 14 to 30 kd, and derives possibly from the prostate. Prausnitz-Küstner tests have been positive in four instances, but IgE antibodies were not identified until now. Use of a condom, but not vasectomy, is helpful for prevention.

3.7.9 Contrast Media

Iodinated organic compounds which are used as X-ray contrast media can cause severe, acute anaphylaxis, with death occurring in from 1:1,400 to 1:60,000 diagnostic procedures. Persistence of radiopaque material, for example in cerebrospinal fluid, may cause urticaria over many years. Because of the pseudoallergic nature of the reactions, these compounds are discussed in detail under the topic of intolerance reactions (Chapter 7, p. 96).

3.7.10 Food

Incidence

Allergic reactions to food cause acute urticaria in up to 44% of children, according to a study by Halpern (1965). In adults, the incidence in all types of urticaria was found to be much lower (8/554, Champion et al. 1969). Small children tend to lose their food allergy with increasing age, possibly due to maturation of the immune system or of the gastrointestinal endothelial lining, whereas the allergy tends to persist in older children and adults (Bock 1982).

Food consists not only of basic nutriants in the form of fats, carbohydrates, and proteins, but it also contains vasoactive amines, histamine liberators (see Table 3.6), toxic products of contaminating bacteria or molds, antibiotics, spices, flavorings, colorings and preservatives. Food additives have received much attention during the past decade as a cause of chronic urticaria, and they are discussed in detail in Chapter 7, p. 96 (anaphylactoid reactions). The incidence of IgE-mediated urticaria due to food is probably low, compared to the non-allergic mechanisms (Hannuksela 1983).

Basic aspects

Most food antigens are heat-, acid-, and enzyme-resistant glycoproteins (18–36 kd) which are unaltered by the digestive enzymes in mouth, stomach, and intestines, and by the highly acidic conditions in the stomach. Smaller molecules can also be allergenic by acting as haptens. Heating inactivates some antigens and activates others, and the same holds for exposure of antigens to digestive enzymes.

Cow milk contains some 25 proteins, the most important antigen being β-lactoglobulin, followed by α-lactalbumin and casein. Its allergenicity can, for example, be enhanced by a reaction with lactose, resulting in an N-glycosidic linkage of the sugar with the protein (Haddad 1982). Similarly, the allergenicity of the sugar D-psicose, a byproduct of high fructose syrup, is also expressed in burned bread and in caramel (Nishioka et al. 1983). Fish can be allergenic in some patients when eaten raw, in others only when dried or cooked (Paulsen 1961).

Pathomechanisms

A basic requirement for the development of food allergy is the absorption of the allergen through the intestinal barrier. Macromolecules, and even pollen grains, starch particles, and *Candida* organisms, can pass inbetween epithelial cells, or they can find access through small defects caused by shedding of epithelial cells. Vasoactive amines or agents in food that liberate mediators from intestinal mast cells cause edema, and thereby enhance the permeability of the gut wall. Mucosal injury due to gastroenteritis, achlorhydria, selective IgA deficiency, immaturity with relative IgA deficiency, and psychogenic factors may temporarily or permanently alter the barrier and immune function of the gut wall and predispose the organism to allergic sensitization (Buckley and Metcalfe 1982).

There are a number of homeostatic mechanisms which make it difficult for primary sensitization to take place (see Fig. 3.5 *A*). Beside the intestinal barrier, the nature and the amount of antigen, and the amount of IgA, its complexing to antigens, and the clearance of these complexes in the circulation, the presence of special adjuvants in the food, the regulation of the

Table 3.6. Foods that cause urticaria, grouped according to their putative mechanism of action.

Probably IgE-(Reagin) mediated	Histamine liberators	Vasoactive amines	Unknown mechanisms
* fish	* egg white (heat labile)	cheese	* cereals
* shellfish	* thiamine (cheese)	beer	* melons
* milk	* strawberries	sausage	alcohol
* nuts		canned food	yeasts
* beans		fish	azo dyes
* potatoes		meat	benzoic acid derivatives
* celery, parsley		tomatoes	salicylates
* spices		pineapple	menthol
rice		wine	mushrooms
bananas		avocadoes	aliphatic aldehydes
-psicose			
tangerines			
pollen			

* more frequent causes; according to Paulsen 1961, Golbert et al. 1969, Much et al. 1978, Atkins 1983.

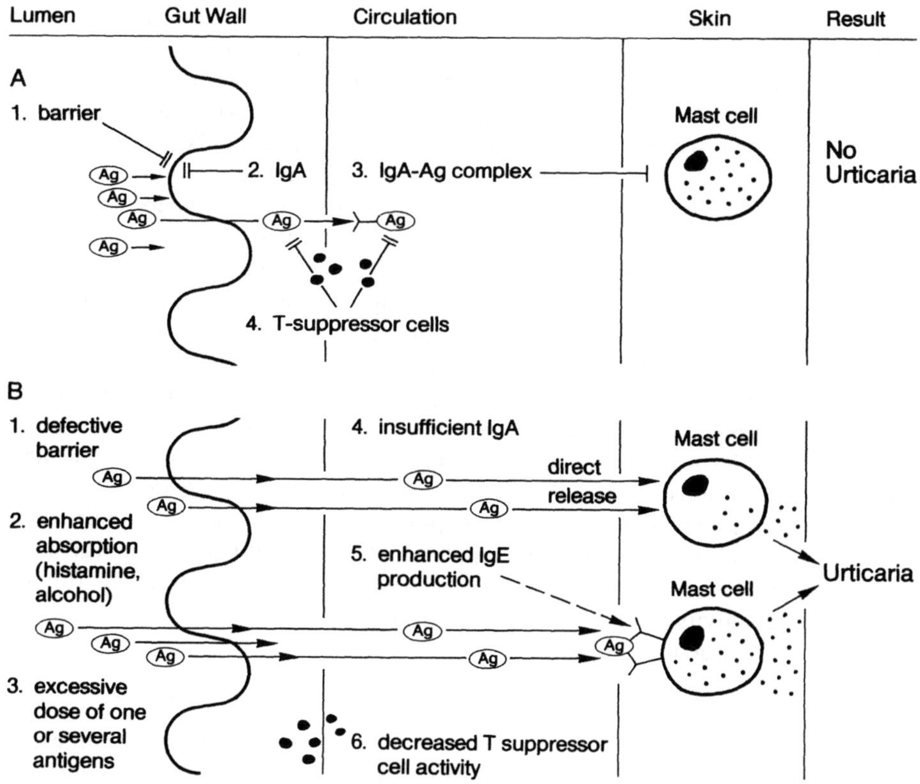

Fig. 3.5. Hypothetical model of immune defense in the normal gut (*A*) and in the gut wall of urticaria patients (*B*) who suffer from food allergy.

immune response by T- and B-suppressor cells, and the genetic make-up of the individual will determine the development of IgE-dependent allergy.

In addition to the factors shown in Fig. 3.5 *B*, another basic defect of immune function which predisposes to food allergy may relate to the immunocompetent epithelial cells overlying Peyer's patches (M cells) which are thought to sample environmental antigens (Owen 1977). A defect might also be present in other immunocompetent cells within the lamina propria such as the mast cells and the lymphocytes.

Histamine, prostaglandins, and most likely also a number of other inflammatory mediators cause increased local vasopermeability, stimulation of mucus production, increased muscle contraction, stimulation of pain fibers, and recruitment of other inflammatory cells which results in the clinical symptomatology of food allergy.

Histamine was considered the most important mediator in IgE-mediated food allergy, until Buisseret et al. (1978) demonstrated prostaglandin E_2 and $F_{2\alpha}$ in stool and plasma of patients after oral antigen challenge. The reaction was depressed by inhibitors of prostaglandin synthetase. Similar mechanisms may be operative in urticarial reactions to alcohol which can be totally suppressed by indomethacin, but also by naloxone and disodiumcromoglycate (Ormerod and Holt 1983).

There are several factors which determine whether food allergy will express itself in a natural setting. Some patients need excessive exposure to antigens. In others, several food antigens must come together, or histamine or alcohol must enhance absorption. Some pollen-allergic individuals will develop food allergy only during the pollen season, and they will then react to food antigens that cross-react with pollens, such as fresh fruits, vegetables, and spices.

Several investigators have reported alterations in gastric acidity, intestinal mobility, and the function of the small intestine and biliary tract in up to 85% of patients with chronic urticaria (Gloor et al. 1972, Husz et al. 1974). The authors imply that these alterations form a pathogenetic basis for the altered handling of food antigens, resulting in increased allergy in these patients. It is equally possible that the changes observed are secondary to massive release of vasoactive amines in association with the urticaria. Furthermore, Schmidl and Kern (1964), in a careful study of 100 patients with urticaria and 100 healthy controls, found no increased gastrointestinal pathology.

Clinical aspects

Following ingestion of food, anaphylactic symptoms can start immediately, as is frequently observed with fish, berries, nuts, and egg white, or they may be delayed for several hours, as with cereals, milk, eggs, chocolate, and vegetables (Paulsen 1961). Symptoms may be limited to the gastrointestinal tract, or they may involve other organs, mostly the skin, less so the respiratory tract. The factors determining the target organ for food allergy in the individual patient are not understood.

While the food is in the mouth, the patient may already experience itching, burning, and swelling of lips, tongue, gums, buccal mucosa, and pharynx. Nausea, vomiting, cramping pain, abdominal distension, and diarrhea may follow soon thereafter. In explosive reactions, systemic anaphylaxis may occur within minutes. Urticaria, angioedema, the flare of an atopic eczema, rhinitis, or asthma may be associated.

For several hours after a reaction, patients can tolerate the food antigen without complaint. This refractory period is often followed by a time of heightened sensitivity, and a period of intermediate reactivity may ensue thereafter.

Causative agents

The list of food ingredients implicated as causes of urticarial reactions is long. In Table 3.6, food allergens are grouped according to their putative pathomechanisms. Some foods contain antigens as well as vasoactive amines and mast cell degranulators. Cross-reactivity exists with some food antigens, and patients react therefore, for example, to several members of the *Umbelliferae* family (parsnip, celery, or mugwort). Some of these same patients also react to carrot, potato, apple, and tomato antigens (Kauppinen et al. 1980). Cross-reactions may also occur with other fresh fruits, vegetables, spices, and pollens (Hannuksela 1983).

Hidden sources of food antigens should always be considered in the search for the cause of urticaria. Pollen-allergic patients may react to pollens in honey (Cohen et al. 1979), or patients with fish allergy may develop symptoms from codliver oil, from meat of chicken or pigs that have been fed with fish meal, from glues that contain fish antigen, and from fish albumin that is used to clear wine in France. Aliphatic aldehydes in garlic and other foods, and menthol in candy and instant iced tea with mint flavor, are further hidden allergens and causes of urticaria (Warin and Champion 1974).

Diagnosis

The diagnosis of food urticaria depends on a meticulous history, with particular attention to temporal relationships between exposure and development of symptoms. Omission of suspected foods from the diet and their gradual addition is a simple way to approach the diagnostic problem (see Chapter 10.4, p. 131). Skin tests can be performed with commonly available food extracts or with whole food in special skin chambers (Hannuksela and Lahti 1977). Oral provocation tests can be done as well, with the suspected food hidden in oblates so that the patient is not influenced psychologically by the taste. These oral tests are more meaningful than skin tests since they also identify allergens that are changed through the digestive process in the gastrointestinal tract. Finally, RAST tests can be done on a number of food allergens to lend support to the diagnosis. They are particularly useful in patients who have experienced anaphylactic reactions, but their value is limited since they are useful only in IgE-mediated reactions (see also Chapter 10, p. 122 for further details).

3.7.11 Infections

Considering the almost continuous exposure of the individual to antigens from infectious agents, the low incidence of urticarial reactions to them is surprising. This may be due to the fact that microorganisms tend to stimulate IgG rather than IgE-antibody production. Immunological tolerance to microbial antigens due to repeated massive exposure may be another reason which would also explain why the incidence of urticaria due to infectious agents is relatively high in children (Kauppinen et al. 1984).

Bacteria

Bacterial infections contribute to urticaria in two major settings: in streptococcal tonsillitis in children and in chronic dental infections in adults. Other rare infectious causes of urticaria include diseases due to *Shigella* (Pollowitz 1980), marine vibrio (Blake et al. 1979), *Vibrio parahemolyticus* (Zide et al. 1974), *Mycoplasma pneumoniae* (Cherry et al. 1975), *Pseudomonas pseudomallei* (Steck and Byrd 1969), and *Campylobacter jejuni* (Bretag et al. 1984).

Schuller and Elvey (1980) took throat cultures and measured serum antibodies against streptococcal exoenzymes in 32 children with acute urticaria, even when an infection was not apparent clinically. Thirteen patients had evidence of streptococcal infection or immunity to these tests. The authors suggest continuing treatment with antibiotics when urticaria supervenes during treatment for streptococcal infections. Clearly, more studies are needed to prove that streptococci play such an important role in childhood urticaria.

More than two decades ago, it was fashionable to implicate a focus of infection as cause for many diverse diseases, and urticaria was one of them. In optimistic studies, such as the one by Castelain and Besson (1961), it was reported that 50 of 70 patients with chronic urticaria cleared when the focus of infection was successfully treated. Schmidl and Kern (1964) found foci of infection in almost 50% of 110 patients with chronic urticaria, but also in the same percentage of an equivalent control group. The overall incidence of sinusitis, tonsillitis, and dental abscesses in different studies was 50% (Resch and Evans 1958), 20% (Fikentscher et al. 1971), 17% (Stemmler and Lischka 1979). Removal of the focus caused regression of the urticaria in 7% and 4% of infected patients, respectively (Rorsman 1962, Stemmler and Lischka 1979). The figures are much better when dental infections are viewed separately. Resch and Evans (1958) observed a prompt cure of urticaria in 17 of 50 patients with dental infections, and Doeglas (1975) reported a cure in 17% of his patients with chronic urticaria and periapical granulomas. A search for bacterial foci in chronic urticaria seems therefore only worthwhile in the teeth.

Viruses

Viral infections frequently cause an exacerbation of chronic urticaria, but they are rarely the primary cause of acute, and even less so of chronic urticaria. Urticaria may develop several weeks before infectious mononucleosis becomes clinically manifest (Africk and Halprin 1969), and its incidence in infectious mononucleosis is 5% (Cowdrey and Reynolds 1969). In Coxsackie A9 infections, three of nine exanthems were urticarial, and urticaria also occurred in a patient with Coxsackie B5 and one with ECHO 11 virus infections (Cherry et al. 1963). Psittacosis causes mostly unspecific and only rarely urticarial rashes (Weber and Stetter 1969). Finally, there are isolated reports of urticaria in the literature in association with smallpox and measles vaccinations (Warin and Champion 1974) and during infections with cytomegalovirus (Humphrey and Myers 1975).

Hepatitis B is the most frequent cause of urticaria due to viral infections and is often preceded or associated with a serum sickness-like syndrome in up to 30% of patients with this infection (Warin and Champion 1974). Vaida et al. (1983) found markers for the virus in 15.3% of their patients with chronic urticaria: 15.3% had anti-hepatitis B surface antibodies and 2.4% had hepatitis B surface antigen in their serum. Histologically, the urticarial lesion is a necrotizing venulitis, with hepatitis B surface antigen in serum cryoprecipitates and vessel walls, and with evidence of alternate and classical pathway complement activation (Dienstag et al. 1978). These pathological findings would argue against a secondary or accidental role of the viral infection in the pathogenesis of urticaria.

Fungi

With the exception of yeast organisms, fungi do not generally play a causative role in urticaria, even though immediate type skin tests may be positive in patients. Exceptions are one case each with dermatophytosis due to *Trichophyton rubrum*, reported by Shelley and Florence (1961) and by Weary and Guerrant (1967). The urticaria disappeared with successful griseofulvin treatment and relapsed when the tinea recurred.

Much has been written about the potential role of *Candida* as an inducer of urticaria. This is an indication of the general confusion on the subject matter. In different populations, infestation with *Candida* varies from 10–70%, being particularly high in hospitalized patients (James and Warin 1971). Schade et al. (1975) isolated different yeast species from the mouth, stool, and bile of 43% of their 108 patients with chronic urticaria, but also from 26% of normal controls. Since the isolation of the organism must thus be incidental, skin tests were performed to assess a possible immunologic response of the host to the yeast as an indicator of a possible causal relationship to the urticaria. The percentage of chronic urticaria patients with positive immediate prick test reactions was 19% (Holti 1967), 35% (Serrano 1975, Numata et al. 1980), 36% (James and Warin 1971), and even 81% (Rives et al. 1972). A total of 71% of these patients with a positive skin test reacted also to oral provocation tests using food prepared with yeasts (Serrano 1975).

Despite these findings, the cure rate of urticaria after treatment with nystatin and proven elimination of the yeast organism is not encouraging. Some authors achieved a cure in only 8% (James and Warin 1971) or 14% (Stemmler and Lischka 1979), others in 55% (Holti 1967), and still others in 75% (Schade et al. 1975) and 92% (Rives et al. 1972). Additional patients improved on a low yeast diet, with avoidance of cheese, chocolate, and nonspecific histamine liberators. Some authors also observed benefit from desensitization to *Candida* (31% cure rate, Vivarelli and Mancosu 1967; 85% cure rate, Westphal et al. 1976). Thus, on the basis of the therapeutic response there is also good evidence for a possible role of candida infections in chronic urticaria.

Parasites

The relationship between protozoal infections and urticaria is unclear, particularly since in endemic regions, patients often carry several types of parasites. For example, the patient with *Giardia lamblia* infection and urticaria reported by Harris and Mitchell (1949) also had amebiasis. *Ameba* and *Trichomonas hominis* have also been implicated in urticaria. Previous reports on the occurrence of urticaria during acute malaria attacks were recently confirmed by the case report on two patients with acute *Plasmodium falciparum* infection (Maru and Mengistu 1979).

Special factors must come together to cause urticaria in patients with intestinal helminths since the load of worms is even slightly lower in urticaria patients than in controls (Pasricha et al. 1972). In only 8% of these patients did the urticaria improve with treatment. The figures are better (16%) after treatment of oxyuriasis (whipworm infections) (Doeglas 1975).

These clinical observations contradict the fact that infestations with helminths are the natural model of IgE-mediated allergy, with massive increase in the serum levels of this tissue-fixing immunoglobulin, positive, specific prick tests to worm allergens, and at times a massive eosinophilia. There is, however, experimental evidence supported by clinical observations that certain helminths can cause all types of rashes, including urticaria. Wheals may be linear, following the subcutaneous migration of *Ancylostoma* or *Strongyloides* worms, or they may be small, possibly polycyclic in outline. Lesions are easily missed in the lichenified, scarred skin of patients with onchocerciasis. Rupture of hydatic liver cysts in echinococcus infections may cause anaphylactic shock. In schistosomiasis, the penetration of the cerceriae through the skin is followed 4–8 weeks later by urticaria, fever, arthralgia, diarrhea, and hepatosplenomegaly. Trichinosis may mimic angioedema with periorbital edema. A maculopapular rash, fever, and muscle pain are other hallmarks of this disease. Trichinosis frequently occurs also in Western civilizations, and the same holds for the liver fluke (*Fasciola*), which has been reported in association with urticaria in an epidemic im Hampshire (Facey and Marsden 1960). *Toxocara* causes urticaria probably only during massive infestations (Rook and Staughton 1972).

Insects

The local, and at times generalized, urticarial reactions to insect stings are discussed in the chapter on contact urticaria. Multiple insect sting reactions present as papular urticaria. Scabies is rarely accompanied by urticaria, and the diagnosis is easily mistaken unless this possible combination is considered (Chapel et al. 1981).

3.7.12 Inhalants

Urticaria is a rare manifestation of inhalant allergy. Asthma and rhinitis are far more frequent, and during exposure to industrial allergens, contact eczema is even more frequent. Nevertheless, there are well-documented case reports and studies on urticaria induced through respiratory exposure. Most of the patients are exquisitely sensitive to their allergens.

Among pollen-allergic patients, Waldbott and Merkle (1952) described 26 subjects with associated urticaria. About half of them developed whealing during the pollen season, and the urticaria persisted thereafter with the other patients. The allergens were mostly ragweed, but also grass and tree pollen. Some patients developed urticaria during nasal provocation. One patient with ragweed allergy lost his urticaria during desensitization (Derbes 1957).

Castberg and Sorenson (1949) observed urticaria due to inhalation in 7 to 130 millers and bakers. A child developed urticaria and angioedema when smelling fried fish, but no shellfish (Derbes 1957). Mite allergens may cause urticaria either through direct penetration through the skin or through inhalation. Thirty of the 52 patients with chronic urticaria studied by Numata et al. (1979) were skin test positive to aqueous extracts of *Dermatophagides farinae*, and the cutaneous response correlated well with in vitro histamine release of the patients' peripheral basophils. A direct causal relationship between this hyperreactivity to the mite allergens and the urticaria was however not proven.

Among industrial workers, inhalant urticaria has been observed with castor bean dust (Kaufmann 1950), castor bean pomade, complex platinum salts, aliphatic polyamines, spices, penicillin, ammonia, sulfur dioxide, formaldehyde, sodium sulfide, aminothiazide, and lindane (Key 1961). The allergen mediating urticaria in castor beans is most likely ricin.

Cigarette smoke can cause urticaria through the action of three major allergens: menthol, nonconjugated aliphatic aldehydes, and a specific glycoprotein.

Menthol is present in menthylated cigarettes, in aerosol room spray, cough drops, paper handkerchiefs, and skin creams (McGowen 1966), and can also cause contact urticaria (see Chapter 6, p. 90). Many cigarettes contain nonconjugated aliphatic aldehydes. In a patient described by Rappaport and Hoffman (1941), tingling in the fingers of the right hand and the lips developed when he started to smoke, and generalized urticaria followed soon thereafter. The chronic urticaria resolved when the patient stopped smoking, and recurred on resumption. No hives developed when cigarettes containing diethylene glycol instead of glycerine were smoked. Skin tests were positive for aldehydes, ranging from formaldehyde to eighteen-chain aldehydes, and to acrolein. These agents are also present in fried and boiled food, in garlic, and in commonly used essential oils. In a patient who was skin test positive to these chemicals (Horsfall 1934), passive transfer tests were negative, indicating that these compounds become antigenic only in vivo.

In cigarette smoke and in saline extracts of cured tobacco leaves, an 18 kd molecular weight glycoprotein has been isolated which causes positive immediate skin tests in one-third of smokers and nonsmokers. The antigen cross-reacts with other members of the *Solanaceae* family, such as green peppers, eggplants (aubergines), potatoes, and tomatoes (Becker et al. 1976). It remains uncertain whether this antigen causes urticaria, although it is conceivable on theoretical grounds.

3.7.13 Hormones and Endocrine Disorders

Acute or chronic urticaria only rarely occurs in association with hormone therapy. Anaphylactic reactions to endogenous hormones and urticaria in association with endocrine disorders are even less frequent.

Insulin and other hormones

Reactions to injectable hormones occur more readily when they are prepared from nonhuman sources, and even then, the degree of analogy of the amino acid sequence will determine whether reactions occur more readily or not. Allergies against beef insulin occur for example much more frequently than against porcine insulin, most likely because the insulin from pigs differs from human insulin only by one amino acid. Depot preparations containing protamine (e.g. isophane insulin) are also more allergenic, and the allergy seems to be due to the protamine itself (Shore et al. 1975). Synthetic hormone preparations are least allergenic, suggesting that contaminants from the tissue extracts contribute to the allergy to insulin from animal sources. Additives and preservatives form an additional source of agents that might cause urticarial reactions.

Reactions against hormones may be IgE- or IgG-mediated (Patterson et al. 1973). Some intestinal enzymes, such as chymotrypsin or dehydrocholic acid, can cause mast cell histamine release directly via nonimmunologic mechanisms (see Chapter 2, p. 5).

Insulin is the hormone most frequently used for therapy, and allergic reactions against it have been studied thoroughly. From 10–56% of diabetics react against insulin at some time. In about 10%, the reactions are serious enough to require modification of therapy (Jegasothy 1980). One-fourth of patients with insulin allergy also have an allergy to penicillin, none are atopics, and allergic reactions appear more readily after injections have been stopped for a brief time. About 40% of diabetics are skin test positive to insulin (Lieberman 1971), and specific IgE may be present at low levels without visible allergic reactions (Velcovsky et al. 1978).

Reactions to insulin injections start mostly with a local erythema, progressing to urtication and possibly also vesiculation. If the timing of development of the lesions is delayed, they will disappear with continued injections. Generalized reactions manifest themselves as erythema, urticaria with or without angioedema, and in rare instances anaphylactic shock. IgE, but also immune complexes, are involved in the pathogenesis. Development of IgG antibodies may result in insulin resistance.

Allergy to hormone preparations can be handled either by searching for an alternative preparation which contains no contaminants, is from a different species, or has no preservatives added. Treatment with diet and oral hypoglycemics may be worth a trial in insulin allergy.

Desensitization, with frequent injections of increasing doses over four days or even every 15, 30, or 50 min within one day, if needed, is a hazardous, but often successful mode of overcoming the immediate immune reactivity and making the patient tolerate his hormone therapy (Lieberman 1971; see also Chapter 11.2.8, p. 141).

Thyroid disease

In recent years, an intriguing relationship has become apparent between chronic urticaria and thyroid disease. Juhlin (1981) found thyroid disease in 6% of 330 patients with chronic urticaria. Hyperthyroidism was reported in isolated cases of urticaria by three different groups (Isaacs and Ertel 1971, Pace and Garretts 1975, Small and Lerman 1981). Midelfart et al. (1983) found elevated antimicrosomal thyroid antibodies in a woman with a 10-year history of severe urticaria and a 3-year history of vitiligo. The same antimicrosomal thyroid antibodies, with titres $\geqq 1:1600$, were found in 17 of 140 (12.1%) consecutive patients with chronic urticaria by Leznoff et al. (1983) and in 8 of 25 patients with chronic urticaria, excluding physical urticaria, by Lanigan et al. (1984). The incidence of this autoantibody in the normal population is 5.6% (Leznoff et al. 1983). Clinically, the patients were either hyper-, hypo-, or euthyroid. They had no evidence of vasculitis on biopsy, and other types of autoantibodies against thyroglobulin or against the thyroid microsomal fraction were not found. Most of the patients were women who also suffered from angioedema. Seven of nine had a remission of their urticaria after a 2–3 month daily treatment with 0.2 mg levothyroxine. Patients benefited even when they were initially euthyroid (Leznoff et al. 1983).

A reason for the association of chronic urticaria and thyroid disease was not found. Doeglas (1975) found vitiligo in five, parietal cell antibodies in two, and thyroid antibodies in one of 56 patients with idiopathic chronic urticaria. Autoimmunity may well be the common denominator between thyroid disease and urticaria.

Progesterone and pregnancy

There are several case reports in the literature of women who developed eczema, erythema multiforme, or urticaria during the mid- and premenstrual period. The condition subsided during treatment with anovulatory agents, but recurred when therapy was discontinued. Immediate skin tests to progesterone were positive, and a passive transfer was accomplished (Farah and Shbaklu 1971), but the exact antibody was never isolated. Most of the women reported by Hart (1977) had previously taken progesterone-containing pills, and a sensitization via antigenically different molecules is thus possible. Paradoxically, these patients may experience relief during pregnancy (Leech and Kumar 1981).

During the third trimester of pregnancy, some women develop highly pruritic papular and plaque-like wheals which start on the lower abdomen and spread to the thighs and occasionally also to the buttocks and arms (Lawley et al. 1979). In contrast to the lesions in the toxemic rash of pregnancy (Bourne 1962), excoriations are rare, and urticae are a constant feature. Newborns may be affected (Uhlin 1981), but there is no increased fetal-maternal risk. The condition, termed pruritic urticarial papules and plaques of pregnancy (PUPPP), occurs in 0.38% of pregnancies and is the most frequent dermatitis during gestation (Noguera et al. 1983). It is seen mostly in primigravidas, and it does not recur during subsequent pregnancies. Local or systemic steroids afford relief (Yancey et al. 1984). The pathogenetic relationship between pregnancy and urticaria is entirely unclear.

3.7.14 Internal Disease

The association of urticaria and internal disease is rare. Two types of disease seem to stand out, the so-called autoimmune or connective tissue diseases, and dysproteinemias with or without malignancies.

In a large series of 520 patients with systemic lupus erythematosus (SLE), Tuffanelli and Dubois (1964) observed urticaria and angioedema in 6.9%, with urticaria as the first symptom in 4%. Urticaria may antidate the onset of SLE by 1 year (Doeglas 1975). O'Loughlin et al. (1978) found a necrotizing vasculitis in 11 of 12 biopsies (see also Chapter 8 on urticarial vasculitis). They observed no consistent relationship between the course of the urticaria-like lesions, the serologic findings, and the clinical activity of SLE.

Urticaria may precede the onset of Still's disease by many months. The rash in Still's disease is described as rarely itchy, fleeting, scattered over the entire body, at times with an urticarial component. It occurs in 25% of the patients, more rarely in adults (Bywaters 1971). Urticaria is also observed in 1.7% of patients with rheumatic fever, primarily in the early stages of the disease. Skin lesions such as erythema multiforme, erythema nodosum, or nonspecific inflammatory lesions may also occur in 10% of patients (Canizares 1951).

Urticarial vasculitis was noted by Callen and Dubin (1978) in association with polymyositis. In all these conditions, urticaria seems a feature of the acute phase of the disease.

The association of cold urticaria with lymphomas and abnormal globulins is discussed in Chapter 5.7.5, p. 71 on the physical urticarias. Barriere et al. (1976) described five patients with nonpruritic chronic urticaria who had monoclonal gammaglobulins and a fulminant clinical picture, with prolonged fever, elevated ESR, lymphadenopathy, and a lethal outcome in some. Clauvel et al. (1982) described five similar patients with monoclonal IgM, four of whom had associated fever, arthralgias, myalgias, leukocytosis, and an elevation of the ESR and the fibrinogen levels. Three of five had a leukocytoclastic vasculitis on biopsy. None had abnormalities of the complement system or evidence of lymphoproliferative disease over a 4–9 year follow-up. Continuous, low-dose steroids controlled the symptoms.

Altmeyer and Welke (1977) described one additional patient with IgM paraproteinemia. There are other scattered observations of urticaria in association with Hodgkin's disease, lymphatic leukemia, lymphosarcoma, reticulosarcoma, and polycythemia vera (Mathews 1974). Resection of a carcinoma of the colon relieved two patients of their chronic urticaria (Sheldon et al. 1954). Two cases of sarcoidosis and chronic urticaria were among the 56 patients of Doeglas (1975) with iodiopathic urticaria. Immune complexes may explain the pathogenesis of the urticaria in some of these cases.

Since the early sixties, a number of families have been described with bouts of urticaria in a dominantly inherited combination of progressive deafness and renal amyloidosis (Muckle and Wells 1962). Toxoplasmosis preceded the syndrome in one family (Campbell and Clifton 1950), but amyloidosis need not always be present (Amblard et al. 1978). The urticarial lesions are typically geographic in distribution, highly pruritic, aggravated by heat and emotion, and they persist for months and years. The analogy to periodic Mediterranean sickness raised the question whether these two conditions are identical (Mamou et al. 1974).

3.7.15 Neurological and Psychic Factors

In the older literature, the possible relationship between whealing and the nervous system was much discussed. The geographic distribution of wheals on the skin which is not yet explained, was thought to depend on peripheral nerves. Such considerations were supported by the observation that urticaria developed after eating fish only on the normal and not on the paralyzed part of the body of a hemiparetic patient (Török 1928). Changes in the tonus of the sympathetic or parasympathetic nervous system were not found by these early workers.

Champion et al. (1969), in their series of 554 patients with urticaria, felt that psychological factors were the main cause in 11.5% and a contributory cause in 24% of patients with chronic urticaria. Rees (1957) concluded that psychological factors were dominant in 39% and subsidiary in 29% of his 100 patients. He described the personality of the chronic urticaria patients as unstable, sensitive, and cyclothymic. They showed more tension, anxiety, and depression than controls. Watzig et al. (1979) recorded merely a variant level of rigidity in his patients which he thought to be related to difficulties in adaption. A further group of workers (Lindemayr et al. 1981) found deviations in established standards with regard to increased introversion, nervousness, and psychosomatic disturbances. Although the patients were not depressed, irritable, emotionally unstable, and unsociable, they were less communicative and aggressive and had more psychosomatic disorders like headaches, chronic gastritis, duodenal ulcers, and migraine headaches.

Stress was identified as a contributing factor in 51% of the patients with chronic urticaria, compared to 8% in controls (Rees 1957). Reinhold (1960) analyzed the type of stress involved in 27 patients and found that 20 had a long history of stress, but no major emotionally stressful crisis. Shoemaker et al. (1962) believed that chronic idiopathic urticaria was a regressive, physiological expression of unconscious conflict, with anxiety being the dominant effect.

The enthusiasm over the role of psychic factors in chronic urticaria derived partly from reports of British workers that wheals in pollen-allergic patients, tuberculin skin test reactions, and even urticaria itself could be inhibited or healed through hypnosis. Levine et al. (1966) were unable to reproduce these observations with histamine or ragweed skin test wheals. Nevertheless, a placebo effect was observed in 12 of 13 patients with chronic urticaria, and whealing restarted when the placebo was stopped (Rudzki et al. 1970). Daniels (1973) reported that behavior therapy resulted in a permanent cure (23-months observation) within 12 weeks of treatment. Koblenzer (1983) considers the psychic component in urticaria so important that all her chronic urticaria patients are treated with hydroxyzine for 1 month after their first visit. She gradually withdraws the drug thereafter and searches for other causes of chronic urticaria only when the urticaria recurs.

There is thus considerable circumstantial evidence for an effect of the psyche on chronic urticaria. This holds also for some of the physical urticarias, particularly for dermographic and cholinergic urticaria, and it fits with the known stimulating and modulating role of neurotransmitters on mast cell release. It remains however unclear to what degree such influences are secondary, due to the chronically vexing itch which wears on the psyche of the patient. Another aspect that has received little attention, is the effect of a constant bombardment of the central nervous system with histamine and other mast cell-derived mediators. The striking cures due to psychotherapy should also be viewed with great caution because chronic urticaria has a high spontaneous cure rate.

3.8 Diagnosis and Differential Diagnosis

(see Chapter 10, p. 122)

3.8.1 General Considerations

The primary lesion of urticaria is so characteristic that a diagnosis is not easily missed. Difficulties arise

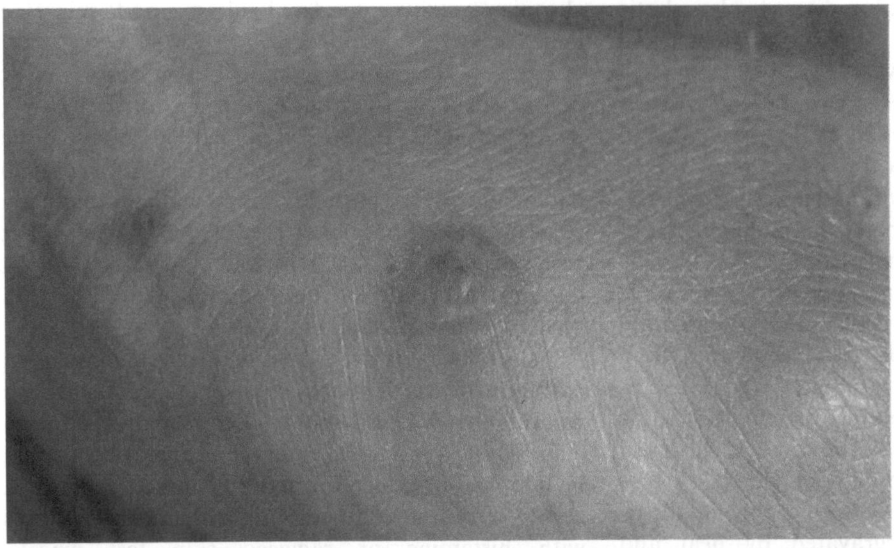

Fig. 3.6. Close-up of a typical target lesion in a patient with erythema multiforme. Note the grayish-white discoloration of the epidermis in the center and the hemorrhagic central punctum.

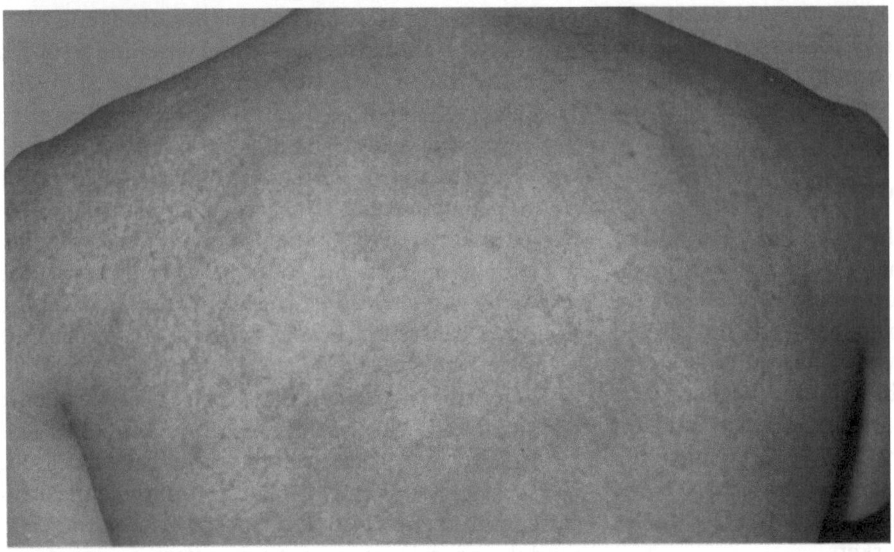

Fig. 3.7. Diffuse, maculopapular rash due to ampicillin. The fine, densely spaced papules which are confluent in the center, the epidermal involvement, and the persistence of the lesions differentiate this exanthem from urticaria.

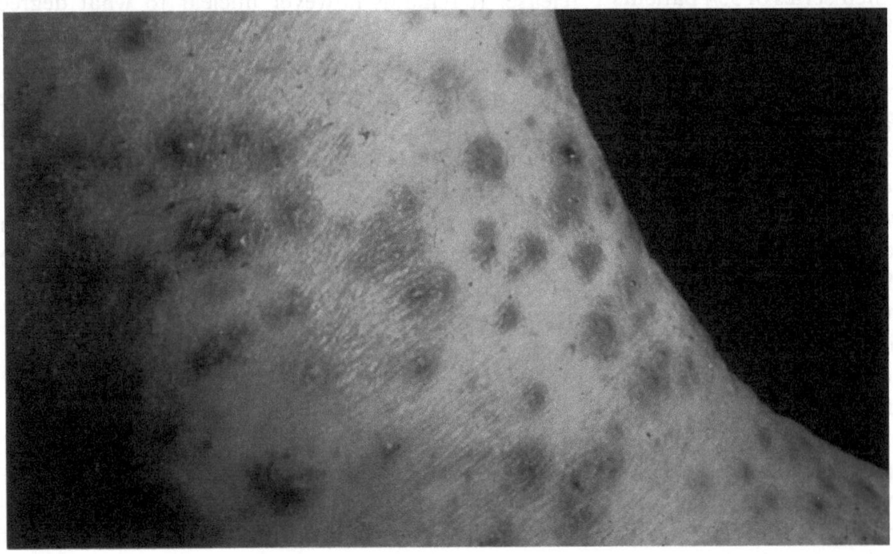

Fig. 3.8. Purpuric macules and papules on the lower leg due to sulfonamides.

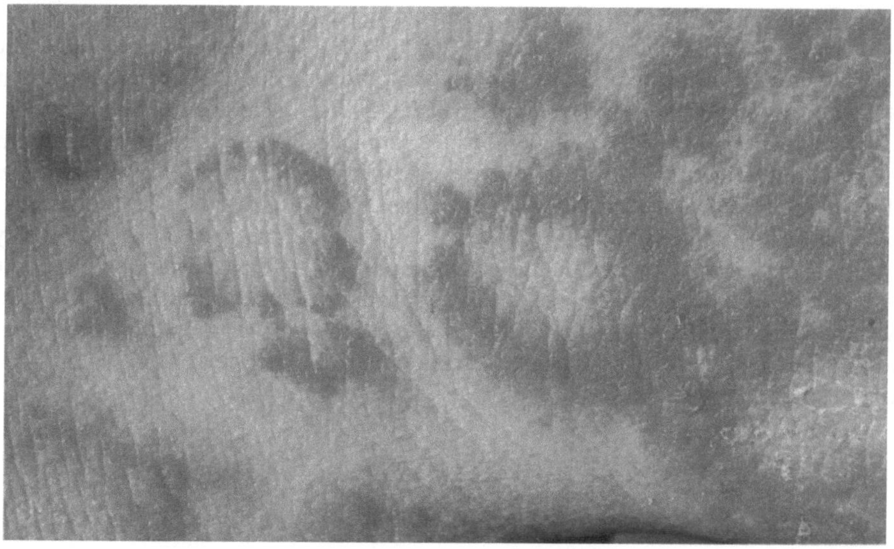

Fig. 3.9. Erythematous papules in an annular arrangement in a patient with bullous pemphigoid. The presence of typical bullous lesions on other parts of the body helped in the clinical diagnosis.

when lesions persist longer than usual or when they are mixed with papular or vasculitic components. Urticarial lesions are also easily overlooked when they coexist with other types of skin lesions in certain systemic diseases or in drug reactions.

It is not meaningful to discuss the diagnosis of acute and chronic urticaria separately at this point since many important differentiating aspects which pertain to a good history, the physical appearance of the lesion, and the diagnostic test methods will be discussed in Chapter 10, p. 122 and in subsequent chapters dealing with the special types of urticaria. A few special dermatological eruption patterns that might present problems in the differential diagnosis shall, however, be briefly discussed here.

3.8.2 Specific Diseases

Erythema multiforme can mimic urticaria, but differs from it by longer persistence of the lesions, the occasional coexistence of erosions of the oral mucosa, and the presence of the classical target lesions on close-up inspection (Fig. 3.6). The lesions of maculopapular drug reactions (Fig. 3.7) are similarly persistent, often have a pronounced purpuric component (Fig. 3.8), and a possible epidermal involvement, with necrosis and crusting. A number of skin lesions present as annular erythemas. They all persist for days and weeks and include erythema marginatum, erythema chronicum migrans, erythema anulare centrifugum, and the annular lesions of granuloma annulare and fungus infections. Even the early lesions of bullous pemphigoid may present as annular, erythematous papules rather than as blisters (Fig. 3.9).

Erythema marginatum does not itch but is otherwise indistinguishable from urticaria. It occurs characteristically during acute rheumatic fever, and because

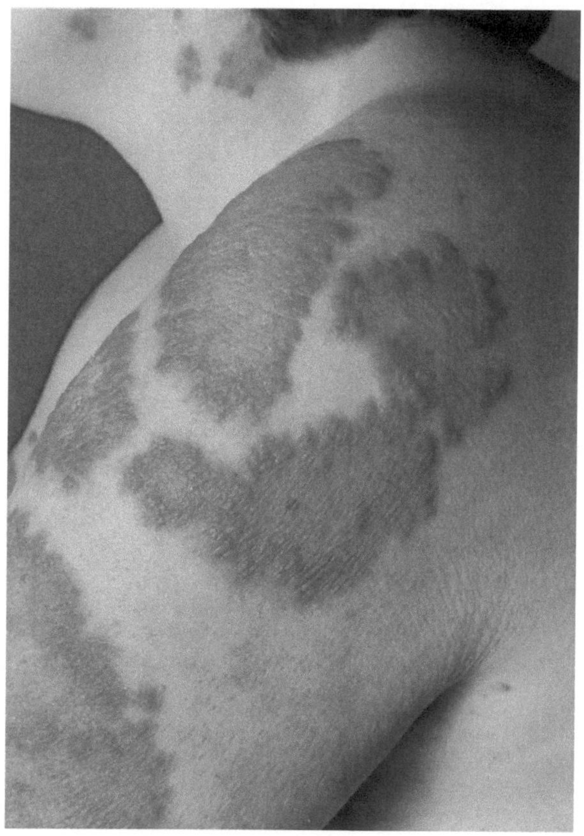

Fig. 3.10. Erythematous plaques, studded with papules, in a woman with acute febrile neutrophilic dermatosis (Sweet's syndrome). The lesions persisted at the same location for several weeks.

of its fleeting nature, it is considered by some to be just a variant form of ordinary urticaria.

Erythema chronicum migrans follows tick bites, and is most likely due to *Borrelia* organisms (lyme disease) (Ackermann 1983). The lesions àre single or multiple and spread centrifugally over several weeks. This slow time course makes differentiation from urticaria relatively easy.

Erythema anulare centrifugum consists of erythematous, ring-shaped lesions which expand by several centimeters during 1 week. The kinetics of the lesions and an occasional scaling on the surface help in the diagnosis of this condition.

Annular lesions due to granuloma anulare or fungus infections never pose a problem in differential diagnosis because of their persistence, the associated scaling, and the crusting of the tinea lesions.

Acute febrile neutrophilic dermatosis (Sweet 1964) (Fig. 3.10) is characterized by painful, symmetric, indurated, erythematous plaques which often spare the trunk. The lesions may be studded with pustules or form blisters on their surface, and persist for weeks and months. These features and the associated symptomatology differentiate this condition from urticaria.

4 Angioedema

4.1 General Aspects and Epidemiology

Angioedema is defined as a circumscribed swelling of the deep cutaneous, subcutaneous, or submucosal tissue. It can involve single or multiple body regions. The lesions develop within minutes, and they usually persist for hours to days. The cutaneous edema causes few symptoms but is disconcerting to the patient because of the physical disfigurement. When vital structures such as the larynx are involved, angioedema poses a life-threatening situation.

There are numerous possible causes for the often massive accumulation of local tissue fluid in angioedema. The condition must therefore be viewed as a symptom of several diseases, including rather well-defined genetic defects.

Several synonyms for angioedema are in common usage, the most important ones being angioneurotic edema and Quincke's edema. The first name derives from the view that the nervous system participates in the development of the edema, a concept that is currently no longer held. Von Quincke (1882) published a very accurate description of the clinical features of several patients with this affliction. A number of patients with similar clinical features had, however, been reported prior to his publication (see Chapter 1, p. 3). It seems therefore more appropriate to call the phenomenon angioedema rather than Quincke's edema since this word encompasses the basic pathological features of the lesions – an edema due to increased postcapillary venular leakage.

Angioedema may occur either alone or in association with urticaria. Champion et al. (1969), in their study of 554 patients with urticaria, observed the simultaneous occurrence of urticaria and angioedema in 49 % of their cases and of angioedema alone in 11 %. Three patients in the latter group had hereditary angioedema.

The sex incidence is about equal in non-hereditary angioedema, with only a slight preponderance of females in hereditary angioedema (Cicardi et al. 1982). Champion et al. (1969) observed a peak incidence of the condition in the third and fourth decades of life, with a spread from childhood to old age. None of the male patients of the latter series who were younger than 15 had angioedema alone, and very few had it in combination with urticaria. In series with hereditary angioedema, two-thirds of the patients were found to have the onset of symptoms before the age of 13 (Frank et al. 1976). The age of onset ranges from 3–79 years (Cicardi et al. 1982).

4.2 Classification

There are two major ways to group angioedema in a meaningful way: on the basis of its pathogenesis or of its mode of genetic transmission. In the first situation, the types with a C1-inhibitor (C1 INH) defect (see Chapters 2.3, p. 19 and 4.7, p. 51) are commonly distinguished from the ones where the biochemical defects are not known. Since the exact pathogenesis of the C1 INH defects are however incompletely understood and, on the other hand, the pathomechanism of certain other types of angioedema without C1 INH defects is partly known, angioedema has been grouped simply on the basis of the non-hereditary or hereditary nature of the disease (Table 4.1).

Non-hereditary angioedema can be associated with many different types of urticaria and shares with them a common basic cause (see Chapter 3, p. 26). Drugs, foods and food additives are the most frequent allergic

Table 4.1. Classification of angioedema.

I. Non-hereditary angioedema
1. allergic causes (drugs, foods, inhalants, contactants, parasites)
2. pseudoallergic causes
3. histamine liberators
4. physical stimuli (cold, heat, pressure, light, water, exercise)
5. urticaria pigmentosa – mastocytosis
6. immune complex diseases (serum sickness, urticarial vasculitis)
7. lymphoproliferative diseases with normal C1 INH
8. acquired C1 INH and protease INH deficiency
9. episodic angioedema with eosinophilia
10. idiopathic angioedema

II. Hereditary angioedema
1. Type I: deficiency of C1 INH synthesis
2. Type II: inactive C1 INH
3. Type III: protein-bound C1 INH
4. familial vibratory angioedema

or pseudoallergic stimuli for angioedema, followed by inhalation antigens and histamine liberators. Ingestion of aspirin and other agents that cause pseudoallergic reactions (Chapter 7, p. 96) can lead to serious edema of the glottis. Angioedema of the tongue can be brought on by direct contact with allergens or histamine liberators in food, by dental fillings, tooth pastes, mouth washes, or insect venoms (see Chapter 6, p. 89). Tannenbaum (1982) described a patient with life-threatening oropharyngeal angioedema which was provoked by diverse olfactory stimuli or by the ingestion of aspirin. The attacks could be stopped by anesthesia of the nasal and sphenopalatine ganglia with 4% cocaine or by intranasal disodiumcromoglycate.

Physical urticarias induced by cold, heat, solar radiation, water, or exercise (cholinergic) can also manifest themselves as deep cutaneous swellings. Cholinergic urticaria may even be associated with abdominal cramps. Angioedema due to vibratory stimuli is very rare, and a hereditary basis has been found in most of the cases reported so far (see Chapter 5.5, p. 64). Physical stimulation of the cutaneous lesions in mastocytosis can also result in extensive cutaneous edema and may, for example, result in massive, painful swellings of the feet after walking, a feature that is also often observed in pressure urticaria (see Chapters 5.6, p. 64 and 9, p. 117).

Defects of the complement system cause several types of angioedema. Immune complex disease, such as serum sickness, rheumatoid arthritis, and certain autoimmune diseases, can have symptoms of urticaria and/or angioedema. These diseases are discussed in detail under the heading of the urticarial vasculitis syndrome (Chapter 8, p. 109).

Since the first report on the association of angioedema with paraproteinemia and acquired C1INH deficiency by Caldwell et al. (1972), the constellation of angioedema and C1INH deficiency has been observed in several other conditions, particularly in association with blood cell malignancies, including chronic lymphatic leukemia, occult lymphoma, autoimmune hemolytic anemia, B-cell proliferative disorders, multiple myeloma, essential cryoglobulinemia, and adenocarcinoma of the rectum (Cohen et al. 1978, Gelfand et al. 1979, Scherak et al. 1979, Gordon et al. 1983).

Despite these intriguing observations, it should, however, be noted that a deficiency of C1INH does not necessarily result in clinically manifest angioedema. This is evident from one of the two patients reported initially by Caldwell et al. (1972).

Both patients had identical complement defects, but the patient with an associated lymphosarcoma had no angioedema. Similar observations were made by Jordon et al. (1974) who reported on an association of normolipemic plane xanthomatosis and C1INH defects without angioedema. Finally, Brasher et al. (1975) examined the incidence of C1INH deficiency and malignancy. They found no complement abnormalities in 50 patients with various malignancies, including Hodgkin's lymphoma and leukemia.

Acquired C1INH defects in association with certain diseases are therefore not only rare, but they need not even result in angioedema. The reverse situation seems to hold as well: Lewkonia and Pineo (1982) reported on seven patients with chronic lymphatic leukemia and one patient with Waldenström's macroglobulinemia who manifested recurrent angioedema in the presence of normal C1INH levels. One patient had increased IgM, another decreased CH50 and three had decreased IgG, IgA, and IgM levels. Unfortunately, the authors failed to exclude a functionally abnormal C1INH (see pathogenesis, 4.7, p. 51), so that further studies must confirm these intriguing findings.

Recently, Gleich et al. (1984) described four patients who suffered from episodic angioedema, urticaria with pruritus, fever, leukocytosis (up to 108000 cells/μl), eosinophilia (up to 88%), and a weight gain of up to 18%. The age of onset ranged from 4–28 years, and one patient had monthly bouts of symptoms for 12 years. The patients did not suffer from parasitosis, their C1INH levels were normal, and their serum C4 levels were low or borderline. Serum IgM was increased in all and IgE in one patient. The authors mention that one other patient with the same symptoms and a convulsive disorder had been reported by Miller and Pepper in 1916.

The hereditary angioedemas (Table 4.1) comprise three clinically indistinguishable variants of C1INH defects. The most common type is due to insufficient synthesis of normal C1INH. About 15 to 21% of the patients (Cicardi et al. 1982) synthesize a dysfunctional inhibitor which is antigenically normal, but immunophoretically abnormal. Finally, a few patients have been described who have an inactive C1INH that is bound non-covalently to albumin (Laurell and Martensson 1971, Rosen et al. 1971, Opferkuch et al. 1974, Gadek et al. 1979).

4.3 Clinical Aspects

4.3.1 Cutaneous Symptoms

One-half to several hours before the appearance of local swellings, some patients note a tingling or tightness at the future site of the lesions. In rare cases, there may also be a prodromal, local, serpiginous, or mottled erythema (Starr and Brasher 1974). This is followed by the sudden appearance of locally limited, but not sharply marginated edema (Fig. 4.1), or by diffuse, soft, doughy tissue swellings which are non-pitting, except at the time of their resolution. The lesions are pale, at times with a red or bluish tinge, and their size varies from a few millimeters in diameter to gigantic plaques. The lesion can even involve an entire extremity. On the mucous membranes, the edema is frequently white, glassy, and transparent. There is no associated pain or pruritus, although a sensation of tightness is noted by many patients. In hereditary angioedema, erythema multiforme-like lesions, macular eruptions, or erythema marginatum (but never urticarial lesions) may be present together with the angioedema. In non-hereditary angioedema, urticaria is the most frequently associated cutaneous lesion.

The duration of local lesions is generally from 24 to 72 h, ranging from 4 h to 1 week. New lesions may evolve, or the swelling can extend over 24–48 h. As with ordinary urticaria, the skin returns to its normal appearance after resolution of the lesions.

Trauma is the precipitating factor of angioedema in 54% of patients with hereditary angioedema, and 43% reported emotional upset or anxiety as provoking factors (Frank et al. 1976).

In 75–86% of the patients, swelling of the skin, especially on the extremities, is the presenting sign of an attack, followed by swelling of face and throat (36–78%) and abdominal pain (52–75%) (Frank et al. 1976, Cicardi et al. 1982). These are also the most frequently involved sites of angioedema, together with those on the genitalia and the gastrointestinal mucosa. In the face, swellings occur frequently in the periorbital region (Fig. 4.1), the nasolabial folds, the lips and the cheeks, usually in a unilateral distribution.

4.3.2 Extracutaneous Symptoms

As with the cutaneous symptoms, there can also be a prodromal general discomfort before an episode of angioedema. Involvement of organs other than the skin is particularly frequent in hereditary angioedema (Table 4.2).

The oral cavity is rarely involved as part of generalized angioedema, and if so, then mostly as a consequence of local, particularly dental procedures. Swellings can be localized to palate, uvula, tongue, cheeks, or floor of the mouth. Dysphagia is a sign of oral cavity, pharyngeal, or esophageal edema. When nose or nasopharynx are involed, there may often be profuse mucus secretion and rhinorrhea.

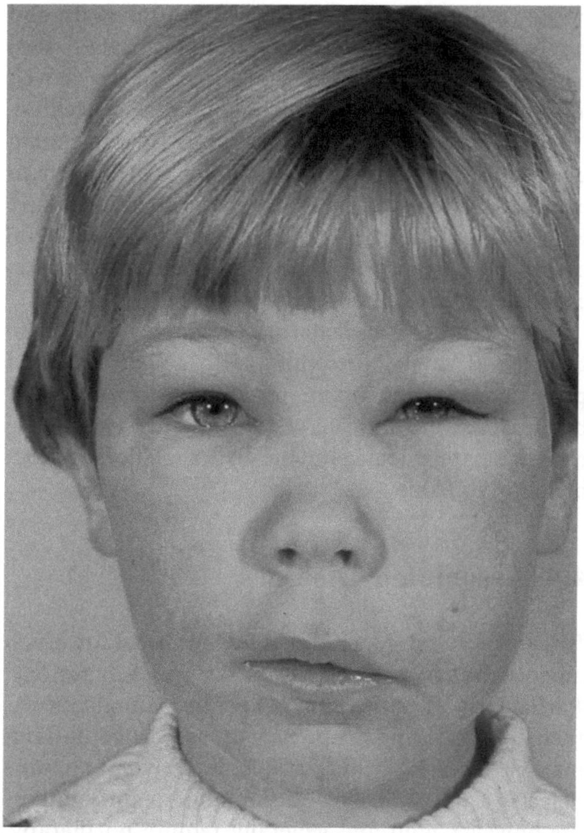

Fig. 4.1. Diffuse facial edema after trauma in a young girl with hereditary angioedema.

Involvement of the pharynx and larynx is particularly feared in angioedema since it has caused death due to suffocation in many patients with hereditary angioedema in the past. Edema has been experienced by 20–30% of the patients at this location at some time in their lives, and about 15% of the patients have to be treated with a tracheotomy (Frank et al. 1976). The entrance to the larynx, the lingual part of the

Table 4.2. Possible site of involvement and symptoms during bouts of angioedema.

Site of involvement	Symptom
Skin	tightness
Oral cavity	dysphagia
Nasopharynx	rhinorrhea
Esophagus	dysphagia
Pharynx + larynx	changes of the voice, shortness of breath, dysphagia
Gastrointestinal tract	pain, diarrhea, vomiting
Pleural cavity	cough, pleuritic pain
Brain	seizures, hemiparesis
Optic nerve	amaurosis, papilledema
Bladder	hematuria

epiglottis, the aryepiglottal folds, the vocal cords, and rarely the subglottis are typically affected sites. Changes of the voice and dysphagia should be viewed as an ominous sign of impending laryngeal swelling.

Recurrent abdominal pain, simulating intestinal obstruction, is a frequent symptom and has led to exploratory surgery in many patients (Warin and Higgs 1982). Diarrhea and vomiting may be severe, causing dehydration and shock and, in rare instances, esophageal tears (Bretza and Novey 1979).

Rarer sites of local edema at extracutaneous sites are the pleural cavity, presenting with cough and mild pleuritic pain; the brain, resulting in seizures and hemiparesis; the optic nerve, causing transient amaurosis and papilledema; and the bladder, inducing gross hematuria (Table 4.2).

4.4 Associated Diseases

In Table 4.1, a number of diseases are listed for which angioedema is part of the basic symptomatology. Particularly in patients with hereditary angioedema, there is a striking frequency of associated inflammatory diseases with possible underlying immune defects (Table 4.3). The autoimmune manifestations are however mild and generally require no therapy. The patients show a higher incidence of the DR3 antigen on HLA typing, compared to ordinary hereditary angioedema patients (Brickman et al. 1984). The increased association of acquired angioedema with lymphoproliferative diseases and malignancies suggests that the immune system plays a special role in the pathogenesis of angioedema.

In this context, the evidence for hormonal influence on angioedema will be briefly discussed. Some female patients have an increased frequency of attacks during menstruation, and worsening of hereditary angioedema has also been observed during treatment with oral contraceptives of the estrogen/progesterone type. Progesterone therapy caused a mild improvement that was not statistically significant. Menopause resulted in improvement of symptoms in only one of four patients. Fewer or no attacks of angioedema were observed in 23 of 25 patients during the last two trimesters of pregnancy, while flare-ups were noted during early pregnancy and again after delivery (Frank et al. 1976). Concurrent with these observations, Beckman et al. (1979) reported that one of their hereditary angioedema patients had two deliveries with episiotomies without complications. There is also a striking improvement of hereditary angioedema with testosterone treatment (to be discussed in detail in Chapter 11.7, p. 149).

Table 4.3. Systemic diseases associated with hereditary angioedema.

Systemic lupus erythematosus
Scleroderma
Thyroiditis
Glomerulonephritis
Sjögren's and sicca syndromes
Juvenile arthritis and IgA deficiency
Rheumatoid arthritis
Inflammatory bowel disease
Partial lipodystrophy
Raynaud's disease
Paroxysmal hemoglobinuria

4.5 Course and Prognosis

The course and duration of angioedema in association with urticaria is similar to that of urticaria alone. In hereditary angioedema, symptoms are usually mild during early childhood, becoming worse during late childhood and adolescence. Most patients improve with increasing age, some male patients already during puberty (Tappeiner et al. 1979). In rare patients, the first clinical signs of their disease become manifest only in the 5th or 6th decades.

Before effective therapy was available, the mortality from hereditary angioedema was about 30%. In a recent analysis of a large group of patients by Cicardi et al. (1982), only 23 of 150 affected family members had died as a result of their disease. In patients with acquired C1 INH deficiency and angioedema, treatment of the underlying disease results in improvement, even though the resection of a tumor need not invariably result in a cure of the tendency to develop angioedema (Gelfand et al. 1979).

4.6 Histology and Ultrastructure

The typical histopathological changes of hereditary angioedema are a separation of the collagen bundles in the skin and an edema of the lamina propria of the jejunum. The submucosal tissue of jejunum, larynx, and even of the urinary bladder may also become edematous (van Dellen and Myers 1980). The ultrastructure shows endothelial gaps and fibrin deposition in the vessel walls, as has been observed in histamine-induced lesions (Willms et al. 1975). In acquired angioedema, there is an additional pericapillary infiltrate of lymphocytes (Lewkonia and Pineo 1982), and in angioedema with eosinophilia, there are also degranulated, diffusely infiltrating dermal eosinophils and degranulated mast cells (Gleich et al. 1984). The presence or absence of a leukocytic infiltrate represents an important distinguishing feature between acquired and hereditary angioedema.

4.7 Pathogenesis

4.7.1 Biochemical Defects in Hereditary Angioedema

Already before the turn of the century, physicians were aware of two different types of angioedema: one was inherited as an autosomally dominant trait and the other not. Two discoveries in the early sixties led to a more exact definition of the specific defect in this condition. First, Landerman et al. (1962) observed that plasma of a patient with hereditary angioedema did not inhibit kallikrein generation of bradykinin. One year later, Donaldson and Evans (1963) succeeded in demonstrating that the affected members of three families with hereditary angioedema had a deficiency of serum C1INH. This defect was not present in several hundred normal controls. Two years later, the same group (Rosen et al. 1965) identified a variant type of hereditary angioedema with an abnormal, nonfunctional, but antigenically normal C1INH protein.

The C1INH protein has a molecular weight of 90,000 d and a sedimentation constant of 4.2 s. It is identical to α_2-neuroaminoglycoprotein, contains 12% hexose and 17% acetylneuraminic acid, is synthesized in the liver, and increases during acute inflammation. Its normal serum concentration is 15.8 ± 1.4 mg/dl (Frank et al. 1976). Johnson et al. (1971) showed that there is a decreased hepatic synthesis of the protein in common C1INH deficiency (see Table 4.1). The serum half-life of the molecule is, however, the same in patients and controls (Brackertz et al. 1975).

In patients with abnormal C1INH proteins, the biochemical defect seems to vary from family to family (Rosen et al. 1971). The patients with the protein-bound, abnormal inhibitor are one such subgroup (see Section 4.2, p. 47 and Table 4.1). Harpel et al. (1975) found an abnormal core protein of the C1INH in one kindred which resulted from a greater number of acidic amino acids and a lower phenylalanine content. The carbohydrate structure appeared normal on the basis of neuraminidase treatment of the molecule.

The C1INH molecule has a controlling function in the intrinsic clotting system, the kinin system, the fibrinolytic system, and the complement system (Fig. 4.2). All these mediator systems are potentially activated through trauma and the Hageman factor (HF). Activated HF and kallikrein continue to stimulate HF in the absence of C1INH (Kaplan 1981), acting thus as feedback for further stimulation of the system. Donaldson (1968) provided evidence that HF plays an important role in the pathogenesis of angioedema.

Of the many potential alterations due to the C1INH defect, the role of the complement and the kinin systems has been studied most thoroughly. C1INH binds irreversibly to activated C1$\bar{s}$ esterase, but it also inhibits C1$\bar{r}$ protease activity, preventing the proteolytic cleavage of C4 and C2 (Gelfand et al. 1979). There is chronic C1$\bar{s}$ generation and therefore increased consumption of C4 even inbetween attacks. During attacks, C1$\bar{s}$ increases markedly, with further decrease of C4 and C2. Several days afterward, these changes revert to normal. C3 levels remain normal during attacks, possibly due to the fact that fluid phase

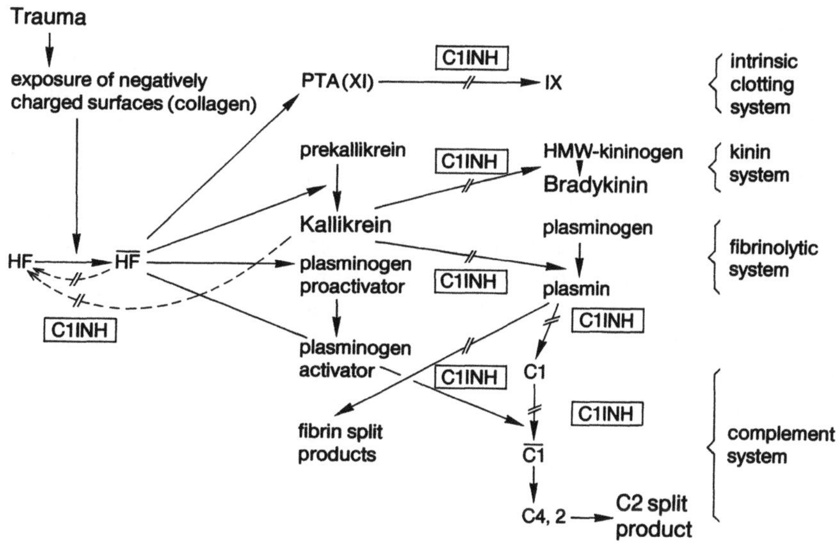

Fig. 4.2. The major pathways of inflammation initiated by physical trauma. The site of inhibition by the C1INH is indicated with *parallel bars* (//). A *transverse bar* over a letter indicates the functionally activated state of the molecule ($\overline{HF}$, $\overline{C1}$). Bradykinin and the C2 split products are increased during attacks as a result of the inhibitor defect in hereditary angioedema, thus explaining the deep tissue edema (after Gelfand et al. 1979 and Kaplan 1981). *HF*, Hageman factor; *PTA*, plasma thrombin activator; *C*, complement, *HMW*, high molecular weight.

$C\overline{142}$ is unable to activate C3 (Frank et al. 1976; see also Section 4.8).

Injection of $C1\bar{s}$ causes angioedema without associated pain or erythema in hereditary angioedema patients, but this does not occur in controls. Complement components beyond C3 are furthermore not necessary to produce the clinical picture of angioedema (Klemperer et al. 1968, Donaldson et al. 1969), and a split product of C2 with kinin-like activity has been found which is thought to explain the effects of the $C1\bar{s}$ injections (Donaldson et al. 1969). C2 kinin is elevated during attacks of angioedema in patient serum. According to recent findings, it must first be cleaved by a process of fibrinolysis before it becomes biologically active (Donaldson et al. 1978). C2 kinin is heat stable and trypsin sensitive, does not cause hypotension on intravenous injection, differs from bradykinin in its chemical structure, and unlike bradykinin does not produce a painful erythematous wheal on local injection (Donaldson et al. 1969). While these findings are intriguing and a potentially plausible explanation for some of the experimental and clinical observations in hereditary angioedema, they have recently been challenged by other workers who found elevated amounts of active kallikrein in suction blister fluid and of low levels of high molecular weight (HMW)-kininogen and increased kinins in the sera of patients with hereditary angioedema (Curd et al. 1980, Cullmann et al. 1982b, Fields et al. 1983). Uninhibited conversion of HMW-kininogen to bradykinin on stimulation by kallikrein (see Fig. 4.2) explains thus a basic aspect in the pathogenesis of C1INH-associated angioedema.

Additional evidence for the role of kinins in hereditary angioedema comes from the observation of a steeper increase and maximum of plasma kinin formation after in vitro activation of factor XII of the coagulation system in four patients studied by Laurberg (1978) as compared to controls. This alteration was partially corrected by therapy with tranexamic acid. Soulier et al. (1981) noted activation of prekallikrein and factor VII during cold storage (0° C for 20 h) of plasma from nine patients with hereditary angioedema.

Evidence for an increased activation of the fibrinolytic system (Fig. 4.2) comes mainly from the therapeutic efficacy of epsilon amino caproic acid in the disease (see Chapter 11.7, p. 151). Bork et al. (1984) have recently shown that several factors of the coagulation system are elevated and that attacks occurred in these patients even in the presence of normal or slightly decreased C1INH levels.

Histamine seems to play no significant role in hereditary angioedema since, although causing wheals and pain on injection, it does not lead to the typical clinical signs of angioedema. Plasma levels have nevertheless been reported to increase during attacks, particularly also in vibratory angioedema (Kaplan 1981). Others have measured slightly elevated levels inbetween attacks (Granerus et al. 1967, Willms et al. 1975). These changes result perhaps from the effect of mediators like C5a on the release of histamine from mast cells.

Recent observations which showed convincingly that androgens raise the serum C1INH levels of patients and also cause a striking clinical improvement, have been considered a further proof that the deficiency of C1INH plays an important role in the pathogenesis of hereditary angioedema (see Chapter 11.7.1, p. 149). The fact that some members of families with the disease have low C1INH levels without symptoms (Röhrich and Endres 1985) and some patients develop their disease only late in life, suggest that additional pathogenetic factors must come into play to explain hereditary angioedema.

4.7.2 Pathogenesis of Acquired Angioedema

The reason why deeper tissue swellings rather than hives develop in allergic angioedema is unclear and has never been studied thoroughly. Possibly, mast cells located in the lower dermis and the subcutaneous fat, rather than those in upper dermal regions, release their mediators on appropriate stimulation. It is also intriguing that an absent functional C1INH and variable hypocomplementemia do not necessarily result in angioedema (see 4.2, p. 47 and Spitzer et al. 1980). This again casts doubt on the theory that C1INH defects alone explain acquired angioedema.

In a recent report of potential interest, Dolovich et al. (1983) observed late cutaneous reactions (at 6 h) in almost half of their eight patients with idiopathic angioedema after intracutaneous histamine and codeine injections. This did not occur in 34 subjects without angioedema in response to histamine and in only three patients of this control group after codeine injections. An explanation for these findings was not offered by the authors, and any interpretation is premature due to our lack of understanding of the pathomechanisms in these reactions.

In acquired C1 INH deficiency, increased catabolism rather than impaired biosynthesis has been shown to be the basic defect (Sheffer et al. 1985).

4.8 Laboratory Findings

The most important laboratory tests (also for diagnostic purposes) involve changes in the serum

Table 4.4. Alterations in serum levels of complement components and the resulting diagnosis (after Frank et al. 1976). Brasher (1977) also found low C1q levels in 21 hereditary angioedema patients.

Serum levels			Diagnosis
C1INH (immuno-chem.)	C4	C1	
↓	↓	–	hereditary angioedema
↓	–	–	very likely hereditary angioedema
–	↓	–	variant type of hereditary angioedema (functionally deficient C1INH)
–	↓	↓/–	SLE[a] or other diseases
↓	↓	↓	acquired angioedema
–(↑)	–(↑)	–	idiopathic angioedema

[a]SLE = systemic lupus erythematosus.

complement components (see Table 4.4). C1INH serum levels are always low in untreated, ordinary hereditary angioedema. During attacks, there is a drop of C4, CH50, and C2, while C1s̄ is often increased and C3 is usually normal (Brasher et al. 1975). C1q was low in 21 patients studied by Brasher (1977), and C4 was chronically decreased, but occasionally it was also normal inbetween attacks. Other possible laboratory changes during attacks are a leukocytosis with a shift to the left, but no eosinophilia. Hypernatremia may develop due to diarrhea and vomiting.

In acquired angioedema with C1INH deficiency, C1 or C1q are markedly reduced, and C4 and C2 are low as well. Cryoglobulins and 7S and 19S paraproteins are often found in the serum of these patients. In chronic idiopathic angioedema, all complement levels remain normal, except in a few patients with associated urticaria (see chapter on the urticarial vasculitis syndrome, p. 109).

During acute abdominal attacks, X-ray studies of the abdomen show a "thumb-printing" pattern, with prominent spiculations and other changes suggestive of mucosal edema and toxic megacolon (Frank et al. 1976).

4.9 Genetics

Since the study of angioedema in five generations of one family by Osler in 1888, the autosomal dominant pattern of the hereditary variant of angioedema is well established. Additional data on the mode of inheritance of the disease have been scanty. Several groups showed that there was no genetic linkage between the disease and the loci for HLA, blood group antigens AB0, or transferrin (Ohela et al. 1977, Jackson et al. 1978).

After the discovery of the C1INH defect, new insights were gained into the genetics of the disease. Shokeir (1973) expressed the belief that because of the variable C1INH serum levels in different patients, the disease was probably not due to a structural gene defect, but to a disorder of gene regulation. An abnormal repressor substance was postulated to exist which caused a chronic repression of the structural gene.

Frank et al. (1976) studied 30 patients with angioedema, seven of whom had a negative family history. The authors concluded that some patients acquire the disease due to spontaneous mutation. Six of the seven patients had kindred with decreased C1INH and C4 levels, suggesting the possibility of complement defects being genetically linked to, but not causative of angioedema.

With the discovery that serum C1INH levels can be raised to normal levels during treatment with testosterone, Rosen and Austen (1976) drew an analogy to other genetic defects that are responsive to steroid therapy. They hypothesized that testosterone might correct a genetic fault which suppresses normal messenger RNA synthesis in the C1INH deficiency type and favors abnormal messenger RNA synthesis in the patients with nonfunctional C1INH. Along these same lines, Ollier et al. (1978) suggested the existence of two varieties of C1INH molecules in the haploid patients which are differentiated on the basis of their complete or incomplete glycoconjugation in the hepatocyte. The defect in hereditary angioedema would thus be related to involvement of the structural gene (s) that control the synthesis of C1INH.

4.10 Diagnosis

The clinical features of hereditary angioedema are so distinctive that one can usually differentiate the disease from the many other types of angioedema listed in Table 4.1 on clinical grounds alone. The most important specific clinical aspects of hereditary angioedema are (1) a history of recurrent cutaneous and oropharyngeal swellings and abdominal pain, (2) a positive family history, and (3) the clinical features of the cutaneous lesions on mere inspection (Table 4.5). The early diagnosis of hereditary angioedema is extremely important because of the serious prognosis of the disease and the relatively effective therapy which is currently available. Surprisingly, the mean duration from onset of symptoms until proper diagnosis in the group of 30 patients studied at the US National Institute of Health was 21 years (Frank et al. 1976).

Table 4.5. Diagnostic features of hereditary angioedema.

History	repeated bouts of non-pruritic cutaneous swellings without urticaria repeated attacks of abdominal pain, diarrhea, vomiting repeated respiratory distress, possibly even with tracheotomy positive family history
Clinical picture	non-pruritic, pale, cutaneous or mucosal swelling, no associated urticaria
Laboratory findings	decrease of C1INH serum levels 1. immunochemically (commercially available) 2. functionally a) inhibition of EAC1$\bar{s}$ b) inhibition of C1$\bar{s}$ esterolysis evidence of complement consumption, reduced C4, C2, C1q serum levels (immunochemically or functionally) lack of an infiltrate on histology of involved skin

EAC1s, a complex of erythrocytes, antibodies against erythrocytes and C1$\bar{s}$.

Once there is a clinical suspicion, the serum C4 and C1INH levels should be measured, since they represent the most reliable screening method. If the C4 level is decreased and the C1INH normal, the functional C1INH test should be done to rule out the variant type of hereditary angioedema. If both factors are decreased and the family history is negative, C1 levels should be measured and a cause for acquired angioedema sought. Table 4.4 provides a simple guideline to the proper diagnosis of hereditary angioedema on the basis of the serum complement changes.

Recently, two simplified laboratory tests have been described as a diagnostic aid for hereditary angioedema. Yelvington et al. (1983) claim that they can differentiate hereditary or acquired C1INH defects from other types of angioedema with urticaria in an immunodiffusion assay. The test is based on the fact that the major antigenic determinants of C1$\bar{r}$ are masked when C1$\bar{r}$ is inactivated by C1INH in the complex of the two components. Another test which measures functional C1INH is performed with an amidolytic assay by monitoring the inactivation of plasma kallikrein (Cullmann et al. 1982a).

Idiopathic angioedema can readily be differentiated from hereditary angioedema by the frequently associated urticarial eruptions, the practically always normal complement levels (Table 4.4), and the presence of a mild to moderate cutaneous infiltrate on biopsy of the lesions (see Section 4.6, p. 50). In episodic angioedema with eosinophilia, the clinical features and the histology are typical (Gleich et al. 1984). Other types of angioedema can be diagnosed by the history of a specific eliciting stimulus (physical urticarias, drug-induced angioedema) and by the associated diseases (urticaria pigmentosa, parasitosis, immune complex disease, lymphoma). Allergic causes should be identified by skin and laboratory tests if the history provides appropriate clues in this direction.

4.11 Differential Diagnosis

There are a number of conditions (Table 4.6) that might be confused with angioedema on first sight. Usually, however, they can be easily differentiated on the basis of a more thorough clinical examination and a good history.

The edema in erysipelas is associated with redness, pain, and fever. The Melkerson-Rosenthal syndrome usually presents with recurrent facial swellings which tend to leave a persistent, granulomatous thickening of the tissue after several bouts of edema. Cheilitis, glossitis, a folded tongue, and facial palsy are other possible features.

Contact urticaria (see Chapter 6, p. 89) could cause confusion with angioedema on inspection, but the history of a specific stimulus and the positive skin test help in differentiation. In contact dermatitis, epidermal changes manifesting themselves as vesicles or fine scales should facilitate differentiation of the conditions.

Tissue edema could be caused by a blockade of the lymphatic drainage, by the superior vena cava syndrome, heart failure, renal insufficiency, and the capillary leak syndrome, to name but a few causes. This type of edema is more diffuse, slowly evolving, more persistent, and it shifts with positioning of the patient. The associated underlying disease will suggest the proper cause of the edema.

Some patients with hereditary angioedema who suffer only from recurrent abdominal pain have been subjected to unnecessary appendectomies in the past. Patients with hereditary angioedema as the cause of the abdominal pain usually show no signs of peritoneal irritation, and the pain disappears after 1–3 days. On the other hand, patients with known hereditary angioedema and an abdominal crisis might also have a normal surgical emergency, and they should be watched accordingly.

Table 4.6. Differential diagnosis of angioedema.[a]

1. Erysipelas
2. Melkerson-Rosenthal syndrome
3. Contact urticaria
4. Lymph and tissue edema due to internal causes
5. Acute abdomen

[a] See also Table 4.1.

5 The Physical Urticarias

5.1 General Aspects

The physical urticarias differ from other types of urticaria in that their eliciting factors are well-defined physical stimuli from the external environment. They also include urticarias due to physical exertion.

The physical urticarias make up the major part of the urticarias for which a cause can be found. Thus, they are a source of satisfaction to the physician who is thoroughly familiar with them. Most subtypes can be readily treated if the patient is able to avoid the eliciting stimulus or if he learns to suppress his symptoms pharmacologically which is possible in almost all cases. Studies of the pathogenesis of physical urticaria, in particular of cold urticaria, have contributed significantly to our present understanding of mast cell-mediated disease.

Duke (1926) used the term physical urticaria synonymously with factitious urticaria, and he divided the physical urticarias into either of two groups: one is limited to the site of contact (light, heat, cold, scratching) and the other is reflex-induced or secondary to changes in body temperature. Duke called attention to the fact that heat tends to induce reflex urticaria (cholinergic urticaria) more frequently than heat contact urticaria, while the reverse is true for cold.

Physical urticarias can also be classified according to the nature of the eliciting stimulus. Such a classification may help to better recall the many possible different types of physical urticaria. Illig and Kunick (1969) differentiated urticaria due to mechanical, thermic, and electromagnetic forces. A fourth group that is elicited by a combination of several stimuli (summation urticaria) was added to these three major categories. It is however difficult to include aquagenic urticaria and exercise-induced anaphylaxis in this scheme, particularly since the exact nature of the eliciting stimulus, whether a chemical agent or a physical force, is not known in these rare disorders. The one patient with decompression urticaria (Warin and Champion 1974) is not easily classified either, although the one urticaria patient who reacted to X-ray and to infra-red light respectively, fits nicely in the group that suffers from urticaria due to electromagnetic radiation (Illig and Kunick 1969).

5.2 Epidemiology and Clinical Aspects

The most important physical urticarias are listed in Table 5.1, according to the frequency of their occurrence (Champion et al. 1969). The patients are generally young adults, some are even children. The condition may develop for no reason at all and may also resolve again spontaneously, although it may persist through life, particularly in the familial urticarias. Women are more frequently affected than men, with the exception of those physical urticarias that become apparent with manual labor and physical exertion (Table 5.1).

The majority of patients with physical urticarias have no personal or family history of atopy. Their disease is mostly idiopathic, and only a few of the associated diseases listed in Table 5.1 have been shown to be of pathogenetic significance. Several types of urticaria often coexist (Table 5.1).

In a well-defined group of patients, there is a genetic basis for their urticaria (Table 5.2). The transmission is usually autosomally dominant.

With almost all types of stimuli, delayed reactions can develop but are probably often missed because they are not looked for. The majority of the lesions develop very rapidly within a few minutes, and they are generally gone by 1 h (Table 5.3). The time course of their development and their clinical appearance can be reproduced during test procedures in the office.

Tiny, pinhead size wheals are typical in the reflex types of urticaria (cholinergic urticaria, cold reflex urticaria) and in urticaria due to water (aquagenic urticaria). Such small lesions can also occur in solar urticaria and exercise-induced anaphylaxis.

The contact urticarias, on the other hand, tend to assume the exact shape of the area where skin and stimulus have touched. Deep tissue edema can develop in cold urticaria and more rarely in cholinergic urticaria. Such deep swellings are also a typical feature of pressure urticaria and vibratory angioedema. In familial cold urticaria, the typical lesions are maculopapular and more rarely urticarial. For this

Table 5.1. Epidemiologic data on the physical urticaria from the literature and our own patients

Type	Relative frequency (%)	Mean age at onset	Mean duration (years)	♂/♀	Associated diseases	
Dermographic urticaria	50	25	6.5	0.4/1.0	*urticarias:*	Chr. U, PU, CU, Chol. U, Aqu. U, angioedema
					other:	parasitosis, hormonal changes, mastocytosis, hypereosinophilic syndrome, neuropsychiatric disorders
Cholinergic urticaria	30	25	5.3	1.4/1.0	*urticarias:*	Chr. U, DU, CU, Aqu. U, vibratory angioedema; exercise-induced anaphylaxis
					other:	asthma, hayfever
Cold urticaria	15	18	4.2	0.5/1.0	*urticarias:*	DU, Chol. U, HU, angioedema, exercise-induced asthma, atopy, infectious mononucleosis, cryoglobulinemia, paroxysmal cold hemoglobulinemia, C2-deficiency
Solar urticaria	3	28	7.1	0.9/1.0	*urticarias:*	DU, CU, HU
					other:	porphyria, lupus erythematosus, drug reactions, peptic ulcers
Pressure urticaria	2	34	6.0	1.7/1.0	*urticarias:*	Chr. U, DU, ASA Intol, angioedema
Heat contact urticaria	rare	37	1.0	0.2/1.0	*urticarias:*	DU, CU, Solar U
					other:	atopy
Aquagenic urticaria	rare	18	not known	0.2/1.0	*urticarias:*	DU, Chol. U
Vibratory angioedema	rare	not known	not known	not known	*urticarias:*	DU, Chol. U
					other:	asthma, allergic rhinitis
Exercise-induced anaphylaxis	rare	24	5.0	1.4/1.0	*urticarias:*	acute U, Chol. U, angioedema
Familial cold urticaria	rare	infancy	life	1.7/1.0		arthritis

Chr. U, Chronic; PU, Pressure; CU, Cold; Chol. U, Cholinergic; DU, Dermographic; HU, Heat; Aqu. U, Aquagenic urticaria.

Table 5.2. Types of physical urticaria that may occur on a familial basis.

Dermographic urticaria
Cold urticaria (11 families)
Delayed cold contact urticaria
Vibratory angioedema
Delayed localized heat urticaria
Solar urticaria with erythropoietic protoporphyria
Exercise-induced anaphylaxis

reason, the inclusion of this disorder among the urticarias has been seriously questioned.

Practically all patients with physical urticaria experience pruritus at the site of their lesions. The nature of this itch makes them rub rather than scratch their skin. For this reason, excoriations are rarely seen in physical urticarias, and their presence suggests other conditions such as eczema.

Some patients experience burning or stinging rather than pruritus at the site of wheals. Itching in the absence of any visible lesions can also occur on contact with cold stimuli, with water, or after stimulation that normally results in cholinergic urticaria. A prodromal itching of the scalp is observed by many patients with cholinergic urticaria, while prodromal itching of the palms has been reported in exercise-induced anaphylaxis. With mild stimulation, only an erythematous response rather than a wheal is observed in some patients.

Table 5.3. Clinical aspects of the physical urticarias (data are summarized from many series in the literature and our own patients).

Type	Eliciting stimulus	Time of onset	Duration of lesions	Diagnostic test	Associated symptoms
Dermographic urticaria (tarda)	stroking, scratching (rubbing for red dermographism)	2–5 min (1/2–8 h)	1–3 h (48 h)	firm stroking of the skin	headache, malaise
Cholinergic urticaria	physical exercise + overheating ± mental stress	2–20 min	30–60 min	bicycling, running, sauna	headache, gastrointestinal upset, wheezing, salivation, lacrimation, syncope
Cold urticaria	cold contact	2–5 min	1–2 h	ice cube, cold arm bath, cold air	wheezing, syncope
Solar urticaria	light of varying wavelengths	2–15 min	15 min to 3 h	phototest	wheezing, dizziness, syncope
Pressure urticaria	pressure	3–8 h	8–24 h	locally applied weights	flu-like syndrome, fever, leukocytosis, arthralgias
Heat contact urticaria	contact with heat	2–15 min	30–60 min	hot arm bath	gastrointestinal upset, dizziness, fatigue, wheezing, dyspnea
Aquagenic urticaria	contact with water	2–30 min	30–60 min	bath, compresses	
Vibratory angioedema	vibration	0.5–4 min	1 h	vibrating motor	faintness, headache
Exercise-induced anaphylaxis	exercise after a previous heavy meal	2–5 min	10–30 min	exercise	flushing, headache, disorientation, glottis edema, dyspnea, collapse
Familial cold urticaria	cold wind, change from cold to warm air	0.5–3 h	48 h	cold wind and subsequent rewarming	tremor, headache, arthralgias, fever

5.3 Pathogenesis

5.3.1 Passive Transfer

While the eliciting stimulus is generally apparent in the physical urticarias, the basic pathologic alterations that lead to the abnormal response are only poorly understood. A passive transfer with the patient's serum has been accomplished in many patients with dermographic urticaria, in a smaller percentage of patients with cold urticaria, and in two subgroups of solar urticaria (Table 5.4). IgE antibodies have been identified in dermographic and in cold urticaria. Illig and Heinicke (1967b) reported finding a relatively heat-stable, transferable serum factor in cholinergic urticaria which, because of its heat-stability, must belong to another group of immunoglobulins than to IgE.

It is not clear whether the lack of these antibodies in the serum of most patients is due to low level production or to highly selective binding of these antibodies to tissue mast cells. Entirely different pathogenetic mechanisms might also be involved in the urticarias where passive transfer is not possible.

5.3.2 Mediators

In all major types of physical urticarias, histamine has been isolated from the lesions in the effluent blood (Table 5.4). Other vasoactive mediators have not been sought in each one of the different types of physical urticaria; but whenever such investigations were done, these mediators were present to a highly variable degree (Table 5.4). The chemotactic factors which have so far been observed include a mixture of low

Table 5.4. Pathogenetic aspects of the physical urticarias.

Type	Positive passive transfer	Histamine	Serotonin	Chemotactic factors	Kinins	Complement
Dermographic urticaria	56–69% IgE	↑	–	–	↑	–
Cholinergic urticaria	?IgG	↑	↑	↑	–	–
Cold contact urticaria (non-familial)	10–30% (IgE, IgM)	↑	–	↑	–	↓
Solar urticaria	only in types included by UVB + vis. light	↑	–	↑	–	–
Pressure urticaria	neg.	↑	–	↑	–	–
Heat contact urticaria	neg.	↑	–	↑	–	↓
Aquagenic urticaria	neg.	↑	–	–	–	–
Vibratory angioedema	neg.	↑		–	–	–
Exercise-induced anaphylaxis	?	↑	–	–	–	–

–, not yet demonstrated; UVB, ultraviolet light-B.

molecular weight eosinophil chemoattractants, high molecular weight neutrophil factors, and chemotactic leukotrienes. These chemotactic factors are important since they play a potential role in the induction of the leukocytic infiltrate that is present in the delayed types of physical urticaria.

5.3.3 Unifying Pathogenetic Scheme

In Fig. 5.1, an attempt is made to elucidate the two major types of lesions due to physical stimuli. In situation A, a mild physical stimulus (e.g. scratching) will induce mast cells to release histamine without causing any major degranulation of the cells; a rapidly appearing, fleeting wheal results. The factor that causes histamine release from mast cells could be an antigen that is generated by the physical stimulus in the dermis which combines with its specific IgE on the cell membrane. Alternatively, a neurotransmitter, released from nerve endings during reflex type stimulation, could also act in this fashion.

In situation B (Fig. 5.1), a delayed wheal develops via the same mechanisms as in situation A, but the stimulus is stronger in intensity or duration. Mast cells degranulate and release chemotactic factors or activate complement, causing generation of chemoattractants. Alternatively, a stimulus-induced neoantigen causes macrophage and lymphocyte stimulation, resulting in the production of chemotactic lymphokines and monokines. As a third possibility, production of antigen/antibody complexes would result in activation of the complement cascade or direct stimulation of mast cells during phagocytosis of the complexes. The elucidation of these processes and their role in the different types of physical urticaria will be the challenge of the future.

5.4 Dermographic Urticaria (Urticaria Factitia)

5.4.1 Clinical Aspects and Epidemiology

Dermographic urticaria is defined as readily elicited whealing of the skin, accompanied by itching, which evolves rapidly at sites of scratching over the skin

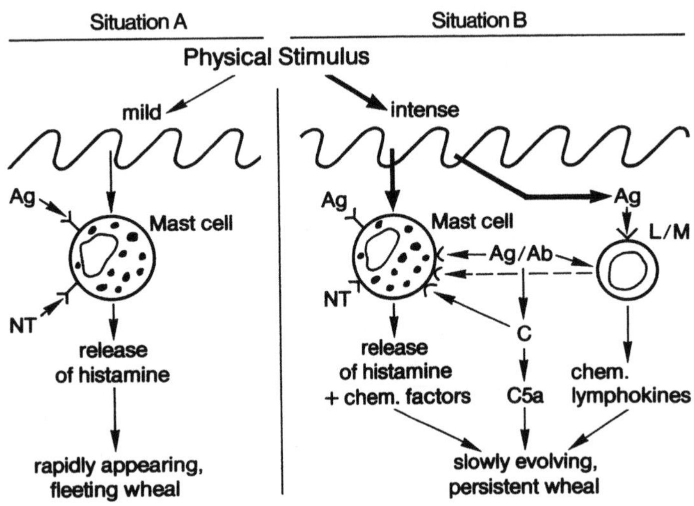

Fig. 5.1 The hypothetical pathological events during physical urticaria. Mild stimulation leads to histamine release and a rapidly appearing, fleeting wheal (e.g., cholinergic urticaria). A more intense stimulus results in release of histamine and chemotactic mediators. Activation of complement or formation of special antigens or antigen/antibody complexes results in generation of other mediators of inflammation which are also chemotactic. A cellular infiltrate will cause a more prolonged persistence of the wheal. *Ag*, antigen; *Ab*, antibody; *C*, activated complement; *L/M*, lymphocyte/macrophage; *MC*, mast cell; *NT*, neurotransmitter; *chem.*, chemotactic.

surface while a moderate pressure is exerted. Its incidence has been estimated at 1.5 to 5% in the general population (Kirby et al. 1971).

Dermographic urticaria is the most frequent type of physical urticaria. It accounts for 8–9% of all cases of urticaria and for 6% of all patients seen in a dermatological referral practice (Champion et al. 1969; own observations). Dermographic whealing occurs in only 1% of patients with generalized pruritus (Marcussen 1950).

In almost all patient groups studied, dermographic urticaria is found twice as frequently in women than in men (Doeglas 1975a, Marcussen 1950) (Table 5.1). The average age of onset is the third decade, but the condition can begin in early childhood or even during the sixth decade. Obese persons who tend to wear tight clothing and persons with a nervous predisposition seem to be more prone to develop the disease. Familial cases have not been reported so far, but Warin (personal communication) has treated several families where virtually all members were affected.

5.4.2 Cutaneous Symptoms

Patients are usually aware that whealing results after localized, mechanical irritation of the skin, such as after stroking, rubbing, scratching, or pinching. Such stimuli can occur in everyday life on contact with furniture, garters, bracelets, towels, or bedding. In some patients, an attack of generalized itching leads to scratching and to typically linear whealing. Inadvertent trauma such as rubbing of the eyes are eliciting causes that are easily missed.

Lesions of dermographic urticaria start within 50–120 s as an erythema which is replaced within 3–5 min by an edema and a surrounding reflex erythema (Fig. 5.2). Maximal edema is reached within 10–15 min, rarely within 20–30 min. The erythema regresses generally within 1 h, whereas the edema can persist for up to 3 h.

Itching can precede erythema, but it usually occurs together with erythema and disappears again suddenly. In one-third of the patients, burning is present together with itching. Pruritus is usually more intense when the patient is tired and stressed, even though the skin lesions are not necessarily larger (Marcussen 1950).

Lesions of dermographic urticaria are observed more frequently over pressure points of the body, such as over bony prominences. Typical localizations are the buttocks (from sitting), the belt region, and the shoulders after carrying shoulder bags. Wheals on the back tend to be larger than on weather-beaten skin such as on the forearm (Matthews et al. 1973). This may be due to constant low-level stimulation and a subsequent refractory state of the tissue. Most patients observe such a refractory period after local stimulation at the site for several days thereafter.

The lesions of dermographic urticaria typically resolve without leaving any changes on the skin. Scratch marks are therefore not typical. Marcussen (1950), however, described the occurrence of excoriations, prurigo and papules, lichenification, and hyperpigmentation in his patients. He attributed these lesions to chronic reactions of the skin to irritation from garments. There was no increased reactivity to contact allergens among his patients; but the high incidence of neurotic and psychiatric disorders in the group may explain this unusual finding.

5.4.3 Systemic Manifestations and Laboratory Findings

Severe headache and malaise are the only major symptoms that accompany severe whealing (Lehner and Rajka 1930). Syncope occurs extremely rarely, unless mastocytosis is present as an underlying disease. Serum IgE and complement levels are normal. Breathnach et al. (1981) reported increased IgM and immune complex levels in 23% and 30% of their patients, respectively. *Candida albicans* was isolated from the gastrointestinal and genital tracts in 30% of their patients with dermographic urticaria. Serum α_1-antitrypsin and α_2-antichymotrypsin levels were decreased. Other specific laboratory alterations occur when an underlying disease, for example hyperthyroidism or parasitic infestation, coexists (see Table 5.1).

5.4.4 Morphological Changes

A very thorough study of the sequential ultrastructural changes in dermographic wheals of one patient has been published by Cauna et al. (1970). In the epidermis, they observed three types of changes:

1) Many keratinocytes developed single, large, membrane-bound vacuoles in the perinuclear region which were maximal at 10 min and vanished by 60 min.
2) The villous processes of some keratinocytes were enlarged and extended.
3) Some basal keratinocytes projected cytoplasmic extensions into the dermis through gaps in the basement membrane.

In the papillary dermis, the endothelial cells of capillaries and venules were filled with vacuoles of varying sizes. The cysternae of granular endoplasmic reticulum of fibrocytes, some smooth muscle cells, and Schwann cells of the nerve endings were distended. In

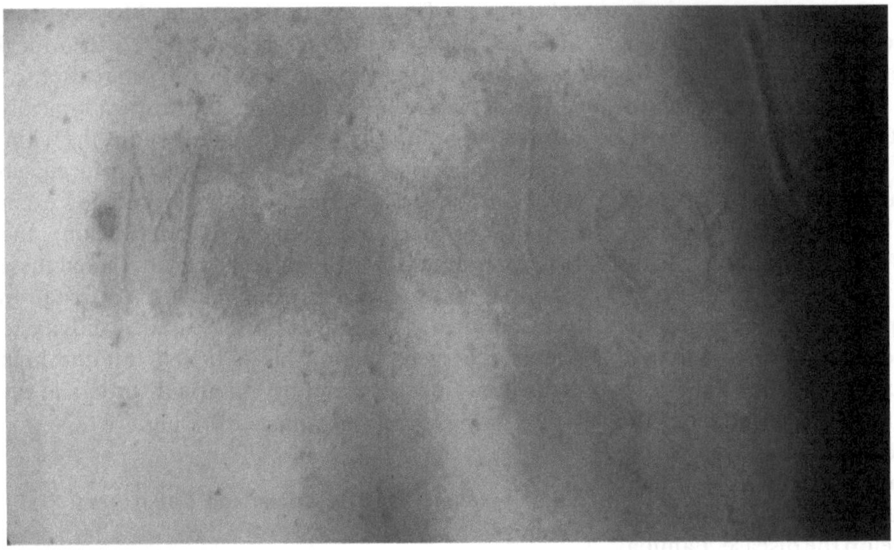

Fig. 5.2. Dermographic urticaria which appeared within seconds after writing with a retracted ballpoint on the patient's back. Note the typical linear wheal and the surrounding erythema. The patient complained of intense pruritus.

the free sensory nerve endings, granular material was deposited between the mesaxons, and the preterminal segments of the horizontal nerve endings were in the vicinity of small blood vessels.

Mast cells were of normal number but varied greatly in shape, size, and texture of their special granules even in normal patient skin. In urticarial skin, the granules were swollen and electron-lucent, but not degranulated.

5.4.5 Special Types of Dermographic Urticaria (Table 5.5)

Delayed dermographism

Kalz et al. (1950) were the first to describe delayed urticarial dermographism in a patient with pressure urticaria. While the condition is not infrequent (see Section 5.6.4, p. 66), delayed whealing is also observed in patients without other types of urticaria.

A frequent association with hypersensitivity to fungi is reported in the older literature. Engelhardt (1961) believes that delayed whealing is induced more frequently after intense dermographic stimulation of the skin. The Prausnitz-Küstner test is always negative, but delayed whealing can be transferred with cantharidin blister fluid from active, delayed wheals to other sites on the patient's skin, but not to controls.

Immediate whealing need not be present in all patients with delayed dermographism and can be inhibited through frequent stroking, while this refractory state does not necessarily occur in delayed whealing. According to Engelhardt (1961), late whealing starts from 1/2 to 9 h after stroking and lasts for 10–72 h, with an average duration of 12–24 h. Immediate wheals can persist in some cases, but usually the immediate wheal disappears after 20 min, and reappears several hours later (Baughman and Jillson 1963). Delayed lesions are usually wider and deeper than the immediate dermographic wheals and need not follow a continuous line. They are often accompanied by burning and tenderness and are depressed by corticosteroids, epinephrine and local warmth, but not by local anesthetics (Engelhardt 1961). Their reduction in response to antihistamines is controversial (Kalz et al. 1950).

Table 5.5. Special types of dermographic urticaria.

Delayed dermographism
Localized dermographism
Cholinergic dermographism
Red dermographism
Transient dermographism
Dermographism is mastocytosis

Localized dermographism

An increased whealing tendency after scratching is frequently observed at sites of insect bites or tattoo marks. This also occurs at sites of recent wheals due to acute but not chronic or physical urticaria and at sites of skin tests with allergens, but not with histamine, for up to 96 h after urticae have subsided (James and Warin 1969). Sites of poison ivy contact dermatitis or skin regions pretreated with tetrahydrofurfuryl ester of nicotinic acid (Trafuril, see chapter 6.6) may also become responsive to whealing. The phenomenon can be blocked by the intake of aspirin 24 h before

Fig. 5.3. Cholinergic dermographism in a patient with cholinergic urticaria. Instead of a linear wheal, punctate wheals arose in a linear distribution, with a marked surrounding erythema and associated pruritus.

application of the agent to the skin, but not 24 h afterward (Winkelmann et al. 1965).

Cholinergic dermographism

In a very few patients with cholinergic urticaria (about 2% of our own patients), scratching trauma results in the development of an erythematous area that is studded with tiny wheals (Fig. 5.3). The wheals can extend beyond the traumatized area into the region of reflex erythema, and the central wheals may become confluent. Itching is intense. In rare cases, this pattern of dermographic whealing also occurs in the absence of generalized cholinergic urticaria (Warin and Champion 1974).

Red dermographism

Warin (1981) described this condition in 40 patients (65% were females) who were older (mean: 41 years) than the patients with dermographic urticaria. The lesions could not be elicited by stretching, but instead only by rubbing. Redness, edema, and pruritus started at 2–3 min after stimulation and were maximal at 5–6 min. The edema had disappeared by 15 min, the redness by 1 h. The whealing was only recognizable by scratching the skin to reduce the erythema. A refractory period was not observed. The condition had lasted for a mean of 1.4 years when the patients were first seen. Within 1 year, 22% of the patients cleared, and 61% improved over the subsequent 8 months of follow-up. Associated diseases were seborrheic eczema (30%), chronic urticaria (10%), and psoriasis (5%). The phenomenon could be reproduced in 2% of normal subjects without associated itching.

Transient dermographism

This condition persists for only a limited period of time. Localized dermographism is one example of transient dermographism (see above). The phenomenon has been described in a generalized from after cutaneous or systemic parasitic infestations (scabies, schistosomiasis), after acute urticaria due to serum sickness, and in association with exercise-induced asthma (Mathews and Pan 1970). Elimination of the parasites does not necessarily coincide with a cure of the dermographic urticaria (Newcomb and Nelson 1973).

Treatment with aspirin, penicillin, or lidocaine can induce generalized dermographic urticaria that can persist for weeks or months (Kalz 1946, Rich 1949, Kalz und Prichard 1952, Chin and Fellner 1980). The reactions developed during or up to 15 days after conclusion of the therapy and were noted in up to 80% of patients treated with penicillin for syphilis.

Dermographism in association with mastocytosis

Whealing and itching in response to scratching or rubbing can be the only sign of mastocytosis in the absence of other cutaneous lesions (Sahihi and Esterly 1972, Ruiz-Maldonado et al. 1975). Rubbing always produces whealing of variable degree over pigmented or nodular skin lesions and is diagnostic of the disease (Darier's sign). Scratching instead of rubbing also produces whealing over the lesions that contain increased numbers of mast cells, and in about 50% of the patients, this stimulus induces dermographic whealing in clinically uninvolved skin (Fig. 9.6, p. 119) (see also Chapter 9, p. 116). In infancy, bullae can develop on top of the urticae.

5.4.6 Other Diseases Associated with Dermographic Urticaria

Several of the conditions occurring with dermographic urticaria have been discussed earlier (Table 5.1) and are listed again in Table 5.6. Marcussen (1950) observed neuropsychiatric disorders in 75% of his patients. Changes of hormone levels in association with hypo- and hyperthyroidism, diabetes mellitus, or pregnancy and menopause have been implicated (Thompson 1968). Three-fourths of the patients with the hypereosinophilic syndrome are reported to have severe dermographic urticaria (Parillo et al. 1979).

Despite the fact that Fisher and Schwartz (1953) found no increased incidence of other urticarias in patients with dermographic urticaria, the condition can arise in certain subtypes of urticaria, such as in association with acute urticaria and at sites of previous whealing due to testing with allergens. Doeglas (1975a) found an association with several physical urticarias and observed angioedema in four of his 25 patients.

An increased incidence of atopy has not been found by patient history (Bart and Ackerman 1966, Doeglas 1975a), and increased reactivity to skin testing, observed on occasion, may well be due to the cutaneous hyperreactivity. An increased frequency of contact allergy is not found (Marcussen 1950), although increased dermographic whealing has been observed at sites of previous poison ivy reactions.

Table 5.6. Conditions associated with dermographic urticaria.

A. Parasitosis
   1. Cutaneous and systemic infestations
   2. Insect bites

B. Neuropsychiatric disorders

C. Hormonal changes
   1. Thyroid disorders
   2. Pregnancy
   3. Menopause
   4. Diabetes mellitus

D. Immunological alterations
   1. After acute urticaria
   2. At skin test sites with allergens (local only)
   3. During or following drug therapy (penicillin)
   4. Contact dermatitis (local only)

E. Miscellaneous
   1. Mastocytosis
   2. Cholinergic, cold, aquagenic, and pressure urticaria
   3. Angioedema
   4. Hypereosinophilic syndrome

5.4.7 Diagnosis

The diagnosis of dermographic urticaria is based on the typical history, which suggests that the lesions are elicited by mechanical trauma, in association with pruritus, and by the reproduction of the rapidly appearing wheals after application of firm pressure and friction on the skin.

Illig and Kunick (1969) caution against using the fingernails or sharp instruments, such as wooden tongue depressors, to elicit the lesions since this might injure the skin. Instead, they recommend the hasp end of a safety-pin as being optimal. They maintain that exact quantitation of the test is not meaningful anyway since friction, speed, and pressure are important for the production of the lesions, and these parameters must vary of necessity from test to test.

Several devices have been constructed for quantitation of the pressure applied during dermographic whealing. They range from a home-made, weighted syringe (Bart and Ackerman 1966) to a weighted knitting needle (Doeglas 1975a) and a sophisticated spring-loaded stylus that is guided through a flat metal template to avoid irregular displacement of the skin (Kirby et al. 1971). Responses to about 200 g are considered diagnostic, with wheals of 1–2 mm width occurring within 10 min. With weights of > 1000 g, whealing is observed in 5–25% of normal subjects (Lewis 1927, Fisher and Schwartz 1953, Kirby et al. 1971). Test sites should be inspected at 1, 4, 8, and 24 h to check for delayed reactions. Tests should be performed on the upper back since the skin of the arms is less responsive.

Besides scratching, the skin should also be routinely rubbed so as not to miss red dermographism which is unresponsive to scratching.

5.4.8 Differential Diagnosis

Simple or physiological dermographism occurs as an incidental finding in certain individuals in all age groups. Greater pressure and a longer time of application are needed until the lesions develop. The wheals are generally smaller and are never accompanied by itching. These criteria should help to differentiate the normal dermographism from dermographic urticaria.

Chronic urticaria, angioedema, and pressure urticaria are conditions which are often confused with dermographic urticaria because of their clinical appearance or a misleading patient history. Routine skin testing with a pulling pressure should help to differentiate these conditions. Lesions on palms and soles of the feet, often occurring in pressure urticaria, are rare in dermographic urticaria, and their absence is another helpful diagnostic sign.

5.4.9 Prognosis

Kirby et al. (1971) carefully studied a group of patients over several months and noted very little variation in the whealing response during the day, from day to day, from week to week, and over several months. After 1 year, 25% of their patients had lost their dermographic whealing. Marcussen (1950) observed a much higher spontaneous rate of remission (35 of his 45 patients) already after 8 weeks. Breathnach et al. (1981), on the other hand, reported spontaneous improvement in only two of their 30 patients, but the time period was unspecified.

5.4.10 Pathogenesis

Immunoglobulin E

A search for pathogenetic factors that might explain the increased whealing in response to shearing trauma of the skin was successful from its onset several decades ago. Walzer (1928) was the first to transfer the condition with serum from an affected to a normal person, and Lehner and Rajka (1930) soon confirmed his observations. More recently, Aoyama (1971) reported a positive transfer in 9 of their 13 patients and Newcomb and Nelson (1973) in 5 of 9 of their patients. Both groups of workers were able to demonstrate that an IgE was the responsible serum factor for dermographic whealing. This IgE from dermographic patients was specific in that myeloma IgE or serum with high levels of IgE from allergic patients was ineffective. Binding of specific IgE to mast cells was necessary for passive transfer since the reaction could be inhibited by excess amounts of non-dermographic IgE.

Dermographic IgE was present at highly variable levels in the serum of the different patients studied. Whealing in response to scratching could be elicited already in normal recipients 10–50 min after serum injections, but the reactions were stronger after 8 h and could be reproduced for up to 10 days. The recipients varied also in that not all of them responded, and if so, not always to the same degree.

A recent study of one patient by Smith et al. (1983) marked further progress in the understanding of dermographic urticaria. The authors identified the dermographic principle in their patient as a heat-labile serum factor. The patient exhibited dermographic whealing only while being treated with penicillin. Both the patient and the passive recipient had negative skin tests to penicillin G, to the minor determinant mixture, and to benzyl penicilloilpolylysine. The passive recipient failed to respond initially to dermographic testing, but he developed dermographic whealing when tested 1 h after ingestion of 500 mg penicillin. An exact identification of the heat-labile serum factor in the patient's serum was not done in this study, even though the authors assumed it was IgE.

Considered together, these studies suggest that the mast cell in dermographic skin reacts only if several factors co-occur: (1) a specific IgE, (2) a sensitizer which must be a chemical such as penicillin or its breakdown products, and (3) mechanical force that acts through the skin on the local mast cell.

Mast cells

There is little doubt that mast cells are the central effector cells in dermographic urticaria, even though their number is not increased in the tissue (Warin 1976, Bart and Ackerman 1966, Cauna et al. 1970). Mast cell granules are not expelled from the cell on stimulation, but instead the granules release their mediators from the cell via diffusion through intracytoplasmic channels that communicate with the cell's exterior. Evidence for this derives from the morphological observations of Cauna et al. (1970). Such a limited mode of mediator discharge would also explain the transient nature of dermographic wheals.

Mediators

The nature of the mediators in dermographic whealing is partly known (Table 5.4). Lehner and Rajka (1930) observed increased serum levels of "wheal-producing" factors after massive dermographic stimulation. Greaves and Sondergaard (1970) identified histamine in skin perfusates from all patients and kinins in two of eight perfusates of their patients. Winkelmann et al. (1965) found kinins in all perfusates of his patients, but failed to measure histamine, apparently because of technical problems. Serotonin was not present in the perfusates, but an additional factor that caused constraction of rat uterus was observed instead. This factor was considered to be neither acetylcholine nor slow-reacting substance because of its organ specificity (Greaves and Sondergaard 1970).

Other pathogenetic considerations

The negative passive transfer test in a subgroup of patients has given rise to the view that there is a second group of patients with dermographic urticaria in which IgE plays no pathogenetic role. Thompson (1968) called this condition the "weak mast cell syndrome", suggesting that the mast cells are weakened by some unknown mechanism and are thus easily triggered by minor trauma. Such a lowered threshold could, for example, be due to modulation of mast cell releasability by hormones.

Vasomotor and neuropathological alterations have been discussed as other possible pathogenetic mechanisms (Kierland 1953). As a final possibility, all pathogenetic IgE in patients without a transferable serum factor could be bound to the mast cells since it is not produced in sufficient quantities to result in a spill-over into the serum. This possibility is all the more likely since specific IgE levels vary considerably from patient to patient (Newcomb and Nelson 1973). Such an explanation is particularly attractive for it eliminates the need to search for diverse reasons to explain the same biological phenomenon. Proof of the validity of the one or the other theory will have to await further experimentation.

5.5 Vibratory Angioedema

This condition was first described as an autosomally dominant transmitted disease by Patterson et al. (1972). Since then, another family with five affected members in two generations has been reported by Highet et al. (1981). Keahey et al. (1984) have observed a case with delayed appearance of the lesions, but a familial occurrence was not mentioned. Kaplan and Beaven (1976) found a positive skin test for vibratory stimuli with an associated flush syndrome and an increased level of histamine in the venous effluent blood in two of their patients who also suffered from cholinergic urticaria.

Patients complain that their lesions develop after massage, vigorous towelling, and running. Taking a shower or even vibrating the lips together can also induce swellings. The patients studied by Highet et al. (1981) developed an immediate, transient erythema on testing, followed by pruritus and progressive edema at the same site 1–1.5 h later, with a peak at 5–8 h. Tests for pressure urticaria were negative.

Histamine has been identified in the serum of all cases studied so far (Kaplan and Beaven 1976, Metzger et al. 1976, Highet et al. 1981, Keahey et al. 1984), and H1 antagonists reduced the swelling (Highet et al. 1981). Mast cell degranulation was observed in the early lesions, and after 5 h, a mixed perivascular infiltrate was observed in the reticular dermis which was replaced by mononuclear cells after 20 h (Keahey et al. 1984).

Routine testing with vibratory stimuli is rarely done in allergy clinics. A careful history and testing might uncover many more cases with this condition than have been reported until now.

5.6 Pressure Urticaria

5.6.1 Epidemiology

Among all patients with chronic urticaria, 2% suffer from pressure urticaria (Champion et al. 1969), and the incidence is about equal to that of cold urticaria (Doeglas 1975a).

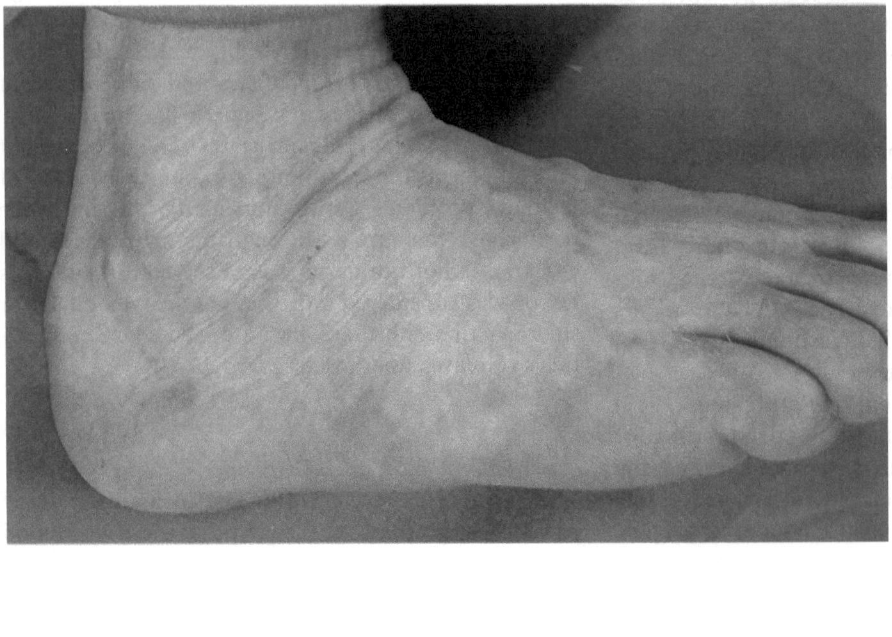

Fig. 5.4. Whealing and redness at sites of pressure from shoes in a patient with pressure urticaria. The soles were also swollen.

Until now, four reports on larger patient groups (up to 17) have appeared in the literature, although a search of our own hospital records yielded a total of 32 patients with proven pressure urticaria over a 4-year period (Czarnetzki et al. 1984b).

In all patient series, there is a predominance of males (65–80 %) (see Table 5.1) and of the younger age group (mean age at onset of the disease 28.2 to 30 years; range 20–44 years) (Sussman et al. 1982, Czarnetzki et al. 1984b). The mean duration of the disease was 8 years in Sussman's and 6 years in our own series (range from 0.3 to 30 years). Most patients belonged to professional groups involved in heavy manual labor.

5.6.2 Clinical Features

Cutaneous symptomatology

The lesions of pressure urticaria develop over body regions that are exposed to heavy pressure, such as the palms, the soles of the feet (Fig. 5.4), the buttocks, the upper back, and more rarely the face (Fig. 5.5). After application of pressure, there is a latency period of 4–8 h (range 1–10 h) before the wheals develop, and the lesions persist for a mean of 20 ± 8 h (range 8–48 h).

The cutaneous lesions present as large, erythematous, deep-seated swellings which may have an area of central pallor. Lesions will rarely extend beyond the exact site of application of pressure (Fig. 5.6). If grasped between finger and thumb, they demonstrate the "peau d'orange" phenomenon as a sign of deep

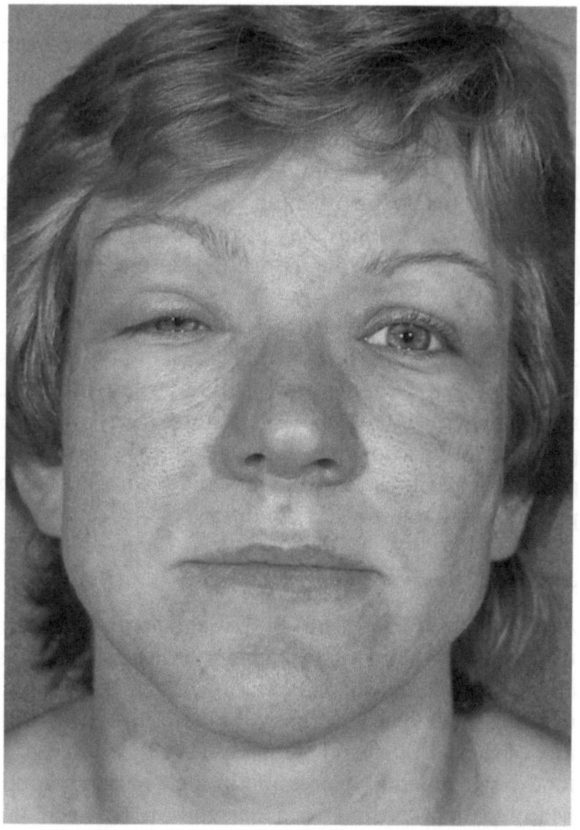

Fig. 5.5. Unilateral swelling of the left side of the face and the periorbital region in a patient with pressure urticaria. The lesions had been present on awakening, and the patient had pressed on this side of her face with her arm during sleep. Note also the papular and annular wheals due to the patient's associated chronic urticaria.

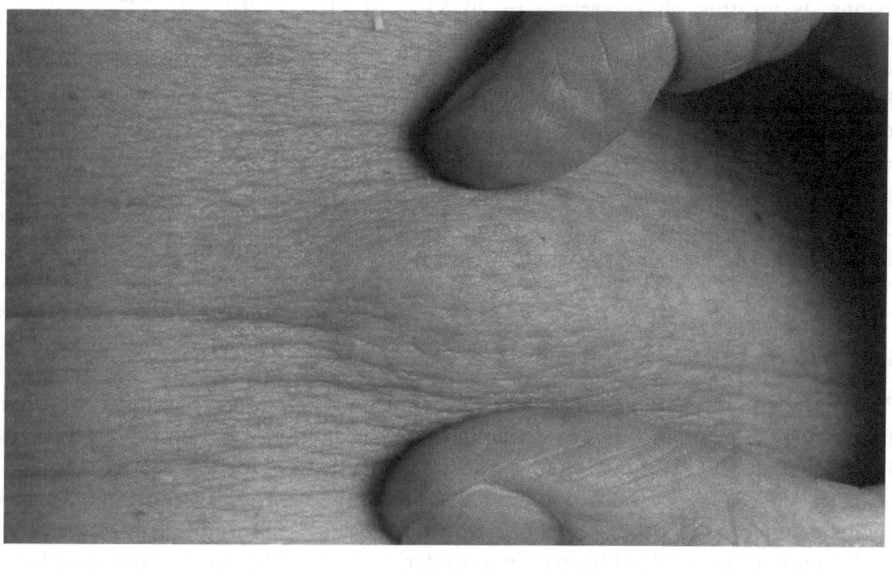

Fig. 5.6. Deep swelling and redness at a pressure test site (1,800 g, 10 min) on the back of a patient with pressure urticaria. The lesions developed 6 h after testing. Note the typical peau d'orange appearance of the lesion when lateral pressure is applied with the fingers.

dermal swelling. They resemble angioedema and erysipelas, conditions for which they have often been mistaken in the past. The skin overlying the swelling appears taught and warm.

Initially, most patients have a sensation of itching at the site of the wheals. Others complain of discomfort, or they notice pain, burning, or stinging. In some patients, deep swellings may also involve the adjacent joints or muscles, with associated severe pain and discomfort.

Immediate pressure urticaria which develops within 2–4 min at the site of a 30-s application of pressure has been reported in patients with the hypereosinophilic syndrome (Parillo et al. 1979). Since many of these patients suffer also from dermographic urticaria, the possibility remains that the immediate whealing with pressure was due to that condition.

Systemic symptoms

Approximately 50% of all patients with pressure urticaria complain of systemic symptoms, such as chills, fever, increased perspiration, dizziness, nausea, malaise, headache, shortness of breath, tiredness, and anxiousness. Illig and Kunick (1969) observed a tendency to mental depression in their patient group. Many patients admit to a correlation between the temporal appearance of lesions and mental as well as physical strain at work or at home. Nevertheless, none of the patients are free of disease during vacation.

5.6.3 Laboratory Findings

On routine testing, up to 70% of the patients will have a slight to moderately elevated erythrocyte sedimentation rate. A fluctuating leukocytosis which does not necessarily correlate with the clinical appearance of lesions, is another characteristic in 20–53% of all patients. Ryan et al. (1968) also reported on a peripheral eosinophilia in two of their 15 patients, a finding that could not be confirmed by others (Czarnetzki et al. 1984b). Other laboratory values, including serum enzymes, immunoglobulins, total serum complement, C1-esterase-inhibitor, α_2-macroglobulin, and α_1-antitrypsin, are within normal range (Doeglas 1975a, Sussman et al. 1982, Czarnetzki et al. 1984b).

5.6.4 Associated Diseases

Patients with pressure urticaria have an unusually high incidence of other types of urticaria (Table 5.1). Sussman et al. (1982) diagnosed an associated chronic urticaria in 94% of their patients, although the incidence is lower in other series (27–82%). Doeglas (1975b) noted that 43% of his patients reacted to oral provocation with aspirin and related chemicals. Very similar observations were made with both skin tests and oral challenges by other groups (Ryan et al. 1968, Czarnetzki et al. 1984b). Urticaria factitia and pressure urticaria coexisted in the first case report on pressure urticaria (Urbach and Fasal 1929) and in the case studied by Kalz et al. (1950). The incidence of coexistent urticaria factitia was 63% in our patient series (Czarnetzki et al. 1984b). In a few patients, the reappearance of swelling and redness at sites of dermographic whealing is observed after a lag period of 2–4 h (urticaria factitia tarda). The dermographic wheals can persist for more than 8 h.

Patients with pressure urticaria have no increased personal or family history of atopy (Doeglas 1975a, Czarnetzki et al. 1984b). Shelley and Florence (1961) reported one case with pressure urticaria and a coexisting mold hypersensitivity. Sussman et al. (1982) noted an increased incidence of atopy (5/16) among their patients. However, since their data came from a referral clinic for allergic diseases, the patient population may have been preselected for allergic diseases. Doeglas (1975a) described an increased incidence of immediate type skin reactions in his patient population, but he interpreted these findings as false positive reactions because of the coexisting dermographic urticaria in many of his patients. Pressure urticaria may indeed be the cause of multiple false positive skin test reactions to allergens since the delayed wheals appear even at sites of NaCl or histamine injections in patients with this condition (own observations).

5.6.5 Histological Findings

Biopsies of wheals show an edematous dermis and a perivascular infiltrate in the mid- and lower dermis which consists primarily of mononuclear cells and occasional neutrophils. In the deep dermis, focal aggregations of the infiltrating cells are particularly prominent around the deeper appendages. Infiltrates may also involve the subcutaneous tissue. In about half of the cases, there is a patchy dermal accumulation of eosinophils. In others, eosinophils are seen scattered inbetween the dermal collagen bundles. Increased numbers of mast cells are seen in the early, but not the late wheals. This phenomenon must be due to immigration of mast cells since they cannot possibly develop from precursors in 4–6 h. The perivascular lymphocytes are predominantly of the helper type, as shown by mononuclear antibody studies (Illig 1973, Czarnetzki et al. 1985).

Immunofluorescence shows no evidence for fibrinogen, immunoglobulins, or complement in the lesions (Ryan et al. 1968). Fibrin deposition was noted by James et al. (1980), but not by Ryan et al. (1968). The histological findings can best be interpreted as signs for a cell-mediated immune reaction to an as yet unknown antigen, with prominent participation of mast cells in the reaction.

5.6.6 Diagnosis

Frequently, the diagnosis of pressure urticaria can be made solely on the basis of a good history. Special attention should be paid to the distribution of the lesions, their delayed onset, and their configuration. The frequent coexistence of dermographic urticaria or chronic urticaria should be taken into account when the patient describes the time course and the clinical appearance of his lesions.

The diagnosis of pressure urticaria is easily confirmed by inspection of the deep-seated, erythematous swellings at their sites of predilection on the skin. In addition, it is mandatory to produce the lesions experimentally. Illig and Kunick (1969) designed a special device by means of which increasing aliquots of weights are applied for various time periods to the back of the patient (Fig. 5.7). A simpler way to obtain the same information is to suspend weights of 2–10 kg by means of a broad strap over the shoulders, or, with the patient in a sitting position, over the thigh. Weights should be left in place for 10–30 min, and readings should be taken immediately after removal of the weights so as not to miss a coexisting dermographic urticaria. Later readings should be taken at 4, 6, and 8 h, and possibly even at 20 h. An additional test for dermographic urticaria should be done at the time of application of the weights, by scratching firmly over the patient's back. This site should also be reexamined at later time intervals in order not to miss a delayed dermographic urticaria.

If the pressure test is negative, despite adequate testing and a highly suggestive history of pressure urticaria, it should be repeated once or even twice at 48-h intervals since it is well known that the lesions cannot always be reproduced in patients with documented pressure urticaria (Estes and Young 1981). The sites of testing should also be changed, in case the test is negative. In some of their patients, Sussman et al. (1982) noted that although the pressure test was positive at the shoulder, it remained negative after application of weights to the abdomen, forearm, and back. Estes and Young (1981), on the other hand, found the back to be the optimal site for testing in their patients.

Reasons for false negative tests may thus relate to

1) the refractoriness of the test site to further stimulation because of previous in vivo exposure,
2) differences or fluctuations in the sensitivity of the patient's skin to pressure,
3) recent treatment with immunosuppressive drugs such as corticosteroids, and
4) insufficient testing; addition of more weights or an extension of their time of application may overcome an increased threshold for wheals in some patients (Estes and Young 1981).

5.6.7 Pathomechanisms

Cells and mediators

Ryan et al. (1968) provided convincing evidence that mast cells are essential for the development of pressure urticaria lesions since depletion of mast cell mediators at pressure sites by injection of the mast cell degranulator, compound 48/80, made the sites refractory to the development of the delayed pressure wheals. Highly variable quantities of histamine and kinins have been extracted from pressure wheals (Winkelmann et al. 1965, Kaplan et al. 1978), but specific therapy, directed against the affected histamine and kinin, has been ineffective (Ryan et al. 1968).

Leukotrienes were not demonstrated in 48/80-induced wheals in patients with pressure urticaria and were only variably present in the delayed wheals induced by the injection of histamine, concanavalin A, and NaCl (Czarnetzki et al. 1984b). It is therefore unlikely that leukotrienes are specifically important as mediators in pressure urticaria.

Leukocytes of patients with pressure urticaria tend to release higher levels of histamine and chemotactic leukotrienes than normal controls (Czarnetzki et al. 1984b). An increased releasability of histamine has also been observed in atopics, and this phenomenon is therefore neither specific for pressure urticaria nor for atopy. Modulation of release of mediators by inhibitors of the lipoxygenase- or cyclo-oxygenase-dependent metabolism of arachidonate is also the same in pressure urticaria patients and controls (Czarnetzki et al. 1984b). However, patients show an increased clinical sensitivity to aspirin and at the same time a good therapeutic response to corticosteroids. Involvement of the arachidonate metabolism is not apparent in vitro, even though the clinical data might have suggested it.

Serum proteins

A possible defect of pathogenetic significance has been sought in serum protease inhibitor levels. Their decrease would result in a prolonged mechanism of action of mediators, thus offering an explanation for

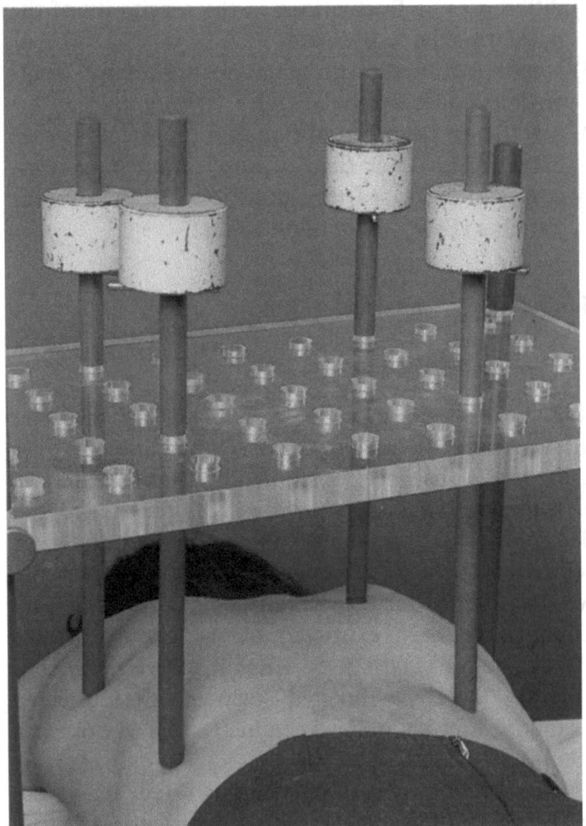

Fig. 5.7. Apparatus designed for pressure testing. Additional weights of 900 g each can be added to increase the pressure that is transmitted through the rods.

the delayed whealing. The serum levels of these enzymes, as measured by Doeglas and Bleumink (1975), were however within normal range.

Because of the striking similarity of the appearance of the large, painful wheals of pressure urticaria to the lesions of hereditary angioedema, complement defects have been sought in the blood of pressure urticaria patients and at the sites of wheals (Ryan et al. 1968, Estes and Young 1981). The results were negative. Similarly, altered serum levels of fibrinogen, fibrin, IgG, IgM, and IgA were not demonstrated (Ryan et al. 1968, Estes and Young 1981, Sussman et al. 1982). A partial deficiency of factor VIII was found in one of our patients whose father was known to have a bleeding disorder, but this defect could not be found in three other patients with pressure urticaria (unpublished observation). The in vitro lymphocyte response to mitogens was within normal range (Czarnetzki et al. 1984b).

Hypersensitivity to food

Recently, delayed whealing in response to compound 48/80 and food allergens has been reported to occur in all of the ten patients with pressure urticaria studied by Davis et al. (1984). The urticaria of these patients cleared completely within 48 h of fasting and after elimination of the specific food antigens from the diet. We have tried to reproduce these findings in five patients, but have been unable to confirm of them (unpublished observations).

Hypothetical pathogenetic events

It one tries to summarize the clinical and experimental observations on pressure urticaria up to this point, the following possible sequence of pathogenetic events seems plausible. On application of pressure to the skin, a factor X is generated in the tissue several hours after stimulation. This factor induces mast cell degranulation and release of histamine, kallikrein, and chemotactic factors which results in wheal formation. An alternate possibility would be that factor X stimulates the production of lymphokines. This would explain the latency period before the development of the wheals since lymphocytes need several hours after stimulation before they secrete these proteins. Lymphokines are able to stimulate histamine release (Thueson et al. 1979), and cause vascular dilatation, tissue edema, and an influx of mononuclear cells, basophils, neutrophils, and eosinophils, alone or in combination with other mediators. Until now, lymphokines have not been demonstrated in lesions of pressure urticaria, but their role in this disease is worth investigating.

The cells which constitute the infiltrate in the lesions of pressure urticaria are thus an additional source of inflammatory mediators, but they can also potentially counteract the effect of the acute phase mediators by secreting anti-inflammatory enzymes. After many hours, the mediators would thus no longer be effective, and the deep wheals would resolve.

5.7 Cold Urticaria

5.7.1 General Aspects

Definition

Cold urticaria is defined as a urticarial and/or angioedematous reaction of the skin to contact with cold objects, water, or air. This pathological hyperreactivity is the epiphenomenon for a number of diseases, and it is due to a wide range of causative factors. In many instances, the reason for this cold hypersensitivity is however unknown.

Classification and frequency

Cold urticaria is relatively common (Table 5.1). It often comes to medical attention only when the symptoms are severely disabling or when the condition is specifically searched for during routine screening for causes of chronic idiopathic urticarias. Duke (1926) differentiated between a local contact type and a systemic, reflex type of cold urticaria. The latter has received little attention in the past and is generally ignored during routine testing. Illig et al. (1980) think that this "reflex" or "cold air and cold water urticaria" occurs as frequently as cholinergic urticaria.

Most types of cold urticaria are idiopathic, and in some patients, more than one type of cold urticaria or of another type of physical urticaria can coexist. Table 5.7 lists all types of cold urticaria known so far. Some of them are very rare.

Cold urticaria occurs most frequently in young adults, but it may also start in early childhood or during the second half of life (Table 5.1). In the familial type, cold sensitivity is noted at or shortly after birth. Women are twice as often affected as men. The condition can last for life in the familial type, and for up to 33 years (mean 4.2 years) in nonfamilial cases.

Cold urticaria is more frequently diagnosed in cold climates and during the cold season, but it has even been observed in the tropics since a drop in temperature rather than the absolute temperature is often the decisive factor for the development of lesions (see Diagnosis, p. 71).

Table 5.7. Classification of urticarial reactions to cold stimuli.

I. Localized contact reactions to cold
   1. Immediate cold urticaria
      a. idiopathic
      b. secondary
   2. Delayed cold urticaria
   3. Cold-dependent dermographism (Summation urticaria)
   4. Localized cold contact urticaria
   5. Localized cold reflex urticaria
   6. Familial delayed cold contact urticaria

II. Systemic reactions to cold (Cold air and cold water urticaria)
   1. Systemic cold urticaria
   2. Cold-induced cholinergic urticaria
   3. Familial cold urticaria (Familial polymorphous cold eruption)

5.7.2 Clinical Features

Elicitation and distribution of lesions

Cold urticaria becomes manifest on contact of the skin or mucous membranes with solid cold objects, cold water, ice, cold air, cold wind, or cold food. Lesions can also develop at sites where water evaporates from the skin. Lowering the body core temperature is a prerequisite for systemic cold urticaria (Illig et al. 1980).

In cold contact urticaria, lesions are generally

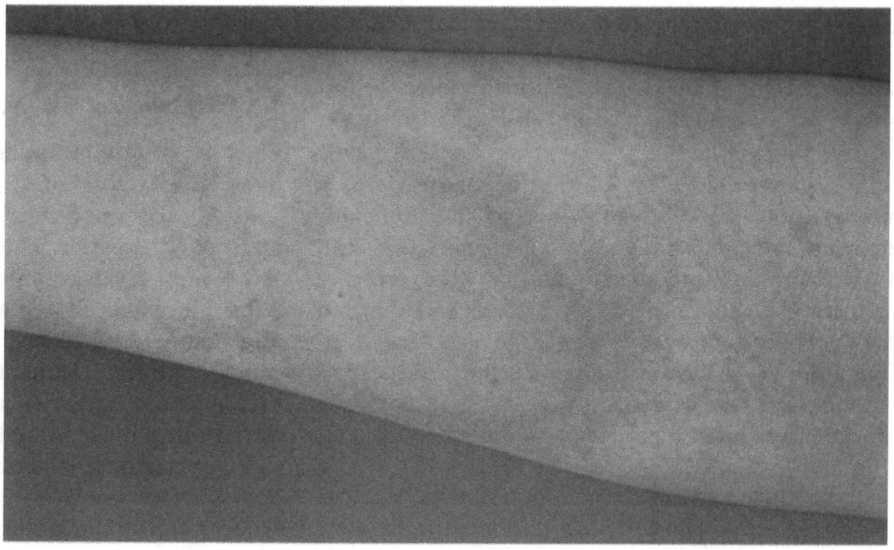

Fig. 5.8. Wheal with surrounding erythema on the forearm of a patient with cold urticaria after local application of an ice cube.

restricted to the area of exposure, and they often develop only after removal of the cold object and on rewarming of the skin. The lesions can become confluent and involve large parts of the body after immersion in cold water during outdoor swimming or during a bath. There is a preference for uncovered parts of the body, including the face and hands. In severe cases, the mucous membranes of the mouth and the tongue can bear lesions, and in rare patients, lesions can be elicited at a restricted part of the body (localized cold contact or reflex urticaria; see Table 5.7).

Cutaneous manifestations

Within a few seconds to minutes after removal of the cooling object, there is erythema at the site of contact, followed rapidly by a wheal, a surrounding flare (Fig. 5.8), and a mild to moderate pruritus. When larger parts of the body have been immersed in cold water, the skin is red, diffusely edematous and often studded with small wheals, exactly as in heat contact urticaria (see Fig. 5.14). The lower the eliciting temperature is, the faster the reactions occur. The swelling clears within $^1/_2$–1 h, maximally by 3 h. Minor purpura can persist at sites of maximal swelling, is seen in 80% of the patients (Eady et al. 1981), and can even be intense and widespread, with ulceration (Koda et al. 1978). Angioedema is observed together with the whealing in up to 73% of the patients (DeLaus and Winkelmann 1973).

In delayed cold urticaria, immediate lesions can persist for many hours (Juhlin 1981), or delayed lesions arise without a preceding immediate reaction, after a lag time of 3–4 h, or even 24 h (Warin and Champion 1974). The swellings are deeper, are not so well confined to the area of contact, and the patients complain of tenderness to touch rather than pruritus.

In localized cold reflex urticaria, small, fleeting wheals develop in the skin region surrounding the test site, but not at the site of contact itself (Czarnetzki et al. 1981).

In systemic cold urticaria, fleeting wheals develop shortly after the onset of shivering. The time for exposure to cold air necessary to elicit the lesions can vary from 5–80 min, depending on the ambient temperature (Illig et al. 1980, Kaplan and Garolfo 1981). Individual wheals have the size and configuration of lesions in ordinary acute urticaria, or pinpoint size wheals develop instead on an erythematous base, as is typical for cholinergic urticaria (Fig. 5.9).

In familial cold urticaria, erythematous macules and urticarial papules develop about 30 min after exposure to cold air, particularly to chilling winds. The lesions last from 48 h up to many days and burn rather than itch. Mucous membranes are generally not involved.

Systemic symptoms

Widespread local exposure and generalized urticaria can be accompanied by flushing, headaches, chills, dizziness, tachycardia, abdominal pain, nausea, vomiting, muscle pain, shortness of breath, wheezing, and unconsciousness. Some of the systemic symptoms can be prevented by placing a tourniquet on the exposed extremity. Death due to drowning has been observed after patients plunge themselves into ice cold water. Swelling of the oral mucosa and the larynx after eating cold food is another, potentially life-threatening situation.

Increased gastric acid secretion has been measured after development of lesions even on local challenge. With a lowering of the core temperature, release of histamine from mast cells in the mucocutaneous organs must also be considered (Lass et al. 1980).

Pinpoint hemorrhages of the retina have been observed in three of 21 patients with cold urticaria. These patients had no circulating cryoglobulins (Floegel and Buchholz 1977). Newman (1981) drew attention to potential changes of central nervous system function in cold urticaria patients due to chronic histamine release which might result in disregulation of body temperature, changes of feeding habits, and feelings of anxiety and depression. Such changes have not been reported, but they have perhaps also not been sought.

In familial cold urticaria, systemic symptoms are prominent and, beside some of the symptoms already mentioned, fever, arthralgia, and swelling of the hands and feet accompany the cutaneous eruption.

5.7.3 Histological Findings

Eady et al. (1981) applied ice for 5 min at 30-min intervals for a total of 4 h to the skin of a patient with cold urticaria and did serial biopsies of the lesions for up to 24 h thereafter. The wheals showed nothing but sparse mast cell degranulation after the first exposure. After 2 h, mast cell degranulation was more intense, and some fibrin deposition was noted. A mixed cellular infiltrate, consisting of neutrophils, mononuclear cells, eosinophils, and erythrocytes had appeared after 3.5 h in and around cutaneous vessels, there was endothelial damage, and clumps of partially degranulated platelets and fibrin filled the vessels. After 24 h, an infiltrate of mononuclear cells was present in the upper and mid-dermis, and the clinical appearance of the lesions was that of a tender, reticulated, erythematous macule.

On immunofluorescence, the same authors noted C3 deposits after the first challenge, and more C3, fibrin, and IgM at later intervals.

No other reports give such detailed, sequential description of the histology of cold urticaria. Mast cell degranulation, although confirmed by several authors, is not an invariable feature (Doeglas and Bleumink 1974, Soter et al. 1977). Neutrophilic infiltrates are prominent in some of the lesions instead.

5.7.4 Laboratory Findings

In idiopathic cold urticaria, a number of significant laboratory changes have been observed. Houser et al. (1970) found an increase of cryoglobulins in 20%, of hemolysins in 5%, and of cryofibrinogen in 3% of their patients, whereas other authors did not observe any abnormal proteins at all (Illig 1973, Pasricha and Nayyar 1975). Leukocytosis is prominent in familial cold urticaria, but is a rare feature of ordinary cold urticaria. Duke (1926) noticed an eosinophilia in 8% of his patients on cold challenge. Changes in levels of mediators, globulins, protease inhibitors, and complement do occur and are discussed under the headings of "associated diseases" and "pathogenesis". These diverse changes underline the heterogeneity of cold urticaria.

5.7.5 Associated Diseases

Cold urticaria can occur in association with several other types of physical urticaria (Table 5.3), such as heat urticaria (Tennenbaum and Lowney 1973), cholinergic urticaria (Sigler et al. 1979), exercise-induced asthma (Mathews and Pan 1970), and dermographism (Illig 1973). Urticarial dermographism can disappear, together with a remission of the cold urticaria (Czarnetzki et al. 1981), but can also worsen after generalized cold urticaria has been elicited (Kaplan 1984).

There is a well-known association between infectious mononucleosis and cold urticaria (Tyson and Czarny 1981, Lemanske and Bush 1982). One patient with cold urticaria had a C2 deficiency, without evidence of a lupus-like syndrome, and vasculitis was present on histology (Sibbald et al. 1979).

While cryoglobulins are found in up to 20% of patients with cold urticaria (Houser et al. 1970), hyperreactivity to cold is seen only in 3.4% of patients with cryoglobulinemia (Costanzi et al. 1969). According to Illig (1973), skin lesions occur only if cryoglobulin levels exceed 500 mg%. Purpura is observed more frequently than in ordinary cold urticaria, and Raynaud's phenomenon, hyperpigmentation, papillomatosis, and hyperkeratosis of the skin may coexist.

Cold urticaria can precede the diagnosis of cryoglobulinemia and myeloma by several years (Thiers and Moulin 1969), and it can disappear, in parallel with a drop in cryoglobulins, on treatment with chemotherapy (Rawnsley and Shelley 1968). Most of the reported cryoglobulins consist of IgG, but IgA-IgG and IgG-IgM mixtures have also been observed. Complement can be activated by some of these cryoglobulins (Wager et al. 1968, Costanzi et al. 1969, Hauptmann et al. 1975).

Cold hemolysins are becoming decreasingly infrequent as a cause of cold urticaria, because of the lower incidence of congenital or tertiary syphilis.

Cryofibrinogemia as a cause of cold urticaria is seen in patients with connective tissue diseases, malignancies, and hemopoietic diseases. Rarely, heparin-inducible cryoprecipitates are found in patients with inflammatory connective tissue diseases. The complexes in the cryoprecipitate consist of a cold-insoluble globulin (fibronectin) and fibrinogen.

DeLaus and Winkelmann (1973) recorded a personal or family history of allergy in 40% of their patients with idiopathic cold urticaria. This association was not found in the Netherlands (Doeglas 1975) or in India (Pasricha and Nayyar 1975a).

5.7.6 Diagnosis

Skin tests

When cold urticaria is suspected on the basis of patient history, a sequence of tests should be performed, as outlined in Table 5.8. The easiest office procedure is to

Table 5.8. Diagnostic tests to determine cold urticaria. The observation time after exposure should be 15 min for immediate and 8 and 24 h for delayed reactions.

1. Cold contact	
Source of cold:	Ice cube in plastic bag, Crushed ice in plastic bag, Chlorethyl spray, or Ice-filled copper cylinder
Exposure time:	3–5 min
2. Cold water contact	
Source of cold:	Arm bath, 8–10° C and 21° C
Exposure time:	5–15 min
3. Cold air contact	
Source of cold:	Cold room, 4° C
Exposure time:	5–10 min, with light clothing

apply an ice cube or crushed ice to the lower forearm for 3–5 min (Fig. 5.8). Wrapping the ice in a plastic bag helps to shield the skin from direct contact and differentiates cold urticaria from aquagenic urticaria. As long as ice is present in the plastic bag, the temperature applied to the skin is 0° C. Patients with sensitivity to higher temperatures are therefore missed.

For office use, chloroethyl can be sprayed on the skin for screening purposes, but more accurate testing is accomplished by using a copper cylinder, filled with ice or with cold water. A thermostat can be attached to the cylinder to keep an even temperature (Illig 1973). This method of testing has the added advantage that only a small area of the skin is necessary for contact and that several temperatures can therefore be tested simultaneously on the back.

Curnow (1978) has described a more sophisticated instrument which allows for the application of temperatures in a close range of 10° C, on a 35–50 mm^2 skin area. This device is too limited in its range of temperatures and far too elaborate for common use.

It should be stressed that whealing usually develops after the skin rewarms, and the test site should be observed for at least 15 min, and again at 8 and at 24 h, in order not to miss delayed reactions. Determination of the threshold temperatures for the production of wheals is useful to follow the course of the disease and the effect of therapy. The upper threshold of the eliciting temperature can be as high as 27–29° C (Illig 1973). In some patients, contact lasting for only a few seconds at 20° C is sufficient to produce cutaneous wheals. There are occasional patients who react to temperatures of 12–14° C, but not to 0° C. Freezing of the skin should be avoided since tissue damage can cause cutaneous edema and thus a false positive reaction.

Regardless of how cold contact tests are conducted, a certain group of patients with cold urticaria will not react to them. Pasricha and Nayyar (1975) observed a positive ice cube test in only one of 43 patients. Sarkany and Gaylarde (1971) reported three patients with a history of cold urticaria and a negative reaction to ice. One of them reacted to cold water, and the other two to body cooling.

Keahey and Greaves (1980) state that when the ice cube or the copper cylinder tests are negative, the cold water test is often positive. The test is conducted by placing one arm for 5-15 min in water at a temperature of 8–10° C, and if the test is negative, also at 21° C. If still negative, patients should take a cold bath. They should be carefully supervised, for if massive histamine release occurs, there is a real danger that they might lose consciousness and drown. It should be kept in mind that this test does not differentiate between cold urticaria and aquagenic urticaria. If both the ice cube and the cold water tests are negative, the patient should sit in a cold room (4° C), with light clothing. If he suffers from cold urticaria, generalized wheals will develop shortly after he starts to shiver. Lesions in this type of cold urticaria will develop even faster at higher temperatures and if a chill factor (cold wind) is added to the cold stimulus (Brehm 1957).

Most clinicians perform only one of these three types of tests on their patients. For this reason, no data are available on the relative incidence of cold contact to ice, cold water, or cold air in larger patient groups. Most studies of the pathogenesis or the treatment of cold urticaria are done with patients who were selected on the basis of their reaction to only one test type. The results should therefore be viewed with caution, and no inferences should be drawn on the entire disease spectrum.

Laboratory tests

Patients with cold urticaria should be checked routinely for lues serology and for possible immunological alterations such as would, for example, be found in systemic lupus. Infectious mononucleosis should be ruled out by physical findings and positive tests for heterophile antibodies. Serum cryoglobulins, cryofibrinogens, and hemolysins should be measured as well.

5.7.7 Differential Diagnosis

Other types of physical urticaria should be ruled out by a careful history, with special attention being paid to the nature of the urticae and the temporal relationship between their development and the exposure to potential stimuli. For example, a patient who notices his urticaria in association with bathing, should be asked whether the wheals occurred while he was swimming in cold water, or immediately thereafter while rubbing himself with a towel. In the latter case, dermographic urticaria or vibratory angioedema should be considered.

Pruritus or prurigo hiemalis is a condition seen mostly in men. Patients with this affliction develop pruritus on rewarming after exposure to the cold, without any visible changes on their skin. There is a preference for the extremities, and the condition is observed mostly in cold seasons. Cold contact tests are negative, but the symptoms are reproducible if the natural eliciting stimuli are imitated.

Pruritus and erythema without whealing in response to cold (Shelley and Caro 1962) may represent an abortive form of cold urticaria. The same holds for cold prurigo, with papules developing also on reheating from cold to warm. Pruritus hiemalis, cold erythema, and papular eruption to cold are extremely rare, having been described mostly in the first half of this century (Illig 1973). Erythema and papules are also a feature of familial cold-induced urticaria.

Cold panniculitis might be confused with cold urticaria on the basis of its clinical appearance (Haxthausen 1941). It occurs frequently in infants, but is also seen in adolescents and adults. The lesions appear with a latency of 6–72 h after cold contact, present as painful, deep swellings, and disappear, leaving a slight hyperpigmentation. Passive transfer tests are negative. Illig (1973) has seen the condition in association with immediate type cold contact urticaria. On histology, there is a marked lymphohistiocytic infiltrate, admixed with eosinophils, in the subcutaneous fat, and there may even be fat necrosis. It is difficult to differentiate this condition from delayed cold urticaria, as described by Juhlin and Shelley (1961).

5.7.8 Prognosis

Very little is known about the natural course of cold urticaria. Many patients improve after a few months or years. Life threatening situations in highly sensitive persons, such as jumping into cold water or eating ice cream, should be avoided.

5.7.9 Pathogenesis

Possible inducing factors

Cold urticaria has been observed to develop after a variety of clinical conditions: after viral infections, infestations with parasites, syphilis, multiple insect bites, sensitivity to eggs, penicillin injections, childbirth, dietary changes, and stress. Pregnancy has no negative effect on already existing cold urticaria and may even cause its improvement. Genetic factors play a role in certain types of cold urticaria (see Table 5.2). In idiopathic cold urticaria, the combination of a mother-son and a mother-daughter involvement has been described (DeLaus and Winkelmann 1973), but such reports are extremely rare.

Immunoglobulins

In 27–50% of the patients with idiopathic cold urticaria, cold sensitivity can be passively transferred, and IgE has been identified as the active principle on gel chromatography (Houser et al. 1970, Kaplan et al. 1981 a). This IgE is not a cryoglobulin, but the specific antigen against which it is directed is not known. It is very possible that this specific IgE is not found in the sera of many patients, but that it is nevertheless bound to its high affinity receptors on tissue mast cells. Such locally sensitized mast cells could also be an explanation for localized cold contact urticaria (see below).

In addition to IgE, several other immunoglobulins have been shown to transfer cold hyperreactivity to normal subjects. Wanderer et al. (1971) described two patients with an IgM, Inou et al. (1980) a patient with an IgA, and Koda et al. (1978) found a transferable IgG cryoglobulin. The antigens and their specificity in cryoprecipitates have not been identified so far.

Mast cells and basophils

Several authors have described mast cell degranulation in biopsies of wheals (Juhlin and Shelley 1961, Fitzpatrick 1963, Costanzi et al. 1969, Eady et al. 1981), whereas others have failed to observe this (Soter et al. 1977, Doeglas and Bleumink 1974). Juhlin and Shelley (1961) observed degranulation of patient basophils after in vivo exposure to cold, but Kaplan et al. (1981 a) could not confirm this with in vitro histamine release studies from the same cells. Instead, they succeeded in demonstrating mast cell degranulation and histamine release after in vitro exposure of tissue biopsies to the cold. Kaplan's patients had cold contact urticaria, with a positive ice cube test. The tissue of these patients may have been particularly sensitive, but blood basophils were not. This might account for the discrepancy between his results and those of previous authors.

Mediators

Mast cells and basophils are the sole source of histamine in skin and peripheral blood. Increased levels of this mediator have been demonstrated in blisters produced at the sites of wheals (Kaplan et al. 1981 a) and after cold challenge of the arm in the effluent blood (Rose 1941) and the urine (Granerus et al. 1969). Beside histamine, the venous effluent was shown to contain eosinophil- and high molecular weight neurophil-chemotactic activity (Soter et al. 1976, Wasserman et al. 1977). Kinins were low or not measurable, and prostaglandins and serotonin failed to be found at all (Kaplan et al. 1975, Bentley Phillips et al. 1976).

All the mediators that have been demonstrated to be released on challenge with cold, occur in mast cells.

But the chemotactic factors may also derive from other cell types, and the mixed infiltrate which is present in later lesions may well be the source of additional mediators of inflammation which cause the protracted duration of some cold urticaria lesions (see Chapter 2.3.8, p. 21).

Studies on the effect of local and systemic therapy have cast doubt on the sole role of histamine in the evolution of early cold-induced wheals. Treatment with prednisone, aminophylline, and salbutamol caused a decrease of histamine release and pruritus but not of whealing (Keaheay and Greaves 1980, Kobza-Black et al. 1981). Local histamine stores were not depleted by this treatment, and another vasoactive mediator was postulated as cause of the edema. Sigler et al. (1980) showed, however, a good reduction of whealing but not of venous histamine levels during therapy with H1 type antihistamines. These apparently conflicting data may be due to the heterogeneity of cold urticaria and the action of diverse vasoactive mediators other than histamine.

Complement and protease inhibitors

Evidence for complement activation is not observed in all patients with cold urticaria and has been found mostly in single case reports. Sibbald et al. (1979) reported on a C2 deficient patient, and Wanderer et al. (1983) described a patient with cold contact urticaria, a serum cryoprecipitate, increased IgE levels, and evidence of alternate and classical pathway complement activation. On histology, features of a fully developed vasculitis were present. Costanzi et al. (1969) identified a mononuclear IgG ($\varkappa$ type) cryoglobulin which passively transferred cold sensitivity and activated complement via C1.

As with the complement system, there are only a few case reports of changes in serum protease levels. Martens and Berrens (1975) described a woman with increased consumption of α-1-antitrypsin, α-2 macroglobulin, and C1 inactivator on cold challenge. Back and Larsen (1978) reported normal C1 inactivator, C3 and C4 levels, but decreased α-1-antitrypsin and even elevated C4 levels in five patients with delayed cold urticaria. Doeglas and Bleumink (1975) studied the question of the role of a defect of protease inhibitors very thoroughly. In 16 patients with acquired cold contact urticaria, they noted a decrease of α-1-antitrypsin and total antitrypsin activity. Nilsson and Bäck (1984) found that total plasma C1-esterase inhibitor concentration was normal in the 20 patients they studied, but that the activity of the enzyme was low. The inhibitor activity dropped in 45% of the patients' plasma during cold-promoted activation of promoted activation of coagulation factor VII. The reasons for these alterations are unclear, and rather than having a pathogenetic significance, the lowering of protease inhibitors could also be due to binding of the inhibitors to other plasma factors or to their increased consumption.

Familial cold urticaria is characterized by normal complement levels, increased trypsin inhibition, as is also seen in severe infections, and decreased chymotrypsin inhibiting capacity of the plasma, suggesting that chymotrypsin-like enzymes are released during the active phase of the disease (Doeglas and Bleumink 1974).

Other theories

A few other pathogenetic factors should be mentioned, although they have not been sufficiently investigated. A defect in central regulation of heat, an instability of vasomotor control, and the occurrence of cold-kinins and cold-lysins have been postulated (Juhlin and Shelley 1961). The degree to which all these factors and mechanisms contribute to the disease will have to be further clarified.

5.7.10 Special Types of Cold Urticaria

The most common types of cold urticaria, including cold contact urticaria, systemic cold urticaria, and familial cold urticaria, have been dealt with in the general discussion.

Since Doeglas and Bleumink published their summary of the clinical data of eight families with familial cold urticaria in 1974, three more families, one from South Africa and two from the United States, have been reported (Vlagopoulos et al. 1975, Commerford and Meyers 1977, Martin et al. 1981). Familial cold urticaria is inherited as an autosomally dominant disease.

Localized cold urticaria

Solomon et al. (1966) described a young man with cold urticaria since early childhood. The disease had disappeared at age 8, but reappeared at the sites of many hyposensitization reactions.

Gerhard and Schöpf (1974) reported a patient with known cold urticaria who developed particularly prominent wheals at sites of previous skin tests with allergens and NaCl.

Roed-Petersen (1978) observed the development of cold contact urticaria which was strictly localized to a previous bite of a ladybird (an insect) in a 6-year-old boy.

Matthews and Warin (1970) could elicit prominent wheals on exposure to cold at sites which had been scratched up to 13 h earlier during dermographic testing.

Kaplan (1984) who coined the word "cold-dependent dermographism", described a phenomenon similar to that found in the patient of Matthews and Warin. Illig (1973) named the same condition "summation urticaria." The common factor in all these cases is a potentially latent cold hypersensitivity which has become manifest due to local alterations of the tissue, regardless of whether they are immunological or simply due to trauma.

Delayed cold urticaria

Several reports of this condition have appeared in the literature. It probably occurs much more frequently but is missed since test sites are generally observed for only a few minutes after stimulation. The time interval until appearance of the lesions and the clinical aspect of the wheals differ from report to report, so that either different pathomechanisms are involved or the lesions vary, depending on the intensity or the type of the cold challenge (Warin and Champion 1974, Back and Larsen 1978). An autosomal dominant inheritance was observed in a patient reported by Soter et al. (1977) whose tissue mast cells were not degranulated on histology. The cold hypersensitivity could not be passively transferred.

Juhlin (1981) tried to differentiate the mediators involved in the immediate and delayed type cold contact lesions in the same patient. Whereas the delayed reaction could not be blocked by antihistamines, the immediate one could. Delayed reactions were dependent on the immediate ones in that they developed only when the preceding immediate reaction had been very intense. Juhlin concluded that the delayed reaction is due to mediators other than histamine.

5.8 Cholinergic Urticaria

5.8.1 Epidemiology

Cholinergic, or heat reflex urticaria, is the second most frequent type of the physical urticarias. Its incidence among a dermatological outpatient population has been estimated at 0.2% (Moore-Robinson and Warin 1968) and 0.7% (Misra et al. 1977). Among the chronic urticarias, it accounts for 5% (Warin 1977) to 8.6% (Misra et al. 1977) of the cases. Kounis and McMahon (1975) have estimated that 15% of normal adolescents suffer from mild forms of the disease.

Cholinergic urticaria primarily affects young patients. The age of onset ranges from 16–35 years, its mean duration being 5.3–7.5 years, with a range of 2–30 years (Warin and Champion 1974). There is a higher incidence among males than among females (see Table 5.1). Two familial cases have been observed: in a pair of twins (Panfilis 1969) and in a brother and sister among 70 patients (Sprekeler and Czarnetzki, unpublished observation).

5.8.2 Local Symptoms

The lesions of cholinergic urticaria consist of pinpoint wheals, surrounded by a more or less pronounced reflex erythema (Figs. 5.9 and 5.10). The wheals arise at or inbetween follicles and develop preferentially on the upper trunk and the upper limbs. Palms, soles, and axillae are generally spared. Only rarely is the face involved and may then appear flushed and swollen, particularly around the eyelids.

Lesions of cholinergic urticaria arise within 2–10 min after provocation and last for only 30–50 min, rarely for up to 3 h.

There are three basic types of stimuli that cause their eruption: (1) passive overheating, (2) physical exercise, and (3) emotional stress. Typical eliciting stimuli noted by the patients are running, swimming, dancing, bicycling, taking a warm tub or a sauna bath, eating of hot spices, or drinking of alcoholic beverages. Fever or intravenous calcium injections can also elicite the reactions, and a stressful situation at school or at work can precipitate the symptomatology as well. Lesions arise only rarely during sleep, and some patients notice remissions during the summer months (Udassin et al. 1981). A refractory period of from one to several days, usually for 8–24 h, is noted by most patients, although some are not aware of it.

Invariably, the onset of lesions is accompanied by intense itching at the site of involvement. Some patients also notice prodromal itching on the scalp.

5.8.3 Systemic Symptoms

In many patients, the symptomatology is restricted to the skin. A variety of systemic symptoms can arise as well, suggesting either a more generalized mast cell release or a systemic effect of the mediators from the cutaneous lesions. Headache is a frequent symptom. Periorbital swelling, lacrimation, and burning of the eyes are observed in about 30% of the patients (Sprekeler and Czarnetzki, unpublished observations). Gastrointestinal symptoms, including hypersalivation, nausea, vomiting, abdominal cramps, and

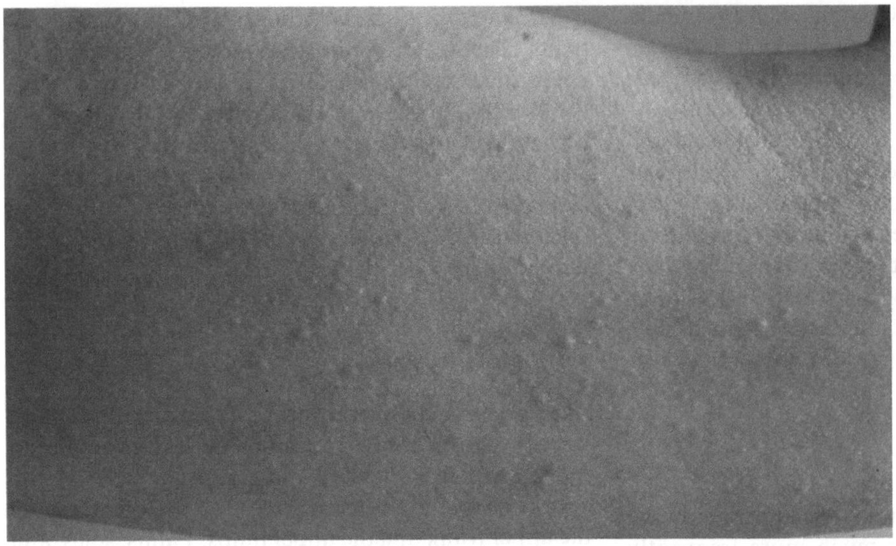

Fig. 5.9. Pinpoint wheals on the upper arm of a patient with cholinergic urticaria 5 min after exercise on a bicycle. The skin was intensely pruritic.

diarrhea, are less frequent. Dizziness and hypotension can proceed to life-threatening anaphylactic reactions, and some patients suffer from wheezing and asthma attacks during the provocation of their lesions.

5.8.4 Laboratory Findings

Except for a rare leukocytosis (Warin and Champion 1974), no laboratory abnormalities have been reported in cholinergic urticaria.

5.8.5 Histology

There are only a few reports on the microscopic morphology of cholinergic wheals. Illig (1967) described an upper dermal, perivascular, cellular infiltrate which consisted of mononuclear cells, neutrophils, and occasional eosinophils. He observed no obstruction or involvement of the sweat ducts. Shelley et al. (1983) described dermal edema and endothelial swelling of the smaller dermal vessels. There was ultrastructural evidence for mast cell degranulation in the one patient studied. We observed this as well in two additional patients, but found no special relationship between nerves and mast cells in the sections studied (Wiesner-Menzel and Czarnetzki, unpublished observations).

5.8.6 Associated Diseases

There is no increased incidence of atopy in patients with cholinergic urticaria (Doeglas 1975a), although patients may suffer from various types of mast cell-related diseases. About 52% react to oral provocation

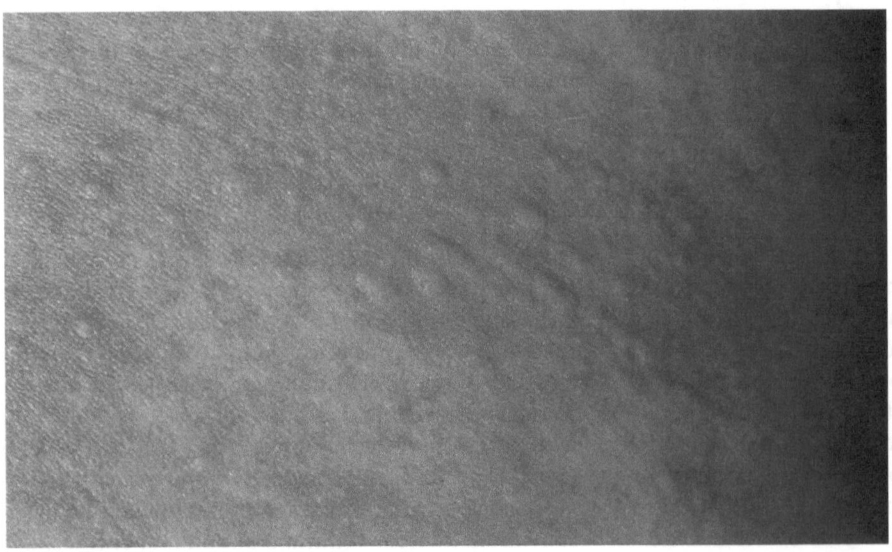

Fig. 5.10. Lesions of cholinergic urticaria which have become confluent. Note also the more intense erythema of the surrounding skin.

with aspirin (Doeglas 1975b). Cold contact urticaria is not infrequent (Illig 1973, Sigler et al. 1979). Smaller numbers of patients suffer from associated dermographism (Morgan 1953, Herxheimer 1956, Mathews and Pan 1970). The dermographic whealing in some of these patients has the special features of starting in a punctate fashion (Fig. 5.3), followed by confluent whealing at the site of contact and typical cholinergic urticae in the immediate surrounding. Angioedema (Hopkins et al. 1938, Lawrence et al. 1981), vibratory angioedema (Kaplan et al. 1975), aquagenic urticaria (Shelley and Rawnsley 1964, Davis et al. 1981), asthma (Mathews and Pan 1970), and very rarely pressure urticaria (Soter et al. 1980) are other associated diseases.

5.8.7 Diagnosis

Once the diagnosis is suspected on the basis of the history, lesions should be provoked and inspected by the physician for confirmation. Intradermal injections of acetycholine or analogues are unreliable diagnostic tests since whealing occurs in all subjects. The typical, satellite, pinpoint wheals around the central large wheal are seen only in patients with severe cholinergic urticaria, according to Commens and Greaves (1978). In addition, they are not reproducible in the same patient. Among our own patients, we have observed satellite wheals in only one of 30 patients, and also in one of 30 controls.

Cholinergic lesions are best reproduced by letting the patient exercise in a warm room and with warm clothing, up to the point of sweating or semi-exhaustion. Riding a bicycle, chair stepping, or rapid bending of the knees are suitable methods. Soter et al. (1980) elicited lesions very reliably by having patients run on a treadmill while wearing an occlusive suit. Illig (1973) also suggested hot baths of both arms (15–20 min, 45° C) or sitting in a hot bath (10–15 min, 40–41° C). These latter methods, however, do not differentiate cholinergic and aquagenic urticaria. Illig et al. (1980) could reliably induce cholinergic whealing at normal ambient temperature by eliciting the gag reflex which also caused sweating and an increased heart rate in his patients, an admittedly unpleasant procedure for both patient and physician.

Application of local heat is ineffective (Illig 1973) since raising the body core temperature seems essential for reproduction of lesions (Illig et al. 1980).

5.8.8 Differential Diagnosis

The cutaneous lesions of cholinergic urticaria resemble those of solar and aquagenic urticaria. The diseases are however easily differentiated by their eliciting stimulus. Cutis anserina might cause confusion, but lack of itching, restriction of the small cutaneous swellings to the follicles, and lack of surrounding erythema differentiates this condition from cholinergic urticaria. In their description of patients with cholinergic erythema, Murphy et al. (1983) reported that their patients had been diagnosed as having urticaria pigmentosa, urticaria vasculitis, and drug eruptions. Careful inspection of the lesions and observation of their time course should rule out these diagnoses.

Cholinergic urticaria should also be differentiated from miliaria. This is easily done by the vesicular appearance of individual miliarial lesions, by their distribution, and by their more persistent time course (Garretts 1958).

5.8.9 Pathogenesis

Basic mechanisms

It is now generally accepted that cholinergic urticaria depends on stimulation of the neuroglandular junction of the sweat glands via cholinergic afferent fibers which receive their impulse from the central nervous system. This results in the release of acetylcholine and the stimulation of sweat production (Grant et al. 1936, Herxheimer 1956). Sweat itself is not essential for the production of lesions since local application of heat and subsequent sweating in the treated area fails to induce cholinergic urticaria (Lorincz 1966). The process of sweating is not important either since rendering one arm anhidrotic by tying it off still causes generalized urticaria of the anhidrotic arm in a sauna bath (Illig and Heinicke 1967a). Thus, the difference between acetylcholine release, with subsequent sweating in normal individuals, and the abnormal response in patients with cholinergic urticaria remain unexplained. The defect could be due to

1) excessive release of acetylcholine or an additional mediator such as ATP which is also released from cholinergic nerve endings. (Either of these mediators could then cause mast cell degranulation);
2) a metabolic product or a carrier product that is formed in the skin. (It could act as an antigen and interact with mast cell-bound immunoglobulin molecules, resulting in mediator release);
3) an increased susceptibility of patient tissue to normally released mediators.

So far, no evidence has been provided for excessive

release of mediators from nerve endings in patients with cholinergic urticaria. During skin testing with acetylcholine and ATP, patients and normal controls develop wheals of about equal size (Czarnetzki et al. 1984a). A passively transferable immunoglobulin which is not IgE because of its heat stability, has been found by Illig and Heinicke (1967b), but not by others (Sigler et al. 1979).

An intriguing explanation for the pathogenesis of cholinergic urticaria was offered recently by Shelley et al. (1983). They reported an increase of specific, cholinergic, muscarinic receptors in cholinergic wheals by measuring ^{3}H-quiniclidinyl benzylate (^{3}H-QNB) binding. After the lesions had subsided, and on rechallenge of previously involved sites 4 h later, binding had decreased. These observations suggest a transient increase of acetylcholine receptor expression in cholinergic wheals and would also offer an explanation for the refractoriness of the tissue in some patients. The exact mechanisms which cause this change in receptor expression are however unclear. Calmodulin which can down-regulate acetylcholine receptor responsiveness (Burgoyne 1981), might be involved. These findings need to be confirmed in more than one patient with cholinergic urticaria.

Mediators

In their one severely affected patient, Shelley et al. (1983) showed that hives induced by acetylcholine were blocked by scopolamine and greatly enhanced by capsaicin, probably because the latter causes the release of substance P, another possible mediator in cholinergic urticaria. Repeated application of capsaicin blocked the erythema around wheals, demonstrating its dependency on axon reflex vasodilatation.

Several authors have measured increases in serum histamine of patients on provocation of their lesions (Mathews and Pan 1970, Kaplan et al. 1975, Sigler et al. 1979, Davis et al. 1981, Lawrence et al. 1981). Histamine levels peak within 7–10 min after challenge, at about the time when the wheals appear. An increase is usually measured over the subsequent 30–40 min, in contrast to other types of physical urticaria where this prolonged histaminemia is not observed. These observations implicate mast cells as central effector cells in cholinergic urticaria, in agreement with the findings on ultrastructure (see Section 5.8, p. 76).

Histamine may not be the only mediator in cholinergic urticaria with smooth muscle contracting activity. One of the three patients of Kaplan et al. (1975) had no increase of blood histamine on exercise challenge, but of serotonin instead. The authors suggest that platelet-activating factor (PAF) might be the link between mast cells and platelet serotonin release in this case (see Chapter 2.3, p. 13). PAF or the SRS-type leukotrienes could also explain the non-histamine serum smooth muscle contracting activity which was measured in two of three patients by Lawrence et al. (1981).

Soter et al. (1980) measured increased eosinophil chemotactic and high molecular weight neutrophil chemotactic activities, together with increased serum histamine, in the sera of patients with severe cholinergic urticaria after challenge. These factors may account for the mixed perivascular cellular infiltrate (see Section 5.8, p. 79). The same authors found, on the other hand, no change of serum CH50 or of individual serum complement components in their subjects so that vasoactive or chemotactic mediators from this source are unlikely to be involved. The same probably also holds for prostaglandins, since indomethacin has no therapeutic effect (Shelley et al. 1983).

Eftekhari et al. (1980) measured decreased α_1-antichymotrypsin levels in the sera of patients with cholinergic urticaria. They suggest that pharmacologically active products of protein digestion might have potential pathogenetic significance in cholinergic urticaria. Another possible explanation of this observation may also simply relate to the fact that all three patients developed angioedema together with their cholinergic wheals. Angioedema, in turn, is frequently linked with changes in protease inhibitors (Doeglas and Bleumink 1975). In contrast to the findings of Eftekhari et al., Doeglas and Bleumink found no alterations of protease inhibitors among their ten patients with cholinergic urticaria.

Pulmonary alterations

The clinical findings of cholinergic urticaria suggest that the basic defects are not limited to the skin. This is supported by in vivo studies which show a drop in pulmonary resistance during exercise challenge in severely affected patients (Soter et al. 1980). Among our own patients, we could demonstrate similar changes on bronchial provocation with acetylcholine (Czarnetzki et al. 1984a), but only in severely affected patients. These patients thus behave like latent asthmatics. A possible explanation may relate to the observation of Ado et al. (1978) who found marked changes in the cholinergic system of patients suffering from both bronchial asthma and chronic urticaria. These alterations depend on type, stage, and severity of the disease.

5.8.10 Variant Types of Cholinergic Urticaria and Related Diseases

Cholinergic itching

Nomland (1944) first described this condition, which seems to be a minimal variant of cholinergic urticaria. The itching appears in the same pattern as in cholinergic urticaria, but there are no clinically evident lesions on the skin. Two such patients presented at the Dermatology Department, University of Münster, within the past 6 years.

Cholinergic dermographism

The phenomenon of cholinergic whealing at sites of scratching trauma is seen very rarely in cholinergic urticaria and is discussed under the heading of dermographic urticaria (Fig. 5.3).

Cholinergic erythema

Murphy et al. (1983) described four patients who suffered from a pruritic, macular, erythematous rash for up to 8 consecutive days. On close observation, the lesions were noted to be of short duration, with continually new lesions appearing at sites adjacent to older lesions. Distribution and size of the eruption was typical for cholinergic urticaria, although wheals were missing. Exercise or a hot bath caused exacerbation, while topical scopolamine blocked the development of new lesions.

Cold-induced cholinergic reflex urticaria

Illig (1973) described a patient who developed a generalized rash identical to that seen in cholinergic urticaria after contact with cold air. No lesions developed at test sites with ice cubes. Kaplan and Garofalo (1981) described four patients with similar clinical features. Sitting in a 4° C room for 5–15 min elicited the eruption in their patients. In three of them, elevated blood histamine levels were measured after challenge.

An additional case with similar features was described by Czarnetzki et al. (1981). The patient had noted small, transient urticae on his legs when bicycling in the cold. The condition disappeared during spring and reappeared in the cold season. On testing with an ice cube, no lesions appeared at the test site itself, but small wheals with surrounding erythema developed rapidly proximally and distally to the site on the forearm. The time course of the lesions was similar to that of heat reflex cholinergic urticaria. The difference between heat and cold reflex urticaria may simply relate to the sensitivity of a putative eliciting agent to different temperatures.

Exercise-induced hypotension and anaphylaxis

Hypotension is a symptom which occurs in almost any type of urticaria and is due to the release of massive amounts of vasodilating mediators such as histamine. It occurs also in severe cholinergic urticaria, and it can even be the major symptom in some patients who have only minor problems with cholinergic whealing and angioedema. In a recent description of two such patients, Kaplan et al. (1981 b) named the disease "exercise-induced hypotension."

Exercise-induced anaphylaxis was known to exist as a separate clinical entity even before the description of exercise-induced hypotension (Sheffer and Austen 1980; Tables 5.1 and 5.3). The associated urticarial lesions are larger than the cholinergic wheals, are often accompanied by angioedema, and may also present only as an itching erythema. Lewis et al. (1981) also noted a cholinergic rash in three of their six patients with exercise-induced anaphylaxis.

Pulmonary symptoms can occur in this syndrome as well. A prodromal palmar itching and a high incidence of familial atopic disease have been reported in afflicted patients (Sheffer et al. 1983, Songsiridej and Busse 1983). Two families have been described in which several siblings had exercise-induced anaphylaxis (Grant et al. 1982, Longley et al. 1982).

In contrast to cholinergic urticaria, exercise-induced anaphylaxis cannot be elicited in all patients at all times (Sheffer et al. 1983). In some patients, ingestion of certain foods such as celery or shrimp is a requirement for provocation of symptoms in addition to exercise (Maulitz et al. 1979, Kidd et al. 1983).

Since the exact mechanisms of cholinergic urticaria and exercise-induced anaphylaxis are unknown, the relationship between these diseases must also remain unclear. Their common denominator is an elevation of plasma histamine during exercise (Kaplan et al. 1981 b, Sheffer et al. 1984). It is not known whether both mast cells and basophils contribute to the elevated serum histamine levels during challenge.

5.9 Solar Urticaria

5.9.1 General Aspects and Epidemiology

Solar, or actinic urticaria, is a relatively rare condition in which urticaria is evoked by electromagnetic radiation of various wavelengths. Reactions to infrared radiation are excluded since they belong to local heat urticaria.

Solar urticaria is mostly idiopathic, but it may also occur secondarily to porphyria, systemic lupus erythematosus, or certain drugs.

Since its first description several centuries ago (see Chapter 1, p. 1), more than 90 cases have been described in the literature (Ive et al. 1965). Twenty-one of these patients were seen in London over a 5-year period (Ive et al. 1965). Among patients referred for a evaluation of a possible photosensitivity, 5% were found to suffer from solar urticaria (Ravits et al. 1982). In Japan, most patients react to visible light while the predominant eliciting wavelength lies below 370 nm in the patients from Europe and North America.

Solar urticaria is found slightly more frequently in females than in males (see Table 5.1) and is normally first noted between the ages of 20–40 years. There is only one report of two siblings who were affected by the disease (Warin and Champion 1974), and there is no increased incidence of allergy.

Harber et al. (1963) have made a major contribution to the proper study and understanding of solar urticaria by classifying the disease according to the eliciting wavelengths and the possible immunological mechanisms involved. Table 5.9 presents a slightly modified classification on the same pathogenetic basis. The numbering system of the types is omitted for the sake of simplicity, and the patients with positive or negative transfer among the reactors to visible light are lumped together, since positive transfer is not a very reliable test. In the individual patient, reactions may be primarily to UV-A, UV-B, visible light, or combinations of either of these spectra. Broad-spectrum reactors may respond to continuous and discontinuous bands of wavelengths.

5.9.2 Cutaneous Reactions

Diffuse erythema and intense whealing, often with a flare, develop rapidly after exposure to the eliciting wavelengths, usually within 30 s–3 min, rarely after a lag time of 20 min. The erythema and swelling is limited exactly to the area of exposure (Fig. 5.11). If the stimulation is less intense or the activity low, diffuse erythema may be the only cutaneous reaction. Smaller wheals, at times even similar to those in cholinergic urticaria, may also appear with mild stimulation (Fig. 5.12) and may progress to diffuse, confluent tissue swelling.

Development of the lesions is generally accompanied by intense pruritus. Sensation of pricking, tingling, and burning may be reported as well. Whealing starts to regress by 15–30 min and usually disappears by 1 h, although an erythema may persist for up to 3 h. Chronically exposed skin such as the face or the dorsa of the hands are usually spared.

Ive et al. (1965) have also described patients who react primarily to UV-B. The lesions became papular or even vesicular after 36–38 h and lasted for 2–3 days. These patients should be grouped with the polymorphous light eruptions.

5.9.3 Systemic Symptoms (Table 5.3)

Fainting, a histamine headache, and even loss of

Table 5.9. Classification of the major types of idiopathic solar urticaria, based on the eliciting wavelengths and possible immunological mechanism. Test methods for the different types and some special features that are helpful for the diagnosis are listed as well.

Type	Eliciting wavelength (nm)	Passive transfer	Reverse passive transfer	Method of testing	Special aspects
Short wave UV-B	280–320	+	+	UV light; neg. with window glass filter	elicited in bright sunlight, not through glass or clothing; sunscreen useful
Long wave UV-A	320–400	–	–	UV light; pos. with or without window glass filter	elicited also in cloudy weather and through clothing
Visible light	400–760	+ or –	–	any good light source (e.g. slide projector, 5–20 min)	elicited in any weather and season, even by artificial light sources
Broad-spectrum light	230–700	–	–	UV light or strong filament bulb	response to wavelengths with discontinuous or continuous bands; sensitivity depends on the wavelengths involved

consciousness can occur when large areas of the body surface are involved with urticarial lesions.

5.9.4 Laboratory Findings

All routine laboratory examinations are within normal limits. In a few patients, increased gastric acid secretion has been observed with bouts of urticaria (Ratanen and Suhonen 1980). The same authors found elevated antinuclear IgM antibodies at a titer of 1 : 1000 in their patients, without other evidence for systemic lupus erythematosus. Baart de la Faille et al. (1975) reported a patient with increased serum lactic dehydrogenase levels and increased fragility of the red blood cells.

5.9.5 Histology

Biopsies of 5-min old wheals revealed only a sparse inflammatory infiltrate around the vessels and appendages. One-half of the cells were mast cells, but the same number of mast cells was also found in normal skin of the patient. Immunofluorescent staining for IgG, IgM, IgA, C3, and fibrin was negative at this time (Rantanen and Suhonen 1980), whereas massive staining for perivascular fibrin was found in 1-h-old lesions (Baart de la Faille et al. 1975). These changes had disappeared by 24 h. On electron microscopy, mast cells were shown to be degranulated (Hawk et al. 1980).

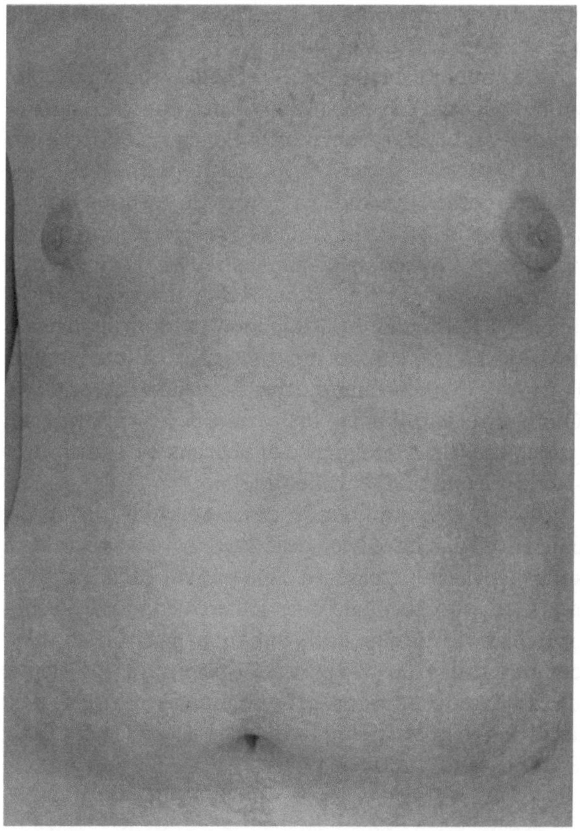

Fig. 5.11. Diffuse whealing and erythema in a patient with solar urticaria who had exposed herself to the noonday sun. The entire upper trunk is involved; only the region covered by bathing trunks is spared.

5.9.6 Underlying and Associated Diseases (Table 5.1)

In most patients afflicted with solar urticaria, there is no underlying cause. The disease may, however, be a manifestation of porphyria cutanea tarda or erythropoietic protoporphyria (Ive et al. 1965), with a peak of the eliciting action spectrum at 405 nm. Similarly, solar urticaria may be an early or late symptom of systemic lupus erythematosus (Delorme and Giroux 1966, Tuffanelli and Dubois 1969). Solar

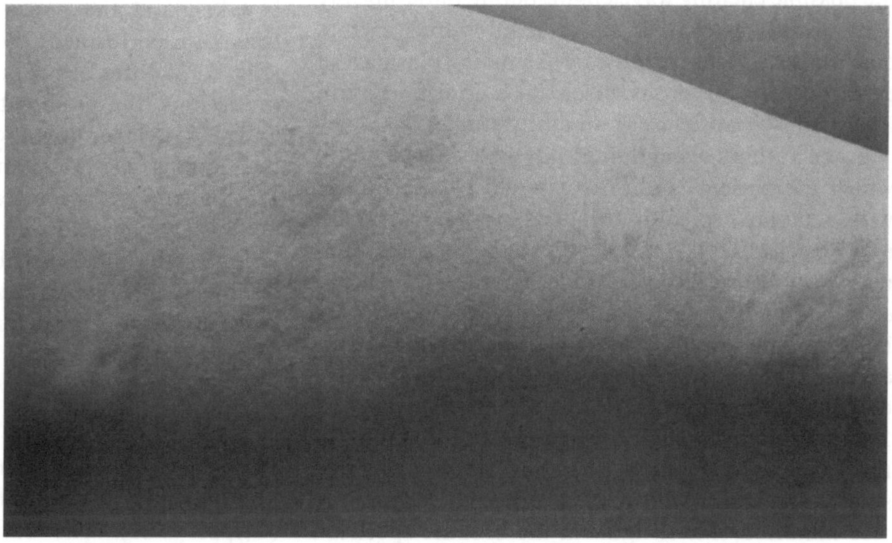

Fig. 5.12. Small, irregularly sized wheals in a patient with solar urticaria after mild exposure to UV light.

urticaria can develop in areas that have previously been exposed to tar or pitch (Crow et al. 1961).

One patient each has been reported who developed solar urticaria during systemic therapy with sulfonamides and chlorpromazine (Lorincz 1964, Horio 1975). Horio's patient also developed an allergic contact dermatitis and a phototoxic reaction to the same drug. Horio was able to transfer the urticaria reaction by injection of the patient's serum into a normal subject's skin. After 24 h, a reaction to light occurred following local injection of chlorpromazine at the same test site. In the discussion of this patient, Horio (1975) mentions another patient of Mizuno and Ohno who had a solar urticaria due to triclocarban (trichlorocarbanilide) and cloflucarban (4.4'-dichloro--3(trifluoromethyl)-carbanalide).

Only a few additional diseases, with no direct causative role, have been described in association with solar urticaria (Table 5.1). One patient each has been reported who had cold contact urticaria and dermographism (Ratanen and Suhonen 1980) and heat contact urticaria (Willis and Epstein 1974). Peptic ulcers may occur secondarily to increased gastric acid secretion in predisposed individuals (Van Hecke 1979, Ratanen and Suhonen 1980).

5.9.7 Diagnosis

Solar urticaria should be suspected when patients observe the rapid development of pruritic, evanescent lesions on exposure to solar irradiation, particularly in springtime during the first days of sunny weather, with an accentuation of skin areas that are not yet "hardened" to the sun. If the patients report that lesions also develop through glass, such as in the car or in rooms with artificial lighting, a clue is provided as to the possible eliciting wavelength. Before initiating any light testing, porphyria and systemic lupus erythematosus should be excluded by examining plasma and erythrocyte protoporphyrin and 24-h urine porphyrin levels, and by antinuclear antibody studies.

Some authors claim that ideally, the wavelength to which the patient is sensitive should be determined with a monochromator (Magnus et al. 1959, Willis and Epstein 1974). A simpler and less expensive alternative is the so-called spectrodermograph (Kochenar et al. 1981). The light source is a 450 W xenon arc lamp, and the spectral output is dispersed by gratings and quartz lenses into 31 slits which allow the passage of 12 nm wide bands from 250–610 nm (Ravits et al. 1982). From a practical viewpoint, determination of the exact wavelength is, however, not so essential since it may shift with time. Furthermore, there are also inhibitory wavelengths in the broader spectrum which can down-modulate the urticarial response to reacting wavelengths (Hasei and Ichihashi 1982, Torinuki et al. 1983). It seems therefore far more meaningful to test the reactivity with less sophisticated methods. A solar simulator is a useful instrument for light testing and is available at most institutions (Willis and Epstein 1974, Ramsay 1980). Glass and other appropriate filters can be inserted to determine narrower wavelength spectra. A slide projector, quite suitable as a source of visible light, should be placed at a distance of 10 cm from the skin.

The skin on the back is usually used for testing. Areas of about 1 cm^2 of skin are irradiated, and the time of exposure is chosen at increasing increments, depending on the specific light source used. The test areas are observed after exposure at 2-min intervals, up to 6 min, then at 5-min intervals for 15 min, and then at 15-min intervals for up to 2 h for the appearance of typical wheal and erythema reactions (Willis and Epstein 1974). Readings at 24 and 48 h should be taken in order not to miss photocontact or phototoxic reactions. For visible light testing, the exposure time should be 10–15 min.

One of the problems with light testing is that the threshold of whealing varies greatly within 2–3 days and that there are also variations in the maximal wavelengths which elicit the lesions (Ive et al. 1965). Skin sites remain refractory to whealing for several days after challenge. Thus, testing should be performed on skin that has been protected from light for a few days.

5.9.8 Differential Diagnosis

Solar urticaria is not easily confused with the conditions mentioned in Table 5.1 if a careful history is taken and the appropriate skin and laboratory tests are performed. Polymorphic light eruptions (Fig. 5.13) differ by the primarily papular character of the lesions, the preferential involvement of the face and neck, delayed evolution (6–8 h), and persistence of the lesions at the same site over several days. Photoallergic contact dermatitis and phototoxic reactions are characterized by eczematous and papular lesions with similar distribution and persistence of the lesions as in polymorphic light eruptions. However, solar urticaria can coexist with these conditions.

5.9.9 Prognosis

Patients with solar urticaria have the highest degree of photosensitivity among the light-associated diseases (Cripps 1981). The condition can be a disabling problem, particularly if eliciting wavelengths in the UV-B and visible light are involved; however, no deaths due to the condition have been reported. The longest persistence of the disease on record is 48 years (Ive et al. 1965), and the mean duration of the cases reported so far in the literature is 7.1 years. Warin and Champion (1974) described one patient who improved over a 3–4 year observation period. There are no reports in the literature on spontaneous remissions.

5.9.10 Pathogenesis

Solar urticaria represents a reaction pattern to multiple causes. This is evident with cases where diverse underlying diseases can be identified (Table 5.1), but it also seems likely in the idiopathic types. In fact, this diversity of possible pathomechanisms led Harber et al. (1963) to classify the disease into different types (Table 5.9). The reason why an increased sensitivity to light develops in idiopathic solar urticaria, is unknown.

The idiopathic types of solar urticaria differ not only in the eliciting wavelengths of the action spectra, but also in the pathogenetic mechanisms involved. A few of them have specific immunologic features. A heat-labile serum factor is consistently found only in the type associated with UV-B. This serum factor elicits wheals even when it is injected into a normal person's skin after the site has been irradiated 5 min earlier (reverse passive transfer). In some of the patients who react to visible light, a heat-labile serum factor has also been demonstrated by passive transfer, but never by reverse passive transfer (Horio and Minami 1977). The exact nature of the serum factors has never been elucidated. They do not belong to the IgG or IgM immunoglobulin class, and their heat lability suggests that they are identical with IgE (Sams 1970, Ramsay 1980).

There is controversy about which mediators are involved in solar urticaria. Ive et al. (1965) found histamine "or a similar substance" in the lesions. Pretreatment of the skin with compound 48/80 or antihistamines reduced the whealing in only one half to two-thirds of their patients. Similar data suggesting that histamine plays only a minor role in solar urticaria, have been provided by several other groups (Sams et al. 1969, Horio 1978, Ichihashi et al. 1985, Torinuki et al. 1983), and the variable, generally poor response to treatment with antihistamines would point in the same direction.

Despite these findings, three different groups have recently found increased levels of serum histamine after local challenge of their patients (Soter et al. 1979, Hawk et al. 1980, Keahey et al. 1981). Peak levels of histamine were reached after 2–5 min; there was a return to baseline after 20 min. Eosinophil and neutrophil chemotactic factors increased by 3–5 fold, with maximal values at 10–20 min and a return to baseline by 60 min (Soter et al. 1979) (Table 5.4). Mast cell degranulation has been demonstrated in these subjects as well (Hawk et al. 1980, Keahey et al. 1981). In two of the four subjects studied by Hawk et al. (1980), serum histamine levels were however only minimally elevated, and the authors suggest that other, not yet identified mediators play a greater role in the evolution of the wheal.

The possible role of an as yet unidentified serum factor causing the induction of the lesions has been suggested, because arterial occlusion blocks or decreases the tendency of the skin to respond to light (Sams et al. 1969, Kobza et al. 1973). Horio et al. (1984) observed that in vitro irradiation of patient serum generated a factor that caused wheal formation on reinjection into patient skin. The nature of this photoallergic product or its mechanism of action is not known. Similarly, the mechanism of action of the inhibitory spectra in patients with reactivity to visible light is unclear.

The sequence of events that leads to solar urticaria may be viewed as follows (Fig. 5.1). A pre-antigen in serum or at tissue sites becomes antigenic after irradiation. This antigen combines with specific IgE on mast cells, causing mast cell mediator release, or it activates complement, causing in either case a venular dilation, an increased leakiness of the vessels, and a cutaneous whealing reaction.

5.10 Heat Contact Urticaria

5.10.1 General Aspects

Heat contact urticaria, or urticaria ab igne (Duke 1924), is extremely rare. Only slightly more than 20 cases have been reported since Duke's first description. We have seen two patients within the last 5 years, and many additional cases are probably not reported or go undiagnosed. Michaelsson and Ros (1971) have described a delayed type of heat urticaria in a kindred, with nine afflicted members involving three generations, and an autosomally dominant inheritance.

The majority of the patients are young adult women (Table 5.1). Symptoms are most apparent in the warmest months of the year (Atkins and Zweiman 1981), and eliciting agents are any stimuli that transfer a sensation of warmth to the skin, such as warm water, warm water bottles, stoves, radiators, fire, sun, hairdriers, and hot drinks or food. The individual patient need not respond to each one of these stimuli.

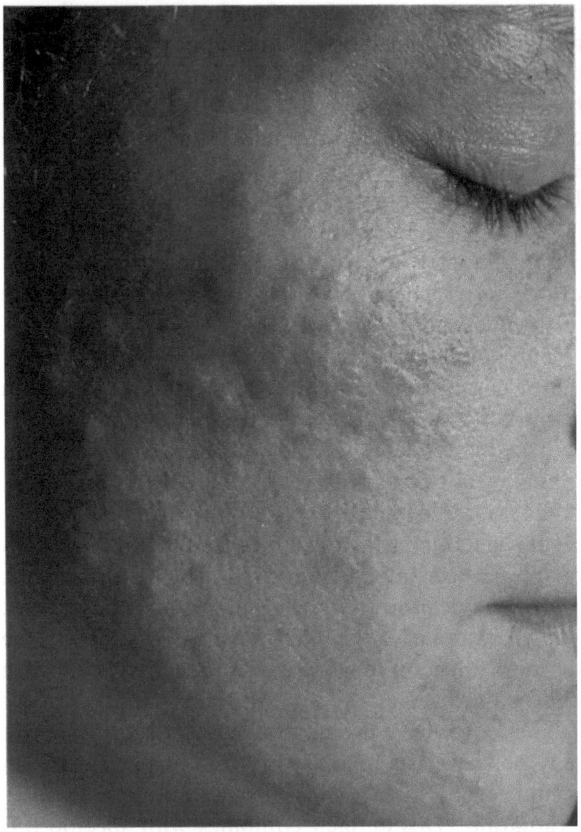

Fig. 5.13. Erythematous papules on the face of a patient with polymorphous light eruption. In contrast to wheals in solar urticaria, these lesions persisted for many days.

5.10.2 Local Reactions (see also Table 5.3)

After local application of heat, lesions develop generally within 3–5 min, rarely within 10 min. In the familial cases (Michaelsson and Ros 1971) and in the first cases described by Duke (1924), wheals developed only after a lag period of 60–90 min. Erythema and whealing are limited to the area of contact, and wheals are small (Fig. 5.14) or confluent. In some patients, a 2–3 cm margin of surrounding erythema has been noted (Hopkins et al. 1938, Lewis 1939, de Moragas et al. 1973), but in others not (Delorme 1969, Michaelsson and Ros 1971, Greaves et al. 1974, Wüthrich 1979). Lesions usually persist for up to 1 h, but occasionally they can last for 6–10 h (Michaelsson and Ros 1971) or even for days (Greaves et al. 1974). The patient of Daman et al. (1978) is unusual in that he exhibited indurated rather than urticarial lesions. Usually, the appearance of the lesions is accompanied by intense local itching or burning. Patients experience numbness and irritation on the tongue after contact with hot food (Leigh and Ramsay 1975). Sensitivity to touch rather than pruritus has also been noted (Daman et al. 1978). The eliciting temperature ranges from 38–56° C. Local sites may be refractory for only 24 h (Michaelsson and Ros 1971) or for up to 3 weeks (Greaves et al. 1974).

5.10.3 Systemic Symptoms

Unless lesions involve extensive areas of the body, the symptomatology remains localized to the exposed site. Generalized symptoms of fatigue, dizziness, headache, facial flush, nausea, diarrhea, abdominal cramps, and loss of consciousness have been recorded (Hopkins et al. 1938, Delorme 1969, Leigh and Ramsay 1975, Grant et al. 1981) (see Table 5.3).

5.10.4 Laboratory Findings

All routine laboratory tests, including exhaustive immunological studies, have been negative until now,

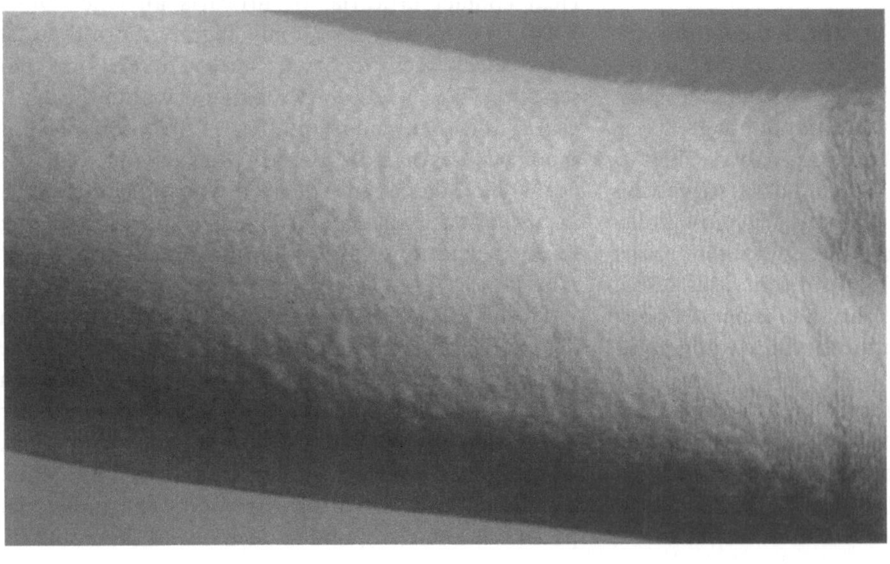

Fig. 5.14. Intense erythema and swelling of the arm, with small wheals in a patient with heat contact urticaria. The arm had been immersed in a bath of warm water.

except for an increased IgM (Greaves et al. 1974) and IgE (de Moragas et al. 1973) in one patient each.

5.10.5 Associated Diseases

There is a relatively high incidence of atopy among the patients and their families (42 %), mostly in the form of allergic rhinitis. One patient each has been described with associated dermographism (Wise et al. 1978), cold urticaria (Tennenbaum and Lowney 1973), and solar urticaria (Willis and Epstein 1974) (see Table 5.1). One young adult, seen at the University Hospital, Münster, had an associated aspirin intolerance.

5.10.6 Histological Findings

Light microscopic examination of early (30 s) and late (180 min) lesions reveals a round cell infiltrate in the upper dermis and around hair follicles, with associated vasodilatation and edema. Mast cells are normal in number and appear either degranulated (Michaelsson and Ros 1971) or intact (Daman et al. 1978). Perivascular fibrin deposition has been observed in 180-min-old lesions, and endothelial swelling after 30 min (Johansson et al. 1984). There are abnormal patterns of immunoglobulin or complement deposition on immunofluorescent examination (Irwin et al. 1984, Johansson et al. 1984).

5.10.7 Diagnosis

Local heating of the skin for 3–5 min, possibly even for 10 min, should be done by immersion of an arm in a warm water bath (Fig. 5.14), or by touching the skin with a metal cylinder containing heated water. The usual eliciting temperature is 38–41° C, but it may have to be raised up to 56° C in individual patients. Delayed reactions should be looked for 2–4 h later.

5.10.8 Differential Diagnosis

Heat contact urticaria must be differentiated from cholinergic (heat reflex) urticaria and from solar urticaria. This is readily done by a negative exercise test and by exposure of the skin to radiation over a wide spectrum of wavelengths. Patients may be confused as to whether heat or cold stimuli elicit the symptoms since wheals occur also after rewarming subsequent to cold exposure (Duke 1926). Skin tests with either cold or hot objects will easily resolve this problem.

5.10.9 Prognosis

Heat urticaria can persist for many years. The 48-year-old patient reported by Michaelsson and Ros (1971) had her disease since late childhood. As no case reports of spontaneous remissions are found in the literature, it is difficult to say anything definite about the duration of the disease. No cases are on record of patients dying from heat urticaria, so that the disease must be viewed as noxious, but with no consequences for life expectancy.

5.10.10 Pathogenesis

Relationship to IgE and allergy

Althoug patients with heat urticaria and their families have an increased incidence of allergy (42 %), there are no indications that allergy and heat urticaria have a common link. Allergic symptoms and increased reactivity to heat do not start at the same time. Serum IgE levels are generally not elevated above controls, and despite numerous attempts, it has never been possible to positively transfer heat urticaria with patient serum to healthy primate subjects (Michaelsson and Ros 1971, de Moragas et al. 1973, Tennenbaum and Lowney 1973, Greaves et al. 1974, Willis and Epstein 1974, Wüthrich 1979). It is therefore unlikely that specific IgE antibodies or other types of antibodies are involved in the pathogenesis of the disease.

There is controversy in the literature even about the possible involvement of mast cells or basophils, of the mediators derived from these cells, and of the complement system. The problem can partly be resolved only by postulating that heat urticaria is evoked by at least two distinct pathomechanisms. The characteristic features of these two types are listed in Table 5.10.

Heat urticaria, type I (mast cells, histamine)

Evidence for in vivo mast cell and basophil degranulation has been provided in the familial type of heat urticaria (Michaelsson and Ros 1971). Morphological examinations of these cells have been done in other patients with elevated serum histamine levels. Greaves et al. (1974) tried to induce basophil histamine release after a 15-min exposure of these cells to 37–49° C temperatures, but he observed no differences between the patient and the controls. This suggests that heat causes the generation of an additional substance in either skin or plasma which is able to cause mediator release from mast cells and basophils.

Table 5.10. Differentiation of heat urticaria into two distinct types, on the basis of the pathomechanisms described in different patients.

Features	Type I	Type II
Effector cells	mast cells and basophils	unknown
Mast cell mediators in serum or tissue	a) histamine b) additional smooth muscle contracting activity (SRS?) c) neutrophil chemotactic factor	none
Change in complement components	none	↓ CH50 ↓ C3 –/↓ factor B –/↓ Cl inhibitor
Response decreased after local 48/80 or after systemic antihistamine treatment	yes	no

Increased levels of histamine have been demonstrated in perfusates of heat-induced urticae (Greaves et al. 1974) and in the venous effluent of a heat-challenged arm, with peak levels at 5–15 min and slight elevations even at 60 min (Irwin et al. 1984). An additional, non-histamine, smooth muscle contracting activity was identified in skin perfusates (Greaves et al. 1974). As a third mediator that may be involved in the pathogenesis, Atkins and Zweiman (1981) measured elevated levels of a high molecular weight neutrophil chemotatic factor which was released, together with histamine, into the venous effluent of a heat-challenged arm.

Further evidence that histamine plays a role in type I heat urticaria comes from a decrease or a suppression of the wheals after prior local injection or systemic therapy with antihistamines (Michaelsson and Ros 1971, Greaves et al. 1974, Wise et al. 1978, Wüthrich 1979, Johansson et al. 1984). Irwin et al. (1984) reported poor control of the whealing with H1 or H2 antagonists alone, but a combination of both was effective.

Some authors took great care to demonstrate that no changes occurred in total hemolytic complement or in the individual components of the complement system in their patients after heat challenge (Grant et al. 1981, Irwin et al. 1984).

Heat urticaria type II (complement-mediated)

In this group of patients, evidence has been provided that mast cell degranulation and release of mast cell mediators might not be involved in heat urticaria. Indirect proof was given by Leigh and Ramsay (1975) when they elicited wheals in response to heat in areas that had been sufficiently pretreated with compound 48/80 to empty mast cell mediator stores. Conversely, 48/80 caused whealing in skin that had been made tolerant to heat stimulation. Additional circumstantial evidence for no mast cell involvement comes from the relative ineffectiveness of treatment with antihistamines (Willis and Epstein 1974, Atkins and Zweiman 1981), even when H1 and H2 antagonists are combined (Starr et al. 1980). Daman et al. (1978) reported on a patient with heat urticaria and unusual clinical features: the lesions showed induration rather than whealing and were sensitive to touch rather than pruritic. Biopsy specimens of the heat-induced lesions showed venular endothelial cell edema and extravasation of red and white blood cells, but the peri-endothelial mast cells were intact. Serial plasma histamine levels of the venous effluent remained within normal limits, whereas total hemolytic complement dropped, reaching a nadir of 24.6 units/ml 15 min after challenge. C3 levels became subnormal, and factor B became undetectable, but C4 and C5 concentrations remained normal. Complement activation via the alternate pathway was therefore the major pathogenetic event in this patient's skin on heat contact.

The patient of Johansson et al. (1984) resembles the patient of Daman et al. (1978) by the rapid drop of serum factor B on heat exposure, although no other changes in complement components or a deposition of such factors in skin biopsies were detected. In contrast, the patient of Wüthrich (1979) had normal C3 proactivator levels and a decrease of total C3, C4, and the C1 inhibitor, suggesting activation via the classical rather than the alternate pathway.

De Moragas et al. (1973) made an additional intriguing observation. They noted that heat contact failed to elicit whealing if the circulation to the challenged skin had been blocked with an inflated cuff. An urticarial reaction developed however at the site 2 min after release of the pressure and return of the circulation. Complement levels were not measured, but some circulating factor was evidently necessary to produce the lesions.

Conclusions

The local application of heat in patients with heat urticaria results therefore in the formation of a new molecule or of a molecule that is altered by heat in the challenged tissue or in the blood. This molecule is in turn able to activate complement via either pathway, resulting in the generation of anaphylatoxins and subsequent tissue edema. In other patients, a molecule is generated after heat exposure that causes primarily mast cell and basophil histamine release, with the same clinical results.

5.11 Aquagenic Urticaria

5.11.1 General Aspects

This type of urticaria develops at sites of contact with water. Since its first description in 1964 by Shelley and Rawnsley, a total of 19 cases have been reported in the literature. The majority of the patients are females, with the age of onset ranging from 7 to 45 years (mean 18 years). The condition can persist for up to 23 years (see Table 5.1).

Predisposing factors or diseases are not known. One older patient developed lesions that were localized to the area of exposure to hydrochloric acid and potash within hours after an industrial accident (Chalamidas and Charles 1971).

In three instances, a familial occurrence was observed (father-son; aunt-niece; three sisters) (Shelley and Rawnsley 1964, Bonnetblanc et al. 1979, own observation).

Associated dermographic urticaria was found in three and cholinergic urticaria in one patient (Shelley and Rawnsley 1964, Bonnetblanc et al. 1979, Davis et al. 1981). Psychogenic influences are not apparent (Chalamidas and Charles 1971).

5.11.2 Clinical Findings (see Table 5.3)

Patients complain about the development of lesions after contact with water while bathing, showering, swimming, or water-skiing. Sweating may also cause the eruption 5–10 min after exposure to water. Highly pruritic, small, papular wheals with surrounding erythema develop exactly at the site of contact. The lesions have an appearance identical to the wheals in cholinergic urticaria. They reach their maximal size and intensity by 30 min and decrease after another 1/2 to 1 h. Some authors have noted a follicular distribution of the wheals, others not. The exposed area remains refractory to further stimulation for a period of several hours. Some patients experience only pruritus without visible lesions on contact with water (Greaves et al. 1981).

The preferential localization of wheals after exposure of the entire body surface is on the trunk and neck, less so on shoulders and thighs, with sparing of palms and soles, exactly as in cholinergic urticaria. All laboratory values are normal, except for an elevated IgM, noted in one patient by Bonnetblanc et al. (1979). Systemic symptoms are not recorded in the literature.

5.11.3 Diagnosis and Differential Diagnosis

There are two methods of testing for aquagenic urticaria. The simplest one is to have the patient take a bath (35–36° C) for 30–40 min. Care must be taken that the urticae are restricted to the area of contact on subsequent examination of the patient.

Illig and Kunick (1969) suggested that a wet compress, such as a towel, soaked preferably in physiologic saline, be placed over the back for 40 min, with a thermometer placed inside its folds and a warm water bottle on top. The temperature should be maintained at 35–36° C. This will help to prevent confusion of the condition with cholinergic, heat contact, or cold contact urticaria.

Tests for other types of physical urticaria should be performed, such as for cholinergic urticaria, heat contact, cold contact, and dermographic urticaria.

5.11.4 Pathogenesis

The cause of aquagenic urticaria, whether physical or chemical, is unknown. An IgE-dependent reaction is apparently not involved since the Prausnitz-Küstner test was negative in the patient examined (Chalamidas and Charles 1971). Initially, the condition was confused with cholinergic urticaria, until Shelley and Rawnsley (1964) showed convincingly that contact with water or sweat was essential. Coating the skin with lanolin prevented the eruption.

The stimulus for elicitation of the lesions seems to be related to water alone, regardless of its source. Distilled water, tap, sea, and spring water were equally effective (Shelley and Rawnsley 1964, Bonnetblanc et al. 1979). The temperature of the water is unimportant (Tronovitch 1967), but pH optima were found at 5.0 and 8.0 in one case (Chalamidas and Charles 1971). Reactions to benzene, ethyl alcohol, or gasoline were negative (Chalamidas and Charles 1971), but acetone was enhancing (Sibbald et al. 1981), probably by improving absorption through the epidermis. The same phenomenon was noted by the latter authors after stripping of the epidermis, probably also due to better penetration of water into the skin. Shelley and

Rawnsley (1964) believed that water had to combine with sebum to produce a histamine liberating substance which would penetrate preferentially through the follicle, accounting for the perifollicular arrangement of the lesions. This concept was supported by the observation of Chalamidas and Charles (1971) that a mixture of sebum and sweat is more effective than sweat alone. Sibbald et al. (1981) proposed instead that acetylcholine is necessary for the production of the lesions since locally applied scopolamine partly suppressed the whealing. This possibility is attractive because of the close morphological resemblance of the lesions in aquagenic and cholinergic urticaria.

Mediator release from mast cells seems to be the final step that results in production of lesions. Increased levels of histamine have been measured in the blood after challenge (Davis et al. 1981, Sibbald et al. 1981), and a variable release of mast cell granules has been observed by the latter authors in lesional biopsies, in association with dermal edema. H1 antihistamines have been found to suppress, at least in part, both the symptoms and the size of the test reactions in all patients, although the participation of other mediators remains a possibility.

6 Contact Urticaria

6.1 General Aspects and Classification

Contact urticaria designates a local immediate and/or delayed urticarial reaction, with swelling and redness at sites of epidermal or transepidermal contact with certain agents. Generalized cutaneous reactions, rhinitis, asthma, or anaphylactic reactions may be associated. Contact urticaria differs thus from other types of urticaria by the route of access of the antigen or the noxious agent to the body: It penetrates transepidermally, whereas the more common mode of absorption of urticarial substances is transmucosal, via the respiratory or gastrointestinal tract.

Although some authors consider contact urticaria rare (Lahti 1980), it is the oldest form of urticaria recorded in writing (the association of nettles and urticaria was discussed in the Greek literature more than 2000 years ago). In the broadest sense, most of the physical urticarias and all immediate type skin test reactions should also be classified as contact urticaria. They, however, are dealt with separately in Chapters 3, p. 26 and 5, p. 55.

In recent years, increased attention has focused on contact urticaria because of its potential significance in occupational medicine and in the drug and food industries. The list of agents that can cause contact urticaria increases from year to year, with the eliciting substances ranging from vasoactive amines in stinging plants and animals, to plant and animal antigens, chemicals, foods, food additives, industrial contactants, and products of the drug and cosmetic industries.

Fisher (1973) classified contact urticaria on the basis of its pathogenesis as either allergic or non-allergic. Maibach and Johnson (1975) added a third category which they designated "uncertain mechanism contact urticaria." The same authors classified contact urticaria on the basis of the extent of its clinical manifestations as: (1) contact urticaria localized to the site of application of the antigen, (2) contact urticaria with angioedema, (3) contact urticaria with asthma, (4) contact urticaria with anaphylactoid reactions. Later on, Von Krogh and Maibach (1981) modified this scheme to include generalized urticaria and rhinoconjunctivitis as a fifth type (Table 6.1). The usefulness of this clinical classification derives from its emphasis on the potentially generalized character of contact urticaria, but it offers no additional help in the understanding of the disease.

Table 6.1. Distribution of symptoms (percent) in 86 patients with contact urticaria (adapted from Von Krogh and Maibach 1981).

	By history	On skin testing
I. Cutaneous reactions		
1. localized urticaria	9%	93%
2. generalized urticaria	41%	9%
II. Extracutaneous reactions		
1. bronchial asthma	8%	2%
2. rhinoconjunctivitis	7%	1%
3. otolaryngeal symptoms	2%	1%
4. gastrointestinal symptoms	8%	3%
5. anaphylactoid reactions	2%	2%

In the subsequent discussion of contact urticaria, it has been considered more expedient to divide the disease into (1) immunologically mediated contact urticaria, (2) contact urticaria induced by histamine liberators, (3) venom-induced contact urticaria, and (4) contact urticaria due to unknown mechanisms.

6.2 Clinical Manifestations

6.2.1 Local Appearance, Time Course, and Histology

The basic clinical appearance of the primary lesion of contact urticaria, a wheal and a surrounding erythema, does not differ from that of other types of urticaria (Fig. 6.1). The conformation of the wheal, however, varies with the type of contactant. Thus, wheals caused by nettles will be linearly arranged if the plant has hit the skin with a stroke. The wheals are punctate and arise exactly at sites where the stinging hairs have penetrated the skin (Fig. 6.2). The shape of the wheals can change with time, very intense reactions resulting in confluent lesions with pseudopods (Fig. 2.1, p. 5). Wheals can also start in a follicular pattern (like goose-flesh) if the contactant penetrates more readily through the hair follicles (Herrmann et al. 1944, Lahti 1980). The associated local symptoms are tingling, itching, and in extremely strong reactions, burning at the sites of the wheal. Burning of the lips may occur when patients react to food (Hannuksela 1980).

Lesions start with redness at the site of contact, followed by whealing at the same site within 10–30 min after contact. The maximal size is reached 45 min afterward, and within 2 h, the swelling disappears, although redness usually persists for up to 6 h. Occasionally, whealing can persist for more than 24 h (Lahti 1980).

As with other types of urticaria, contact urticaria can reappear after 4–6 h. This dual whealing response has been demonstrated experimentally in the ears of BALB/c mice, and only recently in humans (Ray et al. 1983). Delayed onset contact urticaria, as described by Anderson and Maibach (1984), refers to immediate reactions after repeated applications of the agent to the skin over several days.

The time course and intensity of contact urticaria lesions differ depending on the nature of the eliciting agent. This variability may also be due to differences in the reactivity of the cells which secrete the vasoactive amines or to the sensitivity of the target tissue to the mediators or chemicals released.

The histology of the immediate contact wheal has been reported only once in the literature for a case of contact urticaria due to benzocaine gel (Ryan et al. 1980). The authors noted a mild perivascular neutrophil infiltrate in the upper dermis. Immunofluorescence did not reveal deposits of IgG, IgM, IgA, IgE, C3, or fibrin.

6.2.2 Systemic Symptoms

Generalized urticaria occurs in almost half of the patients with contact urticaria (Table 6.1), and an associated eczematous dermatitis is noted with about the same frequency (Von Krogh and Maibach 1981). Only a few patients react with extracutaneous symptoms. Possible sites and the frequency of occurrence of the different types of systemic reactions are listed in Table 6.1. Often, several target organs react simultaneously, the combination of asthma and rhinitis with urticaria being particularly common (Bernstein et al. 1983). Vascular collapse occurs in highly sensitized individuals (Schechter et al. 1984), particularly when the eliciting agent has been applied topically with occlusion (Von Krogh and Maibach 1981). Fortunately, this is an extremely rare event.

6.3 Immunologically Mediated Contact Urticaria

In this type of contact urticaria, the patient's immune system has been sensitized through previous contact with the eliciting agent. Of the many causative agents reported in the literature until now (Table 6.2), involvement of IgE antibodies has been proven in only a few cases by passive transfer of a heat labile serum factor to the skin of a healthy subject or by the RAST technique. The latter provides more exact proof of IgE-dependent mechanisms since cytolytic antibodies of the IgG-type might also yield positive transfer tests.

Non-antibody mediated, delayed type immunologi-

Table 6.2. Causative agents of contact urticaria via proven or strongly implied immunological mechanisms (Lahti 1980, Fisher 1973).

Foods and plants	Textiles	Animals	Medications	Industrial agents
fish, lobster	perlon	hair	estrogen creams	platinum salts
chicken, lamb, turkey	wool	saliva	menthol	acrylic monomers
eggs	silk	danders	ethyl and stearyl alcohols	alipathic polyamide
potatoes		stinging insects	penicillin G	aminothiazole
carrots		cockroaches	gentamicin	ammonia
apples		cow placenta	streptomycin	castor bean
lettuce, endives		seminal fluid (human)	neomycin	lindane
wheat flour			cephalosporins	sodium sulfide
pollens		serum	aspirin	sulfur dioxide
algae, lichens			tetanus antitoxin	formaldehyde
spices			benzophenone	teak
alcohol			mechlorethamine hydrochloride	terpinyl acetate
stinging plants			chlorpromazine	rubber
poison ivy			promethazine hydrochloride	mealworm
perfumes			cod-liver oil	phenylmercuric proprionate
			monoamylamine	exotic woods
			diethyltoluamide	
			aminophenazone	
			polyethylene glycol	
			polysorbate 60	
			bacitracin	

cal reactions can coexist together with contact urticaria and can be diagnosed by the clinical appearance of the reaction and its delayed time course. Ryan et al. (1980) reported the simultaneous occurrence of contact urticaria and delayed dermatitis at skin test sites to ethylaminobenzoate gel and benzocaine; contact urticaria alone developed at test sites to which cyclomethycaine and dibucaine had been applied. Hand eczema was present in three housewives who had positive contact urticaria tests, intradermal tests, and RASTs to raw prawns and shrimp (Nagano et al. 1984). However, the frequent presence of histamine liberators, histamine itself, and antigens in antigen extracts, especially in food extracts and wasp and bee venoms (Jacques and Schacter 1954, Haberman 1972), makes it extremely difficult to decide, on chemical grounds along, whether a true allergy to the antigen exists if the reaction remains localized.

Foods are the most frequent causative agents of immunologically mediated contact urticaria (Hannuksela 1980) (Table 6.2). In two-thirds of the patients who react to birch pollen, a coexistent allergy is found against carrots, celery, potatoes, and apples (Hannuksela and Lahti 1977). The exact antigen in these foods has not been isolated; but a protein and a glycoprotein have been identified as common immunoreactants in apples and carrots (Lahti and Hannuksela 1978). A possible involvement of IgE in potato allergy was shown in 1942 by passive transfer (Tuft and Blumenstein 1942). Even though the allergen extracts from birch pollen, hazelnut, potato, and apple showed no cross-reactivity by immunoelectrophoresis (Anderson and Lowenstein 1978), more recent evidence obtained by IgE RAST technique suggests a cross-reactivity of the antigens (Kalveram et al. 1984). The list of agents which can elicit immunologic contact urticaria is long (Table 6.2). This should however not be misleading as regards clinical significance, since many of them have been described in only one single patient. Agents not mentioned in the exhaustively referenced table by Lahti (1980) include contact urticaria of one patient each to parabens in drugs, cosmetics, and foods (Henry et al. 1979), to most primary alcohols in another patient (Rilliet et al. 1980) and to wheat bran bath (Langeland and Nyrud 1982). Bernstein et al. (1983) described four bait handlers with proven IgE-mediated contact urticaria, asthma, and rhinitis to the exoskeleton of mealworms.

6.4 Contact Urticaria due to Histamine Liberators

For many years it has been established that certain chemicals can induce histamine release from mast cells on direct contact of the cells with the respective substances (Kallos and Kallos 1980). Such reagents include foreign serum, egg white, shellfish, mussel, strawberries, toxins, venoms, mellitin, phospholipase A_2, anaphylatoxins, curare, morphine, codeine, succinylcholine, polymyxin B, bacitracin, and stilbamidine, to name only a few. Some of these agents are only weak histamine liberators, and some are species specific. Only a few of them have any significance at all as causative agents of contact urticaria since their route of administration is not via the skin.

One of the best known histamine liberators is compound 48/80, a condensation product of phenylethylamine (Paton 1951). It is a potent as polymyxin B and acts only on mast cells. In vivo, it can be used to demonstrate whether cutaneous mast cells are able to release histamine and whether mediator stores are intact. A single intracutaneous injection of 0.1 mg of compound 48/80 causes marked whealing, possibly even with pseudopod formation (Fig. 2.1, p. 5), in all normal individuals. If the same do is injected four times daily on two consecutive days into the same skin site, all local histamine stores will be depleted for up to 24 h thereafter.

To prove that an agent that induces contact urticaria is also a true histamine liberator, the following criteria should be met:

1) Whealing should occur in all persons, regardless of previous sensitization, on first contact with the skin.
2) The agent should no longer be effective after application to the skin that has been pretreated by repeated injections of compound 48/80.
3) Whealing of the skin on contact should be diminished or absent after local and systemic treatment with H1 histamine antagonists.
4) A less stringently required criterion is the morphological demonstration of mast cell degranulation.

So far, these criteria have only been met for topically applied dimethyl sulfoxide (DMSO) (Kligman 1965) and for cobalt chloride (Lahti 1980).

6.5 Venom-Induced Contact Urticaria

Plants and animals can elicit wheal and flare reactions on contact with human skin, mostly by piercing the skin with specialized stings or hairs. With rare exceptions, the exact composition of the injected material is not known. Many venoms contain a mixture of substances which belong primarily to the following groups of substances: (1) toxins which can damage muscles or nerves, (2) antigens that affect previously sensitized individuals only, and (3) histamine and other vasoactive amines or histamine

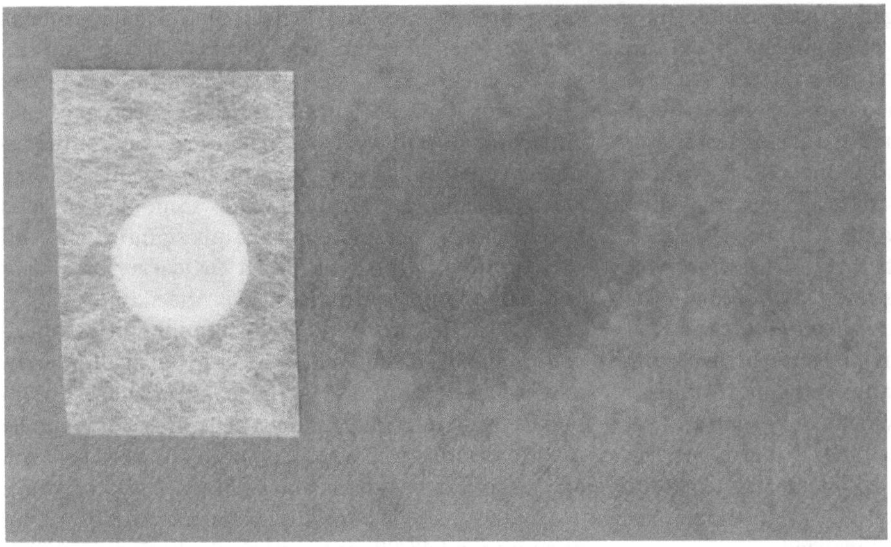

Fig. 6.1. Contact urticaria which developed 30 min after application of dimethylsulfoxide (100%). A Finn Chamber (Hermal Chemie, Hamburg) is in place to illustrate the test procedure.

liberators. The latter group of compounds aids in the transport of antigens and toxins into the body by causing local vasodilatation and increased vascular permeability.

Among the stinging plants, there are four main genera with stinging hairs, the urticaceae (nettles), the euphorbiaceae, the loasaceae, and the hydrophyllaceae. The hairs of nettles have been studies best. Emmelin and Feldberg (1947) isolated histamine, acetylcholine, and an unidentified additional smooth muscle contracting substance from nettle hair. Lower amounts of histamine and acetylcholine were also found in the leaves of the nettle plants. Thurston and Lersten (1969) showed that serotonin, formic acid, acetic acid, tartaric acid, resin acid, and calcium were also present in the stinging hairs of plants. In nettles, only one of three types of hairs contains the vasoactive amines. On contact with skin, the stings penetrate, break off, and inject their contents like a hypodermic needle into the dermis.

A wide spectrum of marine animals and plants can induce localized or generalized contact urticaria. The most well-known are the Portugese man-of-war and a variety of jellyfish which release toxins from their tentacles. IgE is involved in some of these reactions (Burnett and Calton 1981, Togias et al. 1985). Seabather's eruptions in saltwater and schistosome-induced swimmer's itch in fresh water present mostly as pruritic papules, but occasionally also as urticae. Pteropods, sponges, and seaweed are the cause of urticarial eruptions in some regions of the world (Fisher 1973).

Arthropods include a wide array of stinging species. Certain caterpillars, such as the puss caterpillar,

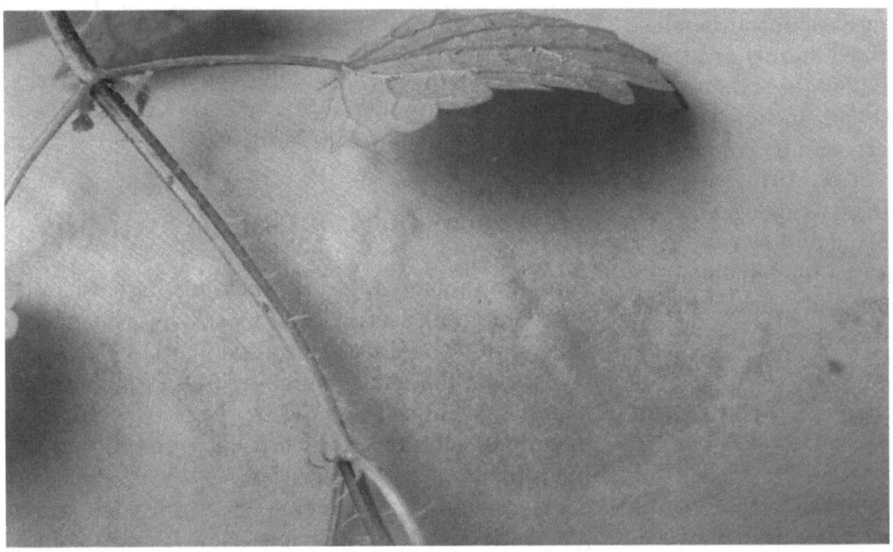

Fig. 6.2. Punctate wheals with surrounding flare after contact with the fine hairs of a nettle.

Megalopyge opercularis, and moths, such as the browntail moth, Euproctis phaeorrhea, have venomous, bristly hairs or spines (Fisher 1973). Bees, wasps, hornets, bedbugs, fleas, mosquitoes, human and animal mites (Dorrestein and Van Bronswijk 1979), and ants produce a wheal at sites of a sting or of the penetration of the animal through the skin. After disappearance of the wheal, a pruritic papule can persist at the sites of bites for many weeks, particularly if foreign material is left behind in the tissue.

6.6 Contact Urticaria due to Unknown Mechanisms

All substances that have been reported to cause contact urticaria which cannot be classified in the three previously discussed groups, are put into this category. None of them shows evidence for a specific immunologically mediated reaction, for a direct release of mast cell mediators, or for a pharmacological effect on the cutaneous vasculature.

The classical chemical among this group is tetrahydrofurfuryl ester of nicotinic acid (Trafuril, Ciba-Geigy, Basel, Switzerland). This agent was used three decades ago as a rubefacient in inflammatory joint diseases. It caused a local hyperemic reaction with or without edema on the skin of almost all subjects to whom it was applied (Schneider 1953, Vaillancourt 1954). The dermal reaction is histamine-independent and possibly due to a direct effect of Trafuril on the dermal vessels (Strehler 1949).

Lahti (1980) published the most thorough, recent investigation on a long list of potentially causative agents of contact urticaria of unknown cause. Although he tried to elucidate the mechanisms involved, many aspects remain unclear (see 6.7). Almost 40% of his 103 test subjects reacted to benzoic acid and to cinnamic acid (5% in petrolatum), while only 14% reacted to the same concentration of sorbic acid. The percentage of persons with immediate urticarial reactions was lower with sodium benzoate, acetic acid, ethyl alcohol, butyric acid, and butyl alcohol.

Benzoic acid is present in balsam of Peru and in many oils, flowers, spices, and berries. Sorbic acid is also found in berries. Cinnamic acid is a constituent of oils of basil, cinnamon, coca leaves, and balsam of Peru. Benzoic acid, sodium benzoate, and sorbic acid are widely used as additives in food and medications and act as preservatives because of their antibacterial and antifungal properties. Cinnamic acid is added to foods for flavoring at lower than 2% concentrations.

Lahti's observations that common food additives and preservatives can cause contact urticaria are supported by a number of case reports in the literature (see Lahti 1980, for review). Other agents that provoke contact urticaria by unknown mechanisms should be mentioned because of their importance in everday life. Ammonium persulfate, used as a bleach by hairdressers, has repeatedly been reported to cause contact urticaria (Calnan and Shuster 1963, Brubaker 1972, Fisher and Dooms-Goossens 1976). Polyethylene glycols of low molecular weight which are used exclusively as solvents in topical medications, can cause contact urticaria or eczema (Fisher 1978). Nickel and components of plastics (polyethylene, polyvinylchloride, and butylhydroxytoluene) have been reported to elicit immediate urticarial reactions (Osmundsen 1980). Ramsay et al. (1972) observed contact urticaria to benzophenones which are used widely as sunscreens in textiles, plastics, paints, and cosmetics, and Bjorkner (1980) reported a patient who reacted to denatonium benzoate (Bitrex) which is added to insecticides and alcoholic skin desinfectants as a denaturing agent. Formaldehyde in leather clothing can present a problem as a contactant with urticarial reactions (Helander 1977). Finally, fiberglass dermatitis should be mentioned because it can be associated with urticaria as well as with a papular rash (Emmett 1983). The same is true for reactions to wool, silk, and nylon (Hatch and Maibach 1985).

6.7 Pathomechanisms of Contact Urticaria

6.7.1 Mechanism of Release

There are three possible major pathomechanisms which underly the development of contact urticaria (see Table 6.3).

As in all types of urticaria, the mast cell is the central effector cell in contact urticaria. Release of its mediators can occur through IgE-dependent mechanisms or through a direct effect of eliciting agents on the mast cell membrane.

Ray et al. (1983) have shown that BALB/c mice

Table 6.3. Possible pathomechanisms underlying the development of contact urticaria.

I. Mast cell-induced contact urticaria
   1. IgE-dependent release of mediators
   2. Non-specific release through histamine liberators
II. Contact whealing through application of vasoactive mediators
III. Mast cell-independent contact urticaria due to release of mediators other than vasoactive amines

which had been passively sensitized with monoclonal IgE-anti-dinitrophenyl antibody 48 h before challenge, developed immediate and delayed ear swelling on application of the reactive hapten, 2,4-dinitrofluorobenzene. IgE dependency in patients with contact urticaria was also proven by the RAST technique, and in former years, by passive transfer of the contact sensitivity with a heat-labile factor from patients' serum to the skin of healthy individuals.

Mast cells also release their mediators through mechanisms other than membrane-bound IgE and its interaction with specific antibody (see Chapter 2.2, p. 6). Basic polypeptides, compound 48/80, and mellitin in bee venom are thought to bind to receptor structures on the mast cell membrane and thus "short-circuit" the complicated IgE-dependent release (Stanworth 1980).

Dimethylsulfoxide acts most likely even less specifically than histamine liberators. It is a potent lipid solvent, a property which facilitates its excellent penetration through the epidermis and also its ability to disturb the lipid bilayer of the mast cell membrane. A rapid and efficient histamine release into the tissue results.

6.7.2 Mediators Involved in Contact Urticaria

Vasoactive mediators are undoubtedly involved in contact urticaria since their direct application to the skin occurs in venom-induced contact urticarias (see 6.5, p. 91). Apart from the classical vasoactive amines, there is recent evidence that contact urticaria can also be induced by mediators from cells other than mast cells. Lahti (1980) showed that after depletion of mast cell mediator stores with compound 48/80, there was still a local urticarial reaction to benzoic acid. Conversely, after repeated application of benzoic acid and a subsequent local unresponsiveness to this chemical, dermographic whealing could still be elicited at the same site. One must assume that mediators with vasoactive properties from sources other than mast cells are generated on contact with benzoic acid. Possible candidates are prostaglandins, bradykinin, leukotriene (SRS-A) and PAF which can be generated from resident cells in epidermis and dermis (see Chapter 2.3, p. 13). C5a or chemotactic arachidonate metabolites may be involved in the rapid accumulation of neutrophils at sites of contact urticaria.

6.7.3 Local Factors Important for Development of Contact Urticaria

A molecule can act not only on vessels directly or through mediator release, but its ability to cause a local wheal and the strength of this reaction depend on a number of other factors:

1) the penetrability of the molecule through the epidermal barrier,
2) the density of local mast cells, and
3) the reactivity of the dermal vessels.

The problem of penetration is circumvented in the case of stinging plants and animals. In all other instances, the epidermal barrier must be overcome. The efficiency of this process depends on the thickness of the epidermis, on the permeability of the skin, and on the vehicle. Contact urticaria can be more easily elicited at sites where the stratum corneum is thinner or where more hair follicles are present (Lahti 1980). The early follicular whealing observed with some chemicals may be due to their more rapid penetration along the hair follicles. A carefully chosen vehicle can result in contact urticarial reactions to allergens which correspond to intracutaneously elicited reactions with aqueous vehicles.

The barrier function of the stratum corneum is not always important for penetration. Lahti (1980) observed that benzoic acid induces contact urticaria equally well in stripped and intact skin. This shows that properties of the molecule itself are important for penetration. Acids are generally better contact urticants than their corresponding alcohols or salts. Not all acids are, however, contact urticants. Wheal and flare reactions are, for example, not elicited by lactic acid or by citric acid (Lahti 1980).

As a final note of interest, the atopic state has no influence on the reactivity of skin to contact urticants such as benzoic acid, in contrast to most other types of contact urticaria (Lahti 1980, Von Krogh and Maibach 1981). Furthermore, a positive oral challenge reaction does not correlate with the cutaneous test reaction of the same patient to agents such as benzoic acid (Lahti 1980).

6.8 Diagnosis of Contact Urticaria

The basic requirement for the recognition of contact urticaria is the appearance of the local reaction and the confirmation of this diagnosis by skin tests.

6.8.1 Clinical Diagnosis

Although the typical wheal and flare reaction is hardly missed by the observer, difficulties in the diagnosis may arise if the patient does not remember that a specific contactant was applied to the skin shortly before the wheal appeared. An associated dermatitis may also hide the whealing reaction. Pressure urticaria and erysipelas have to be considered in the differential diagnosis of contact urticaria, particularly when the lesions are large and the swellings deep. If generalized urticaria or other systemic symptoms are present, contact urticaria is easily missed as the primary eliciting factor, unless the patient recalls the specific event that led to its development.

6.8.2 Diagnostic Skin Tests

The diagnosis of contact urticaria should be confirmed by skin tests with the suspected agent. The technique is the same as for routine patch testing (Fig. 6.1). Antigens need to be applied at times for only 1 min in highly allergic individuals, whereas chemicals need 15–30 min. Readings should be taken immediately, after 30–45 min, and again after 6–8 h in order to diagnose a late urticarial response. A final examination of the test site should occur at 24 and 48 h because of a possibly coexistent allergic contact dermatitis.

Open patch tests should be preferred initially since they yield more positive responses than closed tests (Lahti 1980), and since systemic anaphylaxis is less likely to occur in highly sensitized individuals. Scratch, prick, and intracutaneous tests are recommended when food proteins are suspected as allergens (Hannuksela 1980), but they carry a higher risk of severe reactions, and their clinical relevance is questionable.

If epicutaneous tests are negative on normal skin and if the index of suspicion is high, testing should be repeated on previously involved skin and even on skin that is still inflamed. Two case reports in the literature involved one patient each who responded to meat and flour (Maibach 1976) and to sorbic acid in shampoo and toothpaste (Rietschel 1978) only on the previously involved skin.

Not all regions of the body are equally prone to develop wheals on contact, and for this reason, only the back, the upper arm, the thigh, and the extensor part of the lower arm should be used for testing (Lahti 1980). Furthermore, the vehicle in which the test substance is suspended is important. Alcoholic suspensions yield more rapidly developing, transient wheals, while more lasting reactions are induced when petrolatum is used as a vehicle (Von Krogh and Maibach 1981).

6.8.3 Further Diagnostic Tests

If the mechanism of whealing is suspected to be IgE-mediated and appropriate technology is available, RAST tests can be performed on the serum of the patients to identify specific immunoglobulins of the IgE-type. Total IgE measurements are of little diagnostic help since the incidence of atopy and of elevated serum IgE is not increased in contact urticaria patients (Lahti 1980, Von Krogh and Maibach 1981).

Passive transfer tests (Prausnitz-Küstner reaction) are only of limited interest since they do not allow for the identification of the exact mechanism involved in the urticarial reaction. Furthermore, they carry the risk of transferring infectious diseases to normal persons. Tests to identify the mediators involved by pretreatment of the test site with antihistamines and by depletion of histamine stores with compound 48/80 are also only of scientific interest and do not elucidate the exact pathomechanisms involved.

7 Anaphylactoid Reactions

7.1 Definition

With recent advances in the understanding of the immunological basis of urticaria, it has become apparent that certain chemicals elicit allergic reactions by non-immunological mechanisms (see Chapter 2, p. 5). Since any of the major types of immunological reactions can be mimicked by chemicals, the term pseudo-allergic reactions (PAR) was coined by P. Dukor, P. Kallòs, H.D. Schlumberger, and G.B. West (1980). Their view of this problem is thoroughly discussed in a three-volume series with the same title. In the American literature, the term idiosyncratic has also been used (Farr 1970), but it seems somewhat clumsy. For urticarial reactions of the pseudoallergic type, the term anaphylactoid reactions seems most appropriate since it refers to the specific immunologic type of pseudoallergic reactions that is mimicked clinically. The term intolerance reaction has also been in common usage for many years, particularly in connection with aspirin.

In keeping with their non-immunological nature, a further characteristic of anaphylactoid reactions is the fact that they can be elicited on first contact of the organism with a specific chemical (Table 7.1). A preceding sensitizing period is thus not necessary. The reaction is also not restricted to a specific chemical structure since chemically unrelated agents often cause ("cross"-) reactions in the same individual. Most patients have tolerated the eliciting agents throughout their youth, and many of them go into spontaneous remission after some years.

7.2 Classification

The most common type of anaphylactoid reaction is the intolerance to aspirin and other nonsteroidal anti-inflammatory drugs (Table 7.2). Aspirin intolerant patients also react at times to dyes and preservatives which have been added to or are naturally present in food, although aspirin intolerance is not a prerequisite for anaphylactoid reactions to dyes and preservatives. Other types of agents that cause anaphylactoid reactions are X-ray contrast media, colloidal plasma expanders, anesthetics, and a miscellaneous group of drugs (Table 7.2). Histamine liberators from mast cells should also be classified under this heading, although this is not generally done. These agents have been discussed in Chapter 2, p. 5.

Intolerance reactions can also be classified on the basis of their major organ manifestations (Table 7.3). Some patients react primarily with bronchospasms, and if asthma is already present, it is severely worsened. Up to 10% of these patients also have urticaria and/or angioedema. Patients who react primarily with cutaneous lesions can do so de novo or as an exacerbation of a preexisting urticaria which may be mild or even latent. Szczeklik et al. (1977) further subdivide the patients who react with urticaria into those who respond to either prostaglandin

Table 7.1. Basic characteristics of anaphylactoid reactions caused by certain chemicals.

Clinical signs of anaphylactic reactions
Lack of immunological specificity and transferability (non-IgE mediated)
Dosis dependence
Symptoms can arise on first contact of the chemical with the individual in therapeutic concentrations
Chemically unrelated agents often cause the same reactions in the individual
Skin tests are mostly not of diagnostic value

Table 7.2. Classification of anaphylactoid reactions on the basis of eliciting agents.

Antiphlogistics (prototype: aspirin)
Food additives (dyes and preservatives)
X-ray contrast media
Colloidal plasma expanders
Anesthetics
Miscellaneous drugs

Table 7.3. Classification of anaphylactoid reactions on the basis of predominant organ involvement.

1. Bronchospastic reactions
a. primary, in healthy persons
b. in asthmatics
2. Urticarial reactions
a. primary, in healthy persons
b. in patients with urticaria (simple chronic or physical)

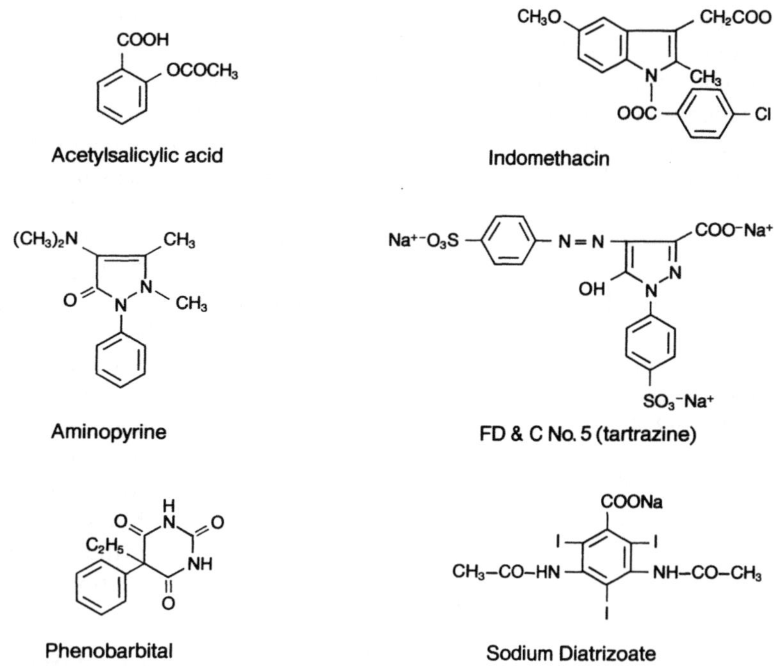

Fig. 7.1. Chemical structure of several types of agents frequently implicated in anaphylactoid reactions. Note that none share common structures even though patients can react to several of them.

synthetase inhibitors, like aspirin and indomethacin, or to pyrazolones, like aminopyrine (Fig. 7.1). In the latter group, the reactions often manifest themselves as cardiovascular shock. Pyrazolones do not "cross-react" with indomethacin or paracetamol. A third group of patients might be called "overreactors" since they react on oral challenge to almost any agent, even to placebo. A strong psychic component seems to be operative in these patients.

Doeglas (1975) made the interesting observation that 52% of patients with cholinergic urticaria, 43% with pressure urticaria, and 14% with dermographic urticaria reacted to oral aspirin challenge. Such reactions were extremely rare (0.01%) in heat contact and cold urticaria. In patients with mastocytosis, there is no increased incidence of aspirin intolerance, according to our own clinical experience, but if present, reactions are unusually severe (Moore-Robinson and Warin 1967, Waldenström 1980).

7.3 Epidemiological Aspects

The incidence of reactions to three major types of chemicals is shown in Table 7.4. Severe, life-threatening reactions occur far less frequently, for example only less than once in 1000 examinations with contrast media, compared to 2–8% of urticarial reactions to the same agents (Ansell 1970, Greenberger et al. 1984). The incidence of urticarial reactions that

Table 7.4. Incidence of anaphylactoid reactions to different agents.

Urticarial anaphylactoid reaction	Incidence	Reference
1. Aspirin-type intolerance		
a. urticaria patients	21–75%	Thune and Granholt 1975, Settipane et al. 1980
b. asthmatics	2–10%	Weber et al. 1979, Chafee and Settipane 1974
c. chronic rhinitis patients	0.7–2.4%	Chafee and Settipane 1974
d. normal population		
adults	3.8%	Settipane et al. 1980
children	0.3%	
2. X-ray contrast media	1.0–10.5%	Greenberger et al. 1984
3. Miscellaneous agents		
local and i.v. anesthetics	0.1–1%	Ring 1981
muscle relaxants	10–30%	
gelatin	1–15%	
fluoresceine and isotopic colloids	1–5%	

develop in patients who are known to suffer from chronic urticaria is strikingly high. Patients with chronic rhinitis, on the other hand, have no more reactions than the normal population. The incidence is however much higher in the so-called aspirin triad, a combination of intrinsic asthma, rhinitis with nasal polyps, and aspirin intolerance.

Table 7.4 also shows that adults react to aspirin more frequently than children. Most patients are 20–40 years old. The sex distribution is normal in children, whereas among adult asthmatics, females predominate (Schlumberger 1980). The data on the sex differences in intolerance urticaria differ from series to series (Doeglas 1975, Ros et al. 1976).

In all published patient series, there is no increased incidence of a positive family or a personal history of atopy. This has also been confirmed with skin tests to a battery of common allergens (Doeglas 1975, Krilis et al. 1981).

A positive family history for aspirin intolerance has been obtained in 3 of 40 patients in one series (Settipane and Pudupakkam 1975). In addition, there have been several reports of families with a markedly increased incidence of aspirin intolerance in more than one generation (Moore-Robinson and Warin 1967, Lockey et al. 1973, von Maur et al. 1974, Settipane and Pudupakkam 1975) (see also Chapter 7.7.4, p. 106 for further discussion of the genetics of anaphylactoid reactions).

Table 7.5. Drugs and chemicals reported to cause intolerance reactions, with agents more frequently implicated in italics (after Schlumberger 1983).

Acetaminophen	*Ketoprofen*
Acetanilid	*Mefenamic acid*
Acetylsalicylic acid free of ASAN[a]	Menthol
Amaranth	*Metamizol*
Aminopyrine	Methysergide
Antazoline	Morphine
Antipyrine	*Naproxene*
Barbiturates	New coccine
Bendroflumethiazole	Novobiocin
Butylhydroxybenzoic acid	Novocain
Butylhydroxytoluene	Parabens
Chloralhydrate	*Paracetamol*
Chlorthalidone	Phenacetine
Cinchophen	Penicillins
Cocaine	Pentazocine
Codeine	*Phenylbutazone*
Diclofenac	Phenylsalicylate
Diphenhydramine	Piroxicam
Dipyrone	Pontocaine
Epinephrine	Potaba
Eucalyptus	Premarin
FD&C red no 3	Probarbital
FD&C red no 4	Probenicid
FD&C yellow no 4	Procaine
FD&C yellow no 5	Prochlorperazine
FD&C yellow no 6	Propyphenazone
Fenoprofen	D-Propoxyphene
Flufenamic acid	Pyribenzamine
Glaphenine	Quinidine
Glutethimide	Quinine
L-Histidin	Quinoline yellow
Hydrocortisone	Recipavrin
4-Hydroxybenzoic acid	Sodium benzoate
2-Hydroxybenzyl alcohol	Sodium dehydrocholate
4-Hydroxybenzyl alcohol	Sodium salicylate
Ibuprofen	Strychnine
Indanthrene blue RS	Sulfamipyrine
Indigotin	Sulfonamides
Indomethacin	Tetrachloroterephthalic acid methyl ester
Iodide	*Tolmetin*
Iodine-containing agents	Xylocaine
Isoniazid	

[a] ASAN = acetylsalicylic acid anhydride.

7.4 Agents Eliciting Anaphylactoid Reactions

7.4.1 Analgesics

The list of drugs and chemicals reported to cause intolerance reactions is long (Table 7.5), although only a few of them can be implicated at a relatively high frequency as causes of clinical disease (in italics in Table 7.5).

The list is headed by aspirin as the most frequent cause of intolerance reactions. The first urticarial reaction to aspirin was observed 3 years after its introduction into clinical practice (Hirschberg 1902). Storm van Leeuwen (1928) noted concomitant reactivity to aminopyrine, antipyrine, and luminal in several of his aspirin intolerant patients. Many of the non-steroidal anti-inflammatory drugs which cause intolerance reactions are also prostaglandin-synthetase inhibitors. Pyrazolones (noramidopyrine, aminophenazones) do not, or only weakly, inhibit this enzyme (Szczeklik et al. 1977).

7.4.2 Preservatives and Colorings

Lockey (1959) made an important discovery which proved to be a valuable aid in the clarification of the etiology of many obscure cases of chronic urticaria. He observed that the analine dye FD & C yellow No. 5 (tartrazine) (Fig. 7.1), present in colored steroid tablets, caused anaphylactoid reactions in three of his patients. Later Juhlin et al. (1972) reported that not only tartrazine, but preservatives in food can elicit and exacerbate urticaria as well. Since then, many food

Table 7.6. Common preservatives and dyes and their place of occurrence.

Agent	Occurrence
Preservatives	
benzoic acid	naturally in berries and spices, added to fruits, vegetables, fish, meat, egg-containing foods
salicylates	naturally in most vegetables, fruits, wine, beer; added to foods, also as flavoring in candy and tooth pastes
ascorbic acid	in wine, tinned food, marmelade, juices
parabens	foods, drugs (local anesthetics)
sulfites	food, wine, drugs
antioxidants (propylgallate, butylhydroxytoluol-BHT, butylated hydroxy-anisole-BHA, tocopherol)	added to fatty foods
Food coloring	ubiquitous in foods and drugs
azo dyes	
tartrazine (orange)	
ponceau (red)	
sunset yellow (yellow)	
amaranth (red)	
non-azo dyes	
brilliant blue (blue)	
erythrosine (red)	
indigotine (blue)	

preservatives and colorings have been identified as causes of urticaria (Table 7.6).

Benzoic acid occurs naturally in many types of berries, in mustard, and in diverse spices. Salicylates are also naturally present in berries, grapes, apples, wine, and beer. The quantities of these chemicals are low in naturally occurring foods, and reactions can be expected in only extremely sensitive subjects. Preservatives and several azo and non-azo dyes are added to numerous foods, including candy, ice cream, fruit juices, pastries, and even tooth paste. The aniline dye tartrazine is not only present in foods, but also in a long list of drugs (Lockey 1971, Smith and Slavin 1976, Lindemayr and Schmidt 1979). Among the chemicals, tartrazine (Fig. 7.1) is unique as it causes anaphylactoid reactions in aspirin-intolerant subjects, even though it is not a prostaglandin-synthetase inhibitor (Gerber et al. 1979). Weliky and Heiner (1980) point out that tartrazine has the following characteristics:

1) It contains benzenesulfonic acid which is found in many detergents, dyes, and pigments.
2) It belongs to the azo compounds which are used as food, paper, and fabric coloring agents.
3) It is related to pyrazolone compounds like antipyrine and phenylbutazone.
4) It belongs to the hydroxy-aromatic acids.

These several chemical properties of tartrazine may explain its high frequency as an inducer of anaphylactoid reactions.

Sulfites are used widely to preserve foods and drugs, particularly solutions of medications. They are implicated in anaphylactic reactions after eating in restaurants, and 5–10% of the asthmatic population reacts to them. Parabens, aliphatic esters of para-hydroxybenzoic acid, have been reported to cause reactions after injections of local anesthetics, although only in rare instances. These compounds are better known as elicitors of severe contact dermatitis reactions (Simon 1984).

7.4.3 Radiocontrast Media

Water-soluble, iodinated radiocontrast media are at present still indispensible in diagnostic radiology. Nearly all of them are triiodinated benzoic acid compounds (Fig. 7.1) which are used mainly as sodium and methylglucamine, but also as calcium and magnesium salts. The first compound with relatively low toxicity was diatrizoate sodium. New contrast media with even lower toxicity (and less basophil histamine release) are sodium salts and low-osmolality media like ioxaglate, iohexol, and iopamidol (Ring and Sovak 1981, Assem et al. 1983).

7.4.4 Plasma Expanders

With the shortage of donor blood and the risk of infections, a number of natural and artificial blood volume substitutes have come into use. They include plasma proteins, particularly human serum albumin, and artificial volume substitutes. To the latter group belong (1) dextrans which are of either low (40000 d) or high (60000 d) molecular weight; (2) modified fluid gelatins which are produced by hydrolysis of animal collagen and have a low antigenicity; and (3) hydroxyethyl starch which is produced by acid hydrolysis of corn and soy beans after hydroxyethyl coupling (Vervloet et al. 1983). Infusion reactions to invert sugars should also be mentioned in this context. Sugars rarely cause anaphylactoid reactions by themselves (1/575000), but their contamination with α-1,6-glucan of bacterial origin increases the incidence more than tenfold (Richter et al. 1976). Unusually high reaction rates to artificial volume substitutes or serum extracts should always arouse suspicion of similar contaminants in the preparations.

Plasma expanders cause reactions that do not differ

from the clinical picture described for anaphylactoid reactions in general. Unique features are the fever accompanying urticarial reactions to human serum albumin and the local irritant reaction with starch along the infused vein (Ring 1980).

7.4.5 Anesthetics

Intravenous or local anesthetics can also be the cause of anaphylactoid reactions. A number of drugs have been implicated, but their exact mode of action is difficult to elucidate since many are administered in rapid succession to induce anesthesia, the time when most reactions occur. Beside anesthetics, muscle relaxants, drugs used during premedication, whole blood, or plasma substitutes might be implicated. Preservatives in the anesthetic solutions might also cause the reactions. Special clinical symptoms of anaphylactoid reactions to anesthetics, in addition to those described below, are a metallic taste, headache, paresthesias, and visual disturbances (Vervloet et al. 1979, Doenicke 1980).

7.5 Clinical Features

7.5.1 Symptomatology

In his first description of an anaphylactoid reaction to aspirin in a patient suffering from rheumatic pain, Hirschberg (1902) gave a very accurate description of the clinical features of the reaction. Three hours after the patient had taken one grain of aspirin, he noticed the onset of rhinorrhea, pruritus of the scalp, dysphagia, facial edema, and a patchy, scarlet-red erythema on face, scalp, neck, and oral mucosa. Trunk and extremities were spared, except for a "5-Mark"-size wheal on the right knee. The doctor told his patient that he suffered from an urticaria and reassured him that this reaction was harmless. Fortunately, he was right in his prognostication.

Illig (1980) points out that the flush reaction, as described above, is typical for reactions to aspirin in the absence of an underlying chronic urticaria. He adds that the patient may experience tightness of the chest, palpitation, dizziness, headache, and fatigue. Conjunctivitis, tachycardia and gastrointestinal symptoms are also common. Wheals, if present, are round and elevated, and they tend to persist longer than ordinary wheals. Convulsions, fever, and angina pectoris are rare. The final outcome of fulminating reactions can be shock and death of the patient.

Anaphylactoid reactions in patients with an underlying urticaria manifest themselves primarily as an aggravation of the preexisting urticarial symptoms (Illig 1980). In asthmatic patients, aggravation of bronchospasms is the major symptom, and a status asthmaticus is easily provoked even with minute doses of the drugs. In view of the threatening nature of these reactions, urticaria is only a minor symptom in aspirin-intolerant asthmatics, and it is either relatively infrequent or overlooked. In normal controls without underlying urticaria or asthma, intolerance reactions are either of the bronchospastic or the urticarial type.

On rare occasions, reactions of the aspirin type present as an erythematous, macular, or papular eruption that has an eczematous character. Purpuric lesions, lesions of fixed drug reactions, and a flare-up of preexisting eczema have also been described in these patients (Schlumberger 1980). Food additives might also be a cause of hyperkinesia in children (Juhlin 1980).

7.5.2 Kinetics of the Reaction

The onset of symptoms after intake of the offending agent varies from a few minutes in highly sensitive patients to 12 h. Most reactions have a latency from 1/2 to 2–3 h. Lesions are usually gone after 1–2 days, but urticae may persist for up to 2 weeks. The cutaneous reactions tend to begin later than the bronchospastic ones.

There is a well-documented refractory period after an anaphylactoid reaction. It usually lasts for 72 h, in rare instances even for a week. This explains why, after a longer period of abstinence, the reactions to the offending chemicals are particularly violent. Patients who react and become refractory to one agent, will tolerate others to which they are intolerant during this refractory period (Schlumberger 1980).

7.5.3 Laboratory Findings

Patients with intolerance reactions have no specific laboratory signs of their disease. Cooke (1919) mentioned that practically all of his patients had an eosinophilia of 10–15%. Almost all of them had bronchospastic reactions. This agrees with the observation (Weltman et al. 1978) that an eosinophilia is observed more frequently in asthmatics (57%) than in urticaria patients (25%) with aspirin intolerance. Settipane et al. (1976) found no eosinophilia at all in their 39 patients with chronic urticaria due to intolerance. IgE levels are normal in these patients.

Fisherman and Cohen (1973a–d, 1976) made the interesting observation that the bleeding time was increased in patients with the aspirin-type reactions on exposure to even subclinical doses of the chemicals. This was not observed in controls.

7.5.4 Prognosis

It is well known that the tendency to develop intolerance reactions can disappear after some time for no apparent reason. Juhlin (1981) found that 50% of the oral challenge reactions were negative after one year. Gibson and Clancy (1980) observed this in only 27%, and Greenberger et al. (1984) cite an incidence of 17–35%. Several other authors have stressed the variability of the response and its tendency to disappear with time (Ros et al. 1976, Lahti 1980, Pleskow et al. 1983).

After a diet and avoiding all known noxious chemicals, 12–24% of chronic urticaria patients are free of symptoms, and 30–57% are much improved (Ros et al. 1976, Wüthrich and Fabro 1981).

7.6 Diagnosis

7.6.1 Patient History

Patients with a history of violent or life-threatening reactions to well-defined, single agents should not be exposed to these chemicals again. When the clinical symptoms during reactions are not as severe and occur later in time, when the symptomatology is of a more subjective nature (see Table 7.7), or when combinations of drugs are involved, the patient is less aware of the eliciting agent.

Ros et al. (1976) observed that 84% of their patients with chronic urticaria reacted to aspirin on oral provocation, but only one-half of them were aware of their intolerance. Along the same lines, Doeglas (1975) found that only 10 of 37 patients with a positive challenge reaction also had a positive history. Lahti (1980) observed no correlation at all between the patient's history and the results of oral challenge tests to salicylates and several other preservatives. Our own findings would agree with this view (Fig. 7.2). Only about one-half of the patients with chronic urticaria and a positive history of aspirin intolerance reacted on oral challenge, while 6.5% of patients with a negative history reacted as well (Ochmann and Czarnetzki, unpublished observations).

There are several possible reasons for the poor correlation between oral challenge tests and patient history:

1) Patients might overinterpret minor clinical symptoms.

Table 7.7. Anamnestic data in patients with anaphylactoid intolerance reactions for which objective signs form a firm diagnostic basis (Michaelsson and Juhlin 1973, after Lahti 1980).

Objective signs	Subjective symptoms
urticaria	tingling
erythema of face and chest	itching
angioedema	headache
hoarseness	palpitation
nasal congestion	shortness of breath
sneezing	perspiration
lacrimation	abdominal pain
wheezing (asthma)	nausea, diarrhea
fall in forced expiratory volume	heat waves
fever	sensations of
syncope	fatigue
	drowsiness
	thirst
	vertigo
	stinging of lips or throat
	pressure across forehead

2) The reaction in a natural setting occurs often under special circumstances, such as during a concomitant viral infection or during the ingestion of agents which enhance mast cell release or the reactivity of the target tissue. Examples would be the consumption of larger amounts of preservatives in a Chinese restaurant, together with alcohol or spices.
3) The patient may have reacted with clinically manifest symptoms or subclinically during the preceding days and would therefore be in a state of tolerance during oral challenge. In case of doubt, the test should be repeated at a later date.
4) The intolerance reactivity to aspirin may have been lost with time.

7.6.2 Skin Tests

The situation is even worse with skin test data. Lahti (1980) found no correlation at all between skin test results and subjective or objective symptoms, and similar observations were reported by others. Hansen-Pruss (1949) found that positive skin tests to aspirin,

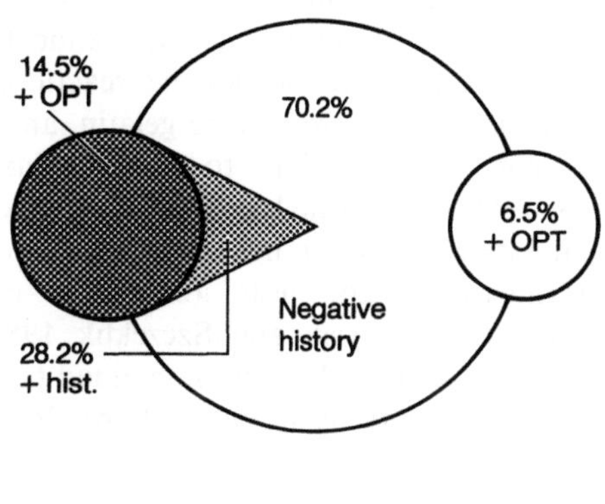

Fig. 7.2. Correlation between the patient history (*hist*) and positive (+) oral provocation tests (*OPT*) to aspirin. Note that only one-half of patients with a positive history will react, while a small percentage of patients will react even if their history is negative.

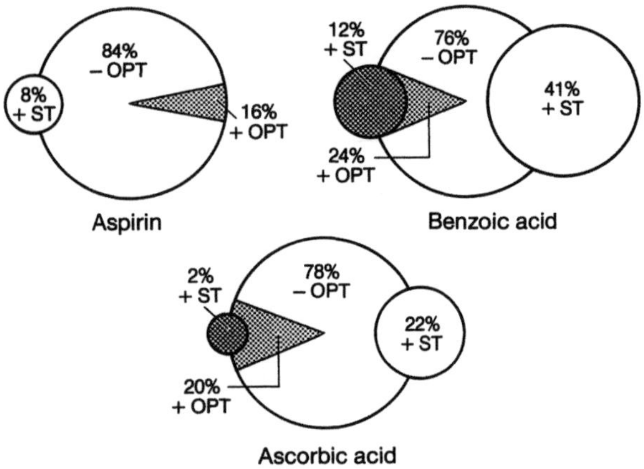

Fig. 7.3. Correlation between skin tests (*ST*) and oral provocation tests (*OPT*) to three different agents. Only one-half to none of the patients who reacted on oral provocation, had positive (+) skin tests, while from 10 to about 50% of patients with negative (–) oral challenge had positive skin tests.

sodium salicylate, and aminopyrine occurred in patients and normal controls. Mathews et al. (1950) had entirely negative skin test results in patients with asthma or urticaria due to aspirin intolerance. Their patients also failed to react to injections of serum from patients who had ingested aspirin. With an aspirin-polylysine conjugate (Krilis et al. 1981), only one of 19 patients with twice proven positive oral provocation tests reacted to this compound, but this patient also responded to the polylysine succinate control. Cooke (1919) finally warned against using intradermal tests with aspirin since minute test doses could cause violent symptoms lasting for 3 days.

Our own patient data also showed no correlation between skin tests and oral provocation tests (Czarnetzki 1983; Fig. 7.3). None of the patients with a positive oral provocation test reacted to aspirin in the skin test, but 8% of those with a negative oral provocation did. Up to one-half of the patients with positive oral tests reacted in the skin test to benzoic acid and ascorbic acid, but the percentage of positive skin tests in the negative oral provocation group was even higher (Ochmann and Czarnetzki, unpublished findings).

According to some reports, skin tests appear to have some value with certain specific chemicals. Vervloet et al. (1979, 1983) found positive reactions in all three patients who had reacted to gelatin, and in all eleven patients with reactions to muscle relaxants, but in none of the normal controls. Practically all the patients with intolerance to pyrazolones had positive intradermal skin tests (Szczeklik et al. 1977, Czerniawska-Mysik and Szczeklik 1981), although Maucher and Fuchs (1984) obtained positive contact urticaria reactions in only 10 of 26 patients and positive scratch test reactions in only 12 of 26 patients. Radiocontrast media caused wheal and flare reactions in normal skin (Rockoff et al. 1970), or none at all according to others (Miller et al. 1975). Skin tests with local anesthetics and dextrans also have only a limited diagnostic value (Ring 1980, Schatz 1984).

7.6.3 Sequential Tests for Vascular Response

In 1966, Quick described a simple test for measuring bleeding time after the intake of aspirin. Using a lancet to cause the ear lobe to bleed, he blotted droplets of blood onto a piece of filter paper at regularly timed intervals. The number of blood stains indicated the bleeding tendency. Fisherman and Cohen (1973a, b, c) claimed in a series of papers that this simple test, performed 2h after oral challenge, provides a fine measuring tool for subclinical intolerance reactions to drugs, chemicals, and foods. Although the test had no value in the diagnosis of urticaria due to physical agents or infectious causes, it presumably identified the causative agent of chronic urticaria in 203 of 215 patients (Fisherman and Cohen 1976). Such high values have not been reached with any other diagnostic tool for chronic urticaria. The test also identifies a number of chemicals to which patients are "cross-sensitive," the pattern being very similar to reports with conventional oral challenge tests by several authors (see below and Fisherman and Cohen 1977). So far, no other group of workers has confirmed these findings, probably also because the reading of the bleeding time is too cumbersome for the nursing or medical staff. In preliminary experiments, we were unable to demonstrate an increased bleeding time in six patients who had intolerance reactions after oral exposure to analgesics.

7.6.4 Oral Provocation Tests

Intolerance reactions are best verified and diagnosed by the route along which the offending agent normally reaches the body. For a few agents, this would mean intramuscular or even intravenous testing. However, the latter is rarely done because of the potentially life-threatening anaphylactic reactions that might result during testing. Many agents that cause intolerance reactions are taken orally. One possible reason why tests along this route have proven to be an important diagnostic tool may relate to the fact that many drugs cause intolerance reactions solely via their metabolic products.

A major prerequisite for oral provocation is freedom of symptoms. Patients are hospitalized and placed on a diet of potatoes and rice to rid them of

Table 7.8. Scheme for oral provocation tests to screen for intolerance reactions to foods and minor analgesics (after Paul and Illig 1983).

Group	Challenge agent	Dosage	Time
I	Tartrazine E102	10 mg	
	Sodium benzoate	50 mg	day 1, h 0,
	Mefenamic acid	250 mg	
II	Food coloring mixture I[a]	25 mg	
	Paracetamol	500 mg	day 1, h 6
	4-Hydroxybenzoic acid	500 mg	
III	Food coloring mixture II[b]	25 mg	
	Sodium benzoate	500 mg	day 2, h 0,
	Sorbic acid	500 mg	
IV	Indomethacin	25 mg	day 2, h 6
	Aspirin	50 mg	day 3, h 0,
		125 mg	subsequent
		250 mg	doses at 2 h
		500 mg	intervals
		1000 mg	each

[a] Consists of 5 mg each of chinolin yellow E104, yellow orange E110; azorubin E122, and amaranth E123.
[b] Consists of erythrosine E127, patent blue E131, indigotine E132, brilliant black E151, pigment brown E172.

their urticaria. Water, possibly also black tea, are allowed for fluid intake. Freedom of symptoms is achieved in 60% of patients by these measures (Paul and Illig 1983). The remaining 40% are subjected to further diagnostic procedures, as outlined in Chapter 10, p. 122. Oral provocation tests are initiated in the patients who are free of symptoms, after ensuring that they have not taken aspirin or other suspected chemicals for several days before. As an exception, oral challenge tests can be done even in the presence of wheals if all other diagnostic procedures fail. Subsequent reactions in such patients should however be interpreted with caution, keeping in mind that they represent mainly an "isomorphic," aggravating reaction and that they do not necessarily uncover the cause of the urticaria.

Prior to testing, an intravenous catheter should be put in place to provide ready access for systemic therapy in case of unexpectedly violent reactions. If the causative agent of the urticaria is not clear, the scheme shown in Table 7.8, which gives a hint of the possible group intolerance within 3 days, can be followed. If a reaction has occurred, testing should be stopped for 2–3 days, or continued with placebo tablets. The individual components of the block where the reaction has occurred can then be tested separately.

The substances to be tested are placed in an oblate or a gelatin capsule so that the patient has no clue as to the nature of the test substance. He is instructed to call the nurse if he notices any of the symptoms and signs listed in Table 7.7, and he is also told that at some time, he will receive placebo tablets. This will lower his level of anxiety and expectation and will make him more critical with regard to his symptomatology. The time until onset of symptoms and their severity depend on the dosage and the individual sensitivity of the patient. Angioedema occurs usually within the 1st h and urticaria often 6–14 h later (Michaelsson and Juhlin 1973). In case of doubtful reactions, the next higher dose should be given or the testing repeated several days later.

In patients who react to just about any of the test substances, including placebo, J. Ring (1985) gives patients a verum and tells them it is a placebo, and he will then give them a placebo and tell them it is the suspected cause of his symptoms ("reversed placebo provocation"). If the patient reacts on the basis of what he has been told, he can then be confronted with the fact that there is a strong psychogenic basis to his reactions. Such a procedure should be followed only in rare situations and when there is a good rapport between patient and doctor. It might also be worthwhile to switch from lactose (100 mg) to starch (100 mg) in the placebo tablet before firm conclusions are drawn about the patient's psyche, since in rare instances, the placebo carbohydrates might be the cause of the urticaria.

In many instances, a rather good history of the patient's reactions to single agents or a combination of agents is available. The oral provocation test is then adapted to the individual situation (Table 7.9). Several alternate antiphlogistic drugs and analgesics are tested to determine which is safe to take. If food intolerance is suspected, preservatives and dyes are tested. Highly suspiciuos agents, particularly aspirin, should always be tested at the end of a test program or on a Friday since, in case of a reaction, testing has to be stopped for 2–3 days because of the refractory period. Condemi (1981) observed that this period can last for up to one week. Doeglas (1975) also stops oral provocation tests for one week after a reaction, however, if symptoms have been only minor, he believes that 2–3 days should suffice.

The agents listed in Table 7.9 should be chosen for testing, depending on the drugs and additives in common usage in the respective country. Each dose is given at 2-h intervals for practical reasons, with the awareness that reactions can also occur at a later period. With asthmatics or highly sensitive subjects, testing should be started at very low dose levels. The concentrations can be increased in small steps at hourly intervals.

Doeglas (1975) tested all his urticaria patients on an outpatient basis, except for patients with asthma,

Table 7.9. Test substances and their dosage for oral provocation tests (after Michaelsson and Juhlin 1973, Doeglas 1975, Thune and Grantholt 1975, Weber et al. 1979, Condemi 1981, Juhlin 1981).

Agent	Dosis (mg)
Antiphogistics and analgesics	
paracetamol	50, 250, 500
phenazone	50, 200, 500
propyphenazone	50, 200, 500
phenacetin	50, 100, 250
metamizol[a]	50, 250, 500
diclofenac	5, 25, 50
phenylbutazon[a]	10, 100, 200
oxyphenbutazon[a]	10, 50, 100
piroxicam	5, 10, 20
pentazocin	10, 25, 50
phenobarbital	10, 20, 100
codeine phosphate	5, 50
indomethacin	5, 25, 50
acetylsalicylic acid	(0.1, 2, 5, 10)[b] 50, 100, 250, 500, 1000
Food additives	
4-hydroxybenzoic acid	50, 200
sodium benzoate	50, 250, 500
BHT-BHA (combined)	10, 50, 125 (each)
sodium salicylate	500, 1000
sodium glutamate	100, 200
phenyl salicylate	500, 1000
sodium nitrite and nitrate	100 (each in sequence)
ascorbic acid	50, 250, 500
sulphanilic acid	50
tartrazine	(0.1)[b] 2, 5, 10
azo dyes (mix No. 1)	(0.1)[b] 2, 5, 10 (each)
amaranth	
ponceaux	
sunset yellow	
non-azo dyes (mix No. 2)	5, 10 (each)
brilliant blue	
erythrosine	
indigotine	
yeast extract	600
caffeine	200

[a] Drugs withdrawn from the general market in some countries due to serious side effects (agranulocytosis).
[b] Lower initial doses in parentheses for patients with asthma or positive history of previous reactions.

rhinitis, and sinusitis. Patients who have experienced an anaphylactic shock because of their intolerance should only be tested on an inpatient basis. McDonald (1972) suggests that severe asthmatics should be kept on their maintenance asthma therapy, to avoid serious reations. The challenge test mimics in this way the natural situation under which reactions occur and gives sufficient information to tell the patient what be should avoid.

There are a number of reports in the literature with listings of the frequency of reactions to different agents on oral provocation. This is helpful in choosing the sequence of the test chemicals and in interpreting the results. The greatest frequency of reactions to oral provocations occurs with aspirin, followed by azo-dyes, particularly tartrazine, indomethacin, and other dyes and preservatives (Doeglas 1975, Thune and Grantholt 1975, Illig 1980, Juhlin 1981, Wüthrich and Fabro 1981). A pattern of cross-reactivity to different drugs is shown for 39 patients from the dermatology department in Münster who had urticaria and intolerance (Fig. 7.4). These data underline the fact that one patient can react to several drugs.

It should be kept in mind that patients who react to low doses of aspirin also tend to react to low doses of other chemicals. "Cross-reactions" imply also "cross-tolerance" to the same drugs after a reaction, as long as the refractory period lasts. This has been shown for aspirin, indomethacin, and other non-steroidal anti-inflammatory drugs (Pleskow et al. 1982). Czerniawska-Mysik and Szczeklik (1981) observed practically no cross-reactions between aspirin and other prostaglandin inhibitors, on the one hand, and pyrazolones on the other. Paracetamol has also only a low cross-reactivity (5 %) with aspirin (Doeglas 1975); it provides a useful alternative in those aspirin intolerant patients who do not react to it on oral provocation.

7.6.5 In Vitro Tests for Lymphocyte Transformation

Valverde et al. (1980) studied the proliferative responsiveness of leukocytes from 258 patients with chronic urticaria during in vitro lymphocyte transformation with food extracts and additives. A total of 35.2% of the patients reacted to food extracts only, 46.6 to both; 25 % responded to aspirin and tartrazine, 25 % to both tartrazine and hydroxybenzoic acid, 11 % to all three componds. A diet on the basis of these results caused a complete remission in 61.6 %, a partial remission in 22 % of the patients, and no improvement in 16.2 %. No mention is made of a correlation of the in vitro data with the patient history. Further data from other laboratories should be awaited to gain more insight into the true diagnostic value of this test.

7.7 Pathogenesis

The basic mechanisms involved in intolerance reactions are not well understood. It is possible that several factors come together to elicit the reactions, whether by enhanced effectiveness of mediators or through their increased production. It is also likely that different chemicals which cause intolerance reactions do so via different mechanisms.

For the prototype of these reactions, aspirin intolerance, Schlumberger (1980) lists several possible

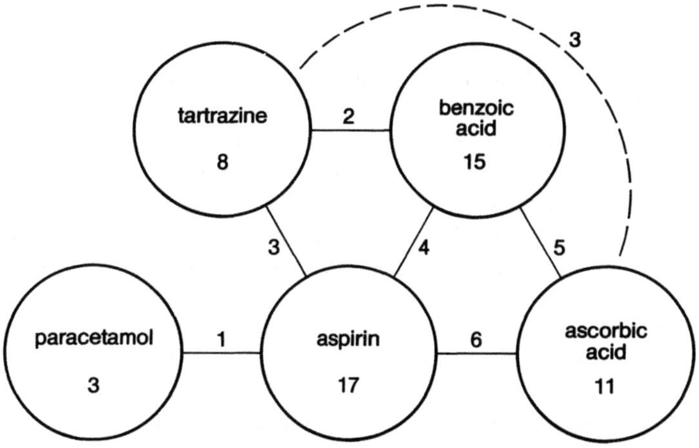

Fig. 7.4. Positive oral provocation tests in 39 patients tested because of positive history of anaphylactoid reactions. The numbers along the connecting lines between circles indicate the number of patients who reacted to both drugs.

causes of the altered reactivity of the patients: paradoxically reactive chemoreceptors; persistent viral infections, changing signal transfer and modulating mediator release or the immune response; a hereditary predisposition; enhanced release of mediators, such as histamine, in the presence of the chemicals involved; an enhanced, compensatory production of leukotrienes as a result of prostaglandin synthetase inhibition; and complement activation at an increase rate, or lack of inhibition, resulting in the production of anaphylatoxins which in turn cause mast cell mediator release.

7.7.1 Immunoglobulins, Mast Cells, Mast Cell Mediators

As mentioned in the introduction to this chapter, a specific immunological mechanism cannot be implicated as a cause of the aspirin type intolerance reactions. This was already recognized by Cooke in 1919. Specific IgE has never been demonstrated despite intensive search by many workers, nor are total IgE levels increased in the patients (Weltman et al. 1978, Settipane 1981). Positive immediate skin test reactions to aspiryl-polylysine in aspirin sensitive patients, as reported by de Weck (1971), were not confirmed by others in aspirin-intolerant patients, nor did these agents cause in vitro lymphocyte transformation in aspirin-intolerant asthmatics (Giraldo et al. 1969). Weliky and Heiner (1980) have reported specific IgD antibodies to a tartrazine conjugate in tartrazine-sensitive patients, with a lowering of nonspecific total IgD. Basophil-bound IgE may be involved in mannitol-induced histamine reactions, since anti-IgE inhibits this reaction in vitro (Findlay et al. 1984). This phenomenon is intriguing and should be looked for with other chemicals that cause intolerance reactions.

Basophil and mast cell involvement and release of histamine from these cells very likely occur during intolerance reactions, although the evidence is not entirely convincing. Cromolyn inhibits mast cell degranulation and intolerance reactions (Settipane 1981), implicating a role of mast cells in the process. Moneret-Vautrin et al. (1984) observed mucosal mast cell degranulation in the intestine after intolerance reactions, but this is the only study that has dealt with this problem until now.

Studies of the whealing reactions to compound 48/80 showed that intolerant asthmatics had larger wheals after aspirin ingestion. This was not seen with histamine wheals and with normal controls after aspirin ingestion, and no increased wheal size was seen in patients with urticaria pigmentosa, dermographic urticaria, cold urticaria, or cholinergic urticaria (Moore-Robinson and Warin 1967).

In vitro rat mast cell and human basophil histamine release was shown to occur with X-ray contrast media (Rockoff et al. 1970, Ring et al. 1978), but not with several food dyes or with sodium benzoate (Kreindler et al. 1980). Wojnar et al. (1980) observed no histamine release by analgesics, food preservatives, or dyes on exposure to basophils in vitro, but there was enhanced antigen-dependent basophil histamine release in the presence of these chemicals from cells of normal donors. In contrast, Bochner et al. (1984) found no increased release in intolerant patients with aspirin plus ionophore, and patients released even less histamine than controls with the ionophore alone.

Increased levels of plasma histamine have been measured after reactions to aspirin (Schlumberger 1983). Wasserman et al. (1978), on the other hand, found no increase of histamine or of neutrophil chemotactic factor levels in sera of patients who had developed bronchospasm after ingestion of aspirin.

7.7.2 Arachidonate Metabolism

Indomethacin and, to a lesser extent, aspirin inhibit the cyclooxygenase enzyme, thus preventing generation of prostaglandins from arachidonic acid

(Fig. 2.11, p. 18). This has attracted the attention of several investigators to the possible role of arachidonate metabolism in the pathogenesis of intolerance reactions. The observation that atropine inhibits the bronchoconstrictor reaction to both $PGF_{2\alpha}$ and aspirin led to the concept of an imbalance of the bronchoconstrictor $PGF_{2\alpha}$ in favor of the bronchodilator PGE_2 (Szczeklik et al. 1967). A drop of serum PGE levels might theoretically explain enhanced histamine release in patients (Schlumberger 1983). Szczeklik et al. (1977) postulated subtypes of intolerance reactions, only some of which are due to cyclooxygenase inhibition.

Siegel et al. (1979) observed that aspirin-related drugs interfere with arachidonate metabolism by inhibiting 12-HETE peroxidase activity. This suggests that products other than the prostaglandins, namely mono-HETEs and leukotrienes, are excessively released in intolerant patients. The inhibition of cyclo-ocygenase might also make more substrate (arachidonic acid) available for the leukotriene pathway (see also Chapter 2.3, p. 13 and Fig. 2.11, p. 18). As the products of this pathway are potent mediators, this could explain the symptomatology in intolerance reactions.

A number of facts argue, however, against an alteration of arachidonate metabolism as a cause of intolerance reactions. Two-thirds of the drugs reported to "cross-react" in aspirin-intolerant patients are not involved in the inhibition of prostaglandin synthesis (Schlumberger 1983), nor do they inhibit lipoxygenation. Tartrazine, one of the most frequent drugs to cause reactions in aspirin-intolerant patients, has no effect at all on the cyclooxygenase in guinea pig lung, human platelets, and sheep seminal vesicles (Gerber et al. 1979). The effect of drugs that elicit intolerance reactions on the cyclooxygenase enzyme, if present, is highly variable on a quantitative basis and does not correlate with the frequency or severity of clinical symptoms (Szczeklik et al. 1977). Furthermore, aspirin and indomethacin inhibit the cyclooxygenase in normal controls as well as in patients. Therefore, this property in itself does not explain the symptomatology of the patients.

All experimental attempts to prove a defect of arachidonate metabolism in anaphylactoid reactions have failed until now. There is no evidence for a difference in prostaglandin inhibition in platelet supernatants of intolerant subjects or controls on exposure to aspirin (Patrono et al. 1978). A change in PGE_2 and $PGF_{2\alpha}$ ratios during aspirin-induced asthma could not be shown by several workers. Inhibition of in vitro release of chemotactic leukotrienes from leukocytes of patients with intolerance and of controls did not differ either (Czarnetzki 1983). Benoxaprofen which has inhibitory activity on lipoxygenase, has no therapeutic effect on intolerance reactions (Lumry et al. 1982).

Thus, while all these findings do not rule out subtle defects along the metabolic pathway of arachidonic acid, possibly even at reaction sites that are as yet unknown, the evidence so far is not convincing. Alterations of the binding of prostaglandins to serum proteins by the drugs (Attallah and Lee 1980) might still be worthwhile examining in this context.

7.7.3 Involvement of the Complement Pathway

An explanation of anaphylactoid reactions was also sought in the complement pathway. Arroyave et al. (1977) observed a drop in CH50 in five of seven intolerant patients on aspirin challenge and in only 20% of normal patients under the same conditions. Since anaphylatoxins can cause basophil and mast cell histamine release and thus mimic the symptomatology of intolerance reactions, a defect in the complement system in these patients is an attractive possibility. Decreases of the C1INH or of the anaphylatoxin inhibitor have also been postulated in intolerant patients (Kallos and Schlumberger 1980), but so far, have been found by only one group, and only for contrast media reactions (Lasser et al. 1979, see below). In fact, a number of other groups could not confirm the decrease of CH50, C3, or C4, as noted above, in bronchospastic patients, urticaria patients, or controls (Doeglas 1975, Delaney and Kay 1976, Weltman et al. 1978, Pleskow 1983). Voigtländer et al. (1980) found a transient drop of serum CH50, C1, C4, and C2 in 19 of 20 normal controls after aspirin ingestion. There is also evidence that salicylates can inhibit C1INH (Hänsch et al. 1980). Since these workers could not demonstrate altered complement activation after aspirin ingestion in intolerant patients compared to controls, a defect in the complement activation pathway of aspirin intolerant patients seems unlikely.

7.7.4 Other Theories

There is good evidence for genetically based variations in the metabolism of drugs in different individuals. Schlumberger (1980) cites arguments why this could also account for the abnormal reactions to drugs in intolerant patients. More than ten reports in the literature describe clustering of aspirin intolerance and asthma in families of different racial groups. Miller (1971) reported the first such family, and Lockey et al. (1973) found affected members in several generations of both a Mennonite and a non-Mennonite family.

Settipane and Pudupakkam (1975) observed 3 in 40 patients with aspirin intolerance with a positive family history, whereas Samter and Beers (1968) found none among 1000 aspirin-intolerant patients, and Delaney (1973) reported only 1 among 34 patients in Liverpool. A genetic predisposition will thus explain the pathogenesis of intolerance reactions in only a small group of patients. Alternately, a predisposing gene might be down-regulated in most cases by an additional gene or need environmental factors for its expression.

Another theory is that an occult, persistent viral infection might change signal transfer, modulating mediator release or the immune response (Schlumberger 1980). So far, no evidence has been provided.

A final theory deals with paradoxically reactive chemoreceptors (Samter and Beers 1967). Aspirin could have a direct effect on kinin receptors, initiating an axon reflex and a subsequent bronchoconstriction, with increased mucus secretion and capillary permeability. Whether any one or several of such mechanisms will explain intolerance reactions, will have to await further experimental evidence.

7.8 Pathogenetic Aspects of Intolerance Reactions to Special Reagents

The reagents discussed here are X-ray contrast media, volume expanders, and drugs used during anesthesia. There is evidence that they operate via other mechanisms than those involved in aspirin intolerance.

7.8.1 Contrast Media

The possible pathomechanisms involved in contrast media reactions have been thoroughly investigated. Histamine release from mast cells and basophils seems to play a major role. Rice et al. (1983) reported that metrizoate and diatrizoate induced non-cytotoxic histamine release from basophils in vitro; this reaction was increased in patients who had reacted to the chemicals. Vervloet et al. (1979) made a similar observation, also that skin basophil release occurred with normotonic solutions. In contrast, Findlay et al. (1981) attributed the release to hypertonicity. Ring et al. (1978) had shown earlier that radiocontrast media cause a dose-dependent in vitro release of histamine from leukocytes and of serotonin from platelets in normal volunteers, and Miller et al. (1975) observed more in vitro basophil release with the reagents that had elicited a reaction in a patient than in normal volunteers. Ring et al. (1978) also had evidence for in vitro degranulation of basophils and platelets and for an increase of plasma histamine in vivo. Finally, Siegle and Lieberman (1976) observed that for up to 3–4 weeks after a reaction to radiocontrast media, in vitro basophil histamine release was increased by 125% in patients and only by 10% after a radiocontrast procedure in normal controls, indicating increased synthesis of histamine or a basophilia after the reaction.

Beside causing a direct histamine release, contrast media could also operate via several other mechanisms. These media are highly reactive chemicals that bind to proteins, resulting in enzyme inhibition, activation of the fibrinolytic and coagulation systems, enzyme secretion from neutrophils, leukocyte aggregation, and changes of endothelial cells. They cause complement activation of normal serum in vitro, but significant quantities of complement are activated in vivo only in patients with clinical symptoms of intolerance (reviewed in Till 1981). Lasser et al. (1979) measured lower baseline levels of functional C1INH and total hemolytic complement levels in reacting patients than in controls. Ring et al. (1978) recorded increased in vitro histamine release from healthy donors due to complement activation via the alternative pathway.

7.8.2 Volume Expanders

Infusions of plasma proteins cause reactions by forming aggregates, producing antibodies of the non-IgE type, and activating complement. Histamine appears to be the major mediator (Ring 1980). Stabilizers in the infusion and not the active compounds themselves could also cause the reaction.

Dextrans of higher molecular weight cause complement activation in vitro via the alternate pathway. They release histamine from mast cells of certain rat strains, cause no lymphocyte activation, and induce antibody formation of the IgG, IgM, and IgA, but not of the IgE type. Aggregate anaphylaxis is the most likely mechanism to explain the reactions, and preinfusion with monovalent dextran effectively prevents them. Atopic patients have a higher incidence of mild reactions, and patients with severe inflammatory diseases have a higher percentage of serious reactions (reviewed by Ring 1980).

Gelatins cause histamine release in reactors and volunteers in vivo, and the level of serum histamine correlates with the severity of symptoms. Anticollagen antibody formation may occur, but IgE antibodies are not involved, based on passive transfer studies and radioimmunoassays (Vervloet et al. 1983).

Hydroxyethyl starch does not cause histamine release, and although low titer antibodies have been found in humans, they probably have no clinical relevance. Although some patients show evidence for complement activation in vivo, the pathogenesis of reactions to starch cannot be explained (Ring 1980).

As regards the pathomechanisms involved in reactions to mannitol, an interesting observation has recently been published by Findlay et al. (1984). They showed that mannitol caused direct in vitro histamine release from basophils in one of their patients which was tenfold higher in the presence of deuterium oxide buffer than in normal control cells. This reaction could be blocked with anti-IgE, suggesting an involvement of basophil-bound IgE antibodies in the patients. It would be fascinating if similar observations could be confirmed with other chemicals that cause intolerance reactions, since it would explain why only certain individuals react and others not.

7.8.3 Drugs for Anesthesia

Studies on reagents used in anesthesia are difficult to evaluate since a number of drugs are usually given at once, and it is not always obvious which one caused the reaction. Vervloet et al. (1979) reported that 11 of the patients studied reacted to muscle relaxants. All had positive immediate type skin tests, in vitro leukocyte histamine release occurred in three cases, and passive transfer with a heat-labile serum factor was positive in one. In vitro lymphocyte transformation tests were negative.

Schatz (1984) gives a critical review of the mechanisms involved in reactions to local anesthetics. He shows that the evidence for IgE-mediated reactions on the basis of passive transfer tests is weak. Immune complex mechanisms, drug-dependent IgM, and subsequent complement activation are more likely. Most local anesthetics induce a delayed-type hypersensitivity reaction which would not cause anaphylactic symptoms.

8 Urticarial Vasculitis Syndrome

8.1 General Aspects

The usual clinical presentation of necrotizing vasculitis is a palpable purpura; other possible features are macules, papules, pustules, ulcers, or scars. A few decades ago, attention was called to the fact that urticaria can also be a manifestation of cutaneous vasculitis (McCoombs 1965). The clinical aspects and underlying pathomechanisms of urticarial vasculitis were studied two decades later (McDuffie et al. 1973, Sissons et al. 1974, Soter et al. 1974, Agnello et al. 1975 and 1976), and by the early eighties, more than 100 patients with the disease had been reported in the literature (Sanchez et al. 1982, Wanderer et al. 1983).

By then, it was apparent that vasculitis can be an accidental finding in chronic urticaria, but that such changes can also be associated with severe disease such as systemic lupus erythematosus (SLE), serum hepatitis, or malignant neoplasms. It is thus appropriate to speak of urticarial vasculitis as a syndrome that encompasses a broad spectrum of systemic symptoms and laboratory changes, with the common features being certain histological alterations and a relative refractoriness to treatment.

Synonyms that have been in use for the disease are vasculitis with urticaria (Feig et al. 1976), hypocomplementemic urticaria (McDuffie et al. 1973), and "unusual SLE-related syndrome" (Agnello et al. 1975).

8.2 Epidemiology

Urticarial vasculitis affects preferably young to middle aged women (range 6–68 years). The incidence is relatively low, but varies widely, depending on how strictly the disease is defined. Jones et al. (1983) diagnosed hypocomplementemic urticarial vasculitis in three of 17,000 referrals to St. John's Hospital. In a prospective study of patients with chronic urticaria, Monroe et al. (1981) found evidence of a leukocytoclastic vasculitis with fibrinoid deposits in and around vessels in 9 of 45 patients (29%). Phanuphak et al. (1980) defined vasculitis less strictly on the basis of a cellular infiltrate within vessel walls. They found an incidence of 52% (22/42) in patients with chronic urticaria. In contrast, Natbony et al. (1983) found leukocytoclastic vasculitis in only one of 43 patients with chronic urticaria, while four had decreased serum complement levels and three had circulating immune complexes. Synkowski et al. (1979) found no histologic evidence of vasculitis at all in 14 randomly selected patients with acute and chronic urticaria. Among 231 patients with chronic urticaria and arthritis, only eight were found to also have vasculitis in urticarial skin lesions (Small et al. 1982).

The incidence of urticaria among patients with proven necrotizing vasculitis is also relatively low. Phanuphak et al. (1980) observed wheals in 12 of 79 patients, Ekenstam and Callen (1984) among 17 of 82 patients in a private practice, and Fauci (1983) reported an incidence of 9%. These authors emphasize that urticaria is typically associated with chronic and not with acute vasculitis.

Urticaria is observed in 0–50% of the patients with systemic lupus erythematosus in different series. Tuffanelli and Dubois (1964) observed it in 7% of their 520 patients and O'Loughlin et al. (1978) more recently in 22% of 54 patients. Urticaria is never a feature of discoid (cutaneous) lupus erythematosus (Provost et al. 1980).

8.3 Clinical Aspects

8.3.1 Cutaneous Manifestations

Urticarial lesions in patients with vasculitis are generalized in their distribution and may even involve the palms and mucous membranes (Soter et al. 1974). Individual lesions are raised, indurated, faintly red (Fig. 8.1), or purple red with an elevated, red margin (Fig. 8.2). A fine, punctate purpura is often observed within the lesions. After healing, a residual slight hyperpigmentation, scaling, or purpura may remain at the site of previous lesions (Callen and Kalbfleisch 1982). Wheals generally persist for 24–72 h, and according to Provost et al. (1980), even up to 1 week. Symptoms can be entirely absent, although most patients experience severe pruritus or even burning at the site of lesions. Hyperesthesia on application of light pressure to the wheals has been noted in some patients (Provost et al. 1980).

Beside urticarial lesions, other types of skin lesions can coexist, such as bullous lesions, erythema multi-

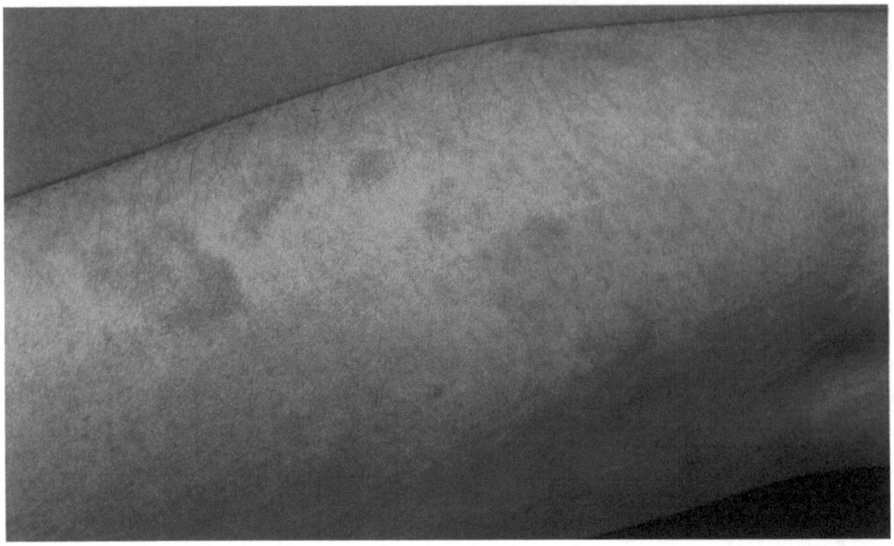

Fig. 8.1. Lesions of urticarial vasculitis in a patient with systemic lupus erythematosus.

forme-like eruptions, or livedo reticularis (Table 8.1). New crops of lesions can appear at daily or monthly intervals.

8.3.2 Systemic Manifestations

Next to the skin, the most frequently involved organs are the joints (Table 8.1). Arthralgias may present as pain, stiffness, or more rarely swelling, may be transient, and may or may not coincide with cutaneous lesions. Symptoms usually last for no more than 72 h; persistent arthritis is relatively seldom. Multiple joints may be affected, with knees, ankles, wrists, and fingers being most frequently involved.

Vascular lesions of the kidneys are often present in urticaria vasculitis, but are missed unless patients are checked for hematuria, proteinuria, or creatinine clearance. Less frequent symptoms and organ involvements are listed in Table 8.1. Mild fever, weight loss, fatigue, pleuritic chest pain, and other symptoms also known to occur in connective tissue diseases are even more rare (Falk 1984).

8.4 Histopathology

There is general agreement that urticarial vasculitis is characterized by the following features: edema of the upper dermis; a neutrophilic infiltrate in and around the walls of the small superficial venules, with scattered nuclear fragments (nuclear dust) and extravasated red blood cells in the dermis; and deposition of fibrinoid material in and around the vessel walls (Table 8.2).

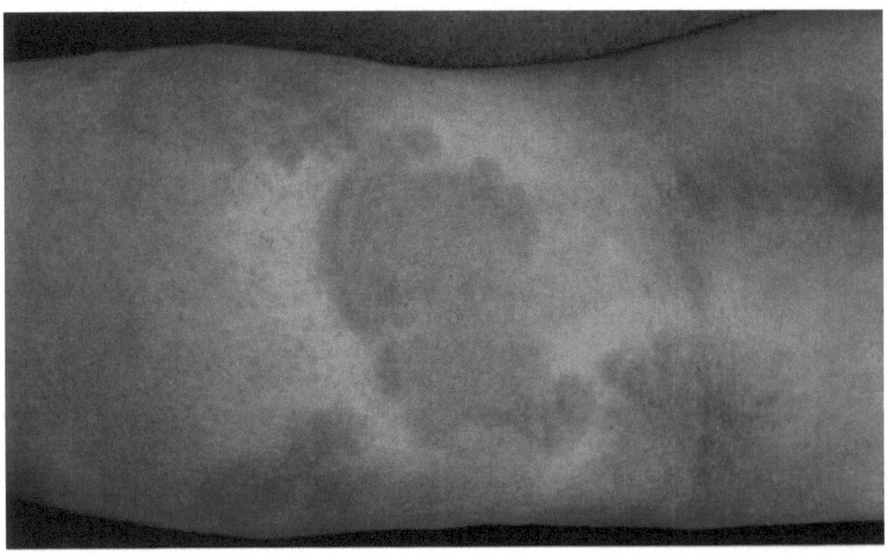

Fig. 8.2. Centrifugally spreading lesions of biopsy-proven urticarial vasculitis. Previously involved skin has a purplish discoloration.

Table 8.1. Clinical symptoms of the urticarial vasculitis syndrome.

Organ	Frequency of involvement	Clinical manifestations
Skin	100%	pruritic or burning wheals, angioedema, bullae, erythema multiforme, livedo reticularis
Joints	75%	arthralgias, swellings, stiffness, arthritis of single or multiple joints
Kidneys	60%	hematuria, proteinuria, decreased creatinine clearance, vasculitis on histology
Respiratory system	55%	chronic obstructive pulmonary disease, pleuritic chest pain, laryngeal edema
Eyes	35%	uveitis, episcleritis
Gastrointestinal tract	30%	nausea, vomiting, diarrhea, abdominal pain
Nervous system	12%	mononeuritis, myositis, seizures, pseudotumor cerebri, increased CNS pressure
Cardiovascular and hematological systems	5%	Raynaud's syndrome, carditis, lymphadenopathy, leukopenia, thrombocytopenia, shock

Differences in the literature regarding these criteria explain the vast variations in the incidence of vasculitis in chronic urticaria.

Other features may or may not be present in skin biopsies. Eosinophils were noted in the infiltrate by most authors (Sissons et al. 1974, Hintner and Tappeiner 1979, Phanuphak et al. 1980, Neumann et al. 1981, Wanderer et al. 1983), but they were conspicuously absent in biopsies of other patient groups (Soter et al. 1974). Mast cells were observed to be increased by one group (Horvath et al. 1981), but not by others (Wanderer et al. 1983).

Sissons et al. (1974) found the distributions of cells to be different from that of other authors, with neutrophils and eosinophils scattered throughout the dermis, and mononuclear cells only in a perivascular distribution. These discrepancies can be explained by the many different causes of urticarial vasculitis, with only some of them stimulating eosinophil production.

Table 8.2. Laboratory changes in patients with urticarial vasculitis.

Histopathology	neutrophilic vasculitis fibrinoid changes edema of upper dermis
Immunopathology (direct IF)	in vessel walls and at the dermoepidermal junction, deposits of a) IgM, IgG, IgA b) C1q, C4, C3 c) fibrinogen
Changes in peripheral blood	↑ ESR ↓↓ CH50, C1q, C4, C3, C5 ↑ circulating immune complexes, mostly normal or decreased immunoglobulins, at times positive: ANF, RF, cryoglobulins, hepatitis B antigen rarely present: leukopenia, thrombocytopenia

ESR, erythrocyte sedimentation rate; ANF, antinuclear factor; RF, rheumatoid factor; IF, immunofluorescence.

The distribution and nature of the infiltrate could also be related to the age of the lesions at the time of biopsy. Soter et al. (1974) removed skin 24 h after the resolution of urticarial lesions and at that time observed only a mild, perivascular, lymphocytic infiltrate. These findings agree with the observations that in experimental Arthus reactions, macrophages replace polymorphonuclear cells to an increasing extent in 12–24 h old lesions (Crawford et al. 1982).

Phanuphak et al. (1980) found a purely neutrophilic infiltrate in only 32% of their biopsies, and Jones et al. (1983) in only 12%. All their other patients with urticarial vasculitis had a perivascular infiltrate of lymphocytes, monocytes, or eosinophils, or a mixture of all of these types. The age of the lesions is not mentioned. Clinically, it is also very difficult to be sure of their duration since they have no distinguishing features (Provost et al. 1980).

Endothelial swelling and necrosis of vessel walls are two features considered an additional essential characteristic of urticarial vasculitis (Soter et al. 1974). However, in a recent, careful study of early lesions from 15 patients, Jones and Eady (1984) demonstrated that endothelial cell necrosis is rarely seen and that endothelial shrinkage as well as hypertrophy can be observed in the same biopsy. Also, in experimental, histamine-induced immune complex vasculitis, endothelial swelling is present to only a slight degree in early lesions (Wolff et al. 1978). One should therefore confine oneself to the criteria listed earlier on for diagnosis.

The histological changes of vessels are basically the same in urticarial vasculitis, irrespective of the underlying cause of the disease, e.g., a drug reaction, hepatitis B, or systemic lupus erythematosus. They are found in involved synovium, renal tissue, or in the skin (Soter et al. 1974, Soter 1977, Neumann et al. 1981, Wanderer et al. 1983).

8.5 Immunopathology

In 30–60 % of patients with leukocytoclastic urticarial vasculitis, fine granular deposits of either C1q, C4, IgM, C3, properdin, IgG, fibrinogen, or IgA are found in decreasing frequency and in various combinations along the dermo-epidermal junction and within blood vessel walls of lesional skin (Table 8.2) (Wanderer et al. 1983, Monroe et al. 1981). Normal skin is only rarely involved. The deposits at the basement membrane are unlike the lupus bands, are nonspecific, and are also seen in many other inflammatory dermatoses. Horvath et al. (1981) also noted deposits of IgA, IgM, IgE, and fibrinogen in the cytoplasm of cells at the dermal infiltrate in their three patients with urticaria, but not in the five patients with urticarial vasculitis and systemic lupus erythematosus.

8.6 Laboratory Findings

8.6.1 Erythrocyte Sedimentation Rate

The most frequent change in the peripheral blood is an elevation of the erythrocyte sedimentation rate (ESR) (Soter 1977), with the incidence varying from 50–90 % (Sanchez et al. 1982, Wanderer et al. 1983). Such elevations are not present in the more common types of urticaria and angioedema.

8.6.2 Immunoglobulins

Serum immunoglobulin levels are normal or decreased in patients with urticarial vasculitis (Soter et al. 1974, Monroe 1981). In a very few patients, cryoglobulins and increased levels of IgG and rheumatoid factor may be found, and up to 30 % of patients have low serum titers against double-stranded DNA (Zeiss et al. 1980, Monroe 1981). Rarely, high antibody titers to single-stranded DNA have also been reported (Monroe 1981). Their pathological significance is uncertain. One patient has been reported with leukopenia and thrombocytopenia (Guillet and Jeune 1983).

8.6.3 Complement System

One of the most striking features in urticarial vasculitis is a consumption of the early components of the classical complement pathway, resulting in a decrease of total hemolytic complement, C1, C1q, C4, and C2, less frequently of C3 and C5. Only rarely was a decrease in factor B found, indicating activation via the alternate pathway. Two of four patients with chronic urticaria and decreased serum complement levels studied by Ballow et al. (1975) had evidence of an unusual type of complement activation via the C1-bypass, with decreased levels of C1, C1q, C1s, properdin and factor B, and with normal C4 and C2. All in all, evidence for complement activation and decrease of the different components varies from 41 to 100 % (Wanderer et al. 1983).

8.6.4 Immune Complexes

A plausible reason for complement activation has been sought by measuring serum immune complexes in these patients. As with the evidence for serum complement activation, their presence has been demonstrated to a variable degree. Wanderer et al. (1983) measured complexes in 44 % of his patients by the C1q assay and in 22 % by the monoclonal rheumatoid factor assay, Phanuphak et al. (1980) in 56 % by the C1q assay, and Provost et al. (1980) in nine of his ten patients with urticarial vasculitis and systemic lupus erythematosus by the Raji cell assay. The latter test can give false positive values because it also measures antilymphocyte antibodies. Thus, disease activity as well as the assay used determines whether circulating immune complexes can be detected or not.

There have been attempts to identify the composition of the immune complexes in sera of patients with urticarial vasculitis. Agnello et al. (1976), Marder et al. (1978), and more recently Zeiss et al. (1980) were able to isolate a 7S protein that is partly IgG and that precipitates with C1q in agarose. This molecule has been considered a hallmark in chronic urticaria with vasculitis (Marder et al. 1978), but too few patient sera have yet been examined to be certain of this assumption.

8.7 Diagnosis

Considering the broad spectrum of possible clinical and laboratory abnormalities in patients with urticarial vasculitis, an agreement on the basic features necessary for diagnosis must be reached. This will also help to define the disease and to eliminate some of the confusion in the literature with regard to the pathogenesis and proper management of urticarial vasculitis.

Small et al. (1982) have rightly pointed out that no single test or clinical parameter is diagnostic for urticarial vasculitis. Many patients with urticaria and circulating immune complexes have no evidence of vasculitis at all. Other patients have decreased serum CH 50, urticaria, and arthritis, but no leukocytoclastic vasculitis and circulating immune disorders. Small et al. (1982) suggested therefore that the syndrome of urticarial vasculitis should encompass not just one but several parameters. These include (1) the basic clinical aspects, (2) a variety of possible immunological changes, and (3) certain well-defined pathological alterations.

Table 8.3 is an attempt to outline the clinical and pathological spectrum of changes that define urticarial vasculitis. At the one extreme are minor changes that may be found accidentally in chronic urticaria and should not suffice for the diagnosis of urticarial vasculitis. At the other extreme are the hallmarks of systemic lupus, as defined in more detail by the American Rheumatism Association (in Wechsler 1983). Urticarial vasculitis should, in the latter case, be regarded as only one of the many clinical aspects of this disease.

8.8 Differential Diagnosis

Serum sickness is the classical clinical counterpart of the Arthus reaction and of immune complex vasculitis.

Table 8.3. Diagnostic criteria of chronic idiopathic urticaria, the urticarial vasculitis syndrome, and systemic lupus erythematosus.

Clinical signs	Diagnosis
1. Idiopathic chronic urticaria lasting > 24 h 2. Leukocytoclastic vasculitis on histology	chronic urticaria
	↓
3. Purpuric or erythema multiforme-like lesions 4. Clinical signs of multisystem disease (see Table 8.1) 5. ↑ ESR, circulating immune complexes, pos. direct immunofluorescence, ↓ serum complement (see Table 8.2) 6. Resistance to therapy with antihistamines	urticarial vasculitis syndrome
	↓
7. Serologic evidence of connective tissue disease (+ double-stranded ANF; + lupus band on immunofluorescence)	SLE

SLE, systemic lupus erythematosus; ESR, erythrocyte sedimentation rate; ANF, antinuclear factor.

In contrast to the findings in the urticarial vasculitis syndrome, the urticaria and angioedema of serum sickness are usually triggered by an acute event, e.g., an injection with serum or penicillin. They subside again, but only slowly (Fellner 1976). The urticarial vasculitis syndrome might be viewed as the chronic counterpart of serum sickness, with the elicting agent being generally unknown.

Infectious mononucleosis can be observed in association with urticarial vasculitis (Wands et al. 1976) as well as the prodromal phase of viral hepatitis B, during which a necrotizing vasculitis (Dienstag et al. 1978) and a perivascular infiltrate of lymphocytes and eosinophils have been demonstrated, respectively (Neumann et al. 1981). The latter types of urticaria run a more acute course than the urticarial vasculitis syndrome. Disease-specific serological tests are available to aid in their proper diagnosis.

Physical urticarias, in particular cold and pressure urticarias, can have features of leukocytoclastic urticarial vasculitis, with an increased ESR, arthralgias and involvement of organ systems other than the skin (Monroe et al. 1981, Wanderer et al. 1983) see also Chapter 5, p. 55). Mixed IgG-IgM cryoglobulinemia can be associated with urticaria, vasculitis, and decreased serum complement. The presence of cryoglobulins and the diagnostic cold contact and pressure tests should help to differentiate these diseases from the chronic idiopathic urticarial vasculitis syndrome.

Wüthrich (1979) screened 169 patients with chronic urticaria and found decreased levels of C3 in 10 %, of C4 in 9.4 %, and of the C1-inhibitor in 12.9 %; 24 % of his patients had at least one of these three factors decreased. This points to difficulties in sorting out the chronic urticarias, and patients should be examined more carefully for specific causes of their urticaria and for other features of the urticarial vasculitis syndrome before they are assigned to this latter category.

The differentiation of systemic lupus erythematosus from the urticarial vasculitis syndrome is not difficult if the typical clinical and pathological features of lupus erythematosus are present. There are, however, reports of patients with urticarial vasculitis and transient, low serum antinuclear factors (ANF) titers (Gammon and Wheeler 1979). It is thus possible that a gray zone exists between the two diseases, and that patients will have to be observed carefully over an extended period for other signs of lupus before a diagnosis of the one or the other disease is made.

A familial deficiency of C3 can present with cutaneous vasculitis and an SLE-like syndrome (McLean et al. 1980). Similarly, C1q inhibitor deficiency can be associated with urticarial vasculitis, systemic lupus erythematosus, rheumatoid arthritis, chronic liver disease, and a decrease of C4. These diseases can be differentiated by their special clinical and laboratory aspects. In allergic angioedema, all complement components are within normal range (Brasher et al. 1975).

8.9 Prognosis

The urticarial vasculitis syndrome can last for up to 10 years (Guillet and Jeune 1983), although 30–40% of the patients stop having their lesions within a year. No deaths have yet been reported due to the disease alone, and it runs a relatively benign course.

If patients have proven systemic lupus erythematosus, associated urticarial vasculitis may worsen their prognosis. Horvath et al. (1981) reported a fatal outcome for all four patients with this combination who had lupus nephritis in addition. Sanchez et al. (1982) observed a less severe clinical course in patients with the normocomplementemic urticarial vasculitis syndrome despite signs of systemic involvement. They also believe that cutaneous deposits of IgG and IgM and decreased complement levels may be an indicator of renal disease.

8.10 Pathogenesis

8.10.1 Immune Complexes

Vasculitis is a reaction pattern of the cutaneous vasculature caused by a wide variety of substances. Therefore, more than one pathogenetic mechanism is involved. There are a number of indications that immune complexes are invariably present during the induction phase of urticarial vasculitis. They are not always measured, possibly because even in experimental immune complex disease, complexes are no longer detectable in the serum 2 and 18 h after their injection (Cream et al. 1971, De Shazo et al. 1972). Variability in the severity of disease may be another reason, and Pussell et al. (1978) have noted a correlation between disease severity and detection and level of immune complexes.

8.10.2 Mediators

Figure 8.3 depicts the possible pathogenetic events that lead to immune complex vasculitis. Immune complexes stimulate the formed elements of the blood and the tissue, inducing secretion of histamine, serotonin, platelet activating factor, prostaglandins and leukotrienes. These mediators cause vasodilatation, increased vascular permeability, and the deposition of circulating immune complexes within the walls of the capillary venules. Immune complexes can also activate complement and cause the generation of vasoactive and leukotactic complement fragments, like C5a. Fluid- and cell-derived leukotactic factors in the blood induce neutrophil adherence to the vessel walls and the subsequent emigration of leukocytes into the perivascular tissue. Thus, immune complexes initiate a complex sequence of events that results in the

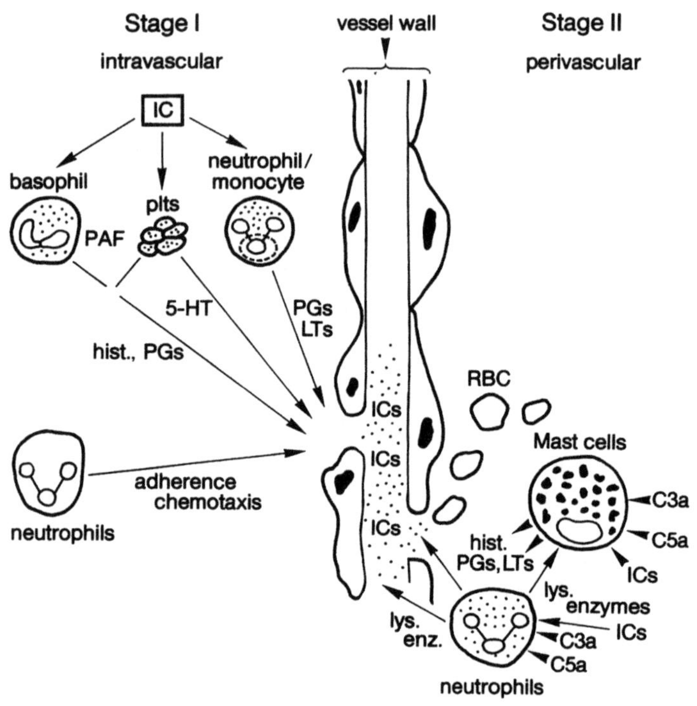

Fig. 8.3. Schematic outline of the possible events initiated by immune complexes with their deposition in the vessel walls, leading to the development of urticarial vasculitis.
Hist, histamine; *5-HT*, 5-hydroxytryptamine; *IC*, immune complex; *LTs*, leukotrienes; *lys. enz.*, lysosomal enzymes; *plts*, platelets; *PAF*, platelet-activating factor; *PGs*, prostaglandins; *RBC*, red blood cells.

clinical and histopathological picture seen in urticarial vasculitis.

8.10.3 Relationship to the Arthus Reaction

Neutrophils have been shown to be essential for the development of the Arthus-type vasculitis. Neutrophil infiltration reaches a peak 2–4 h after immune complex injection into perivascular tissue. Phagocytosis of immune complexes and stimulation of the neutrophils by C3a and C5a induces the secretion of prostaglandins, leukotrienes, and lysosomal enzymes from cells. The enzymes cause vascular injury and hemorrhage which peaks in 6-h old lesions. Macrophages are seen in increasing number in 12–24 h old Arthus lesions (Crawford et al. 1982).

Many of these features of the Arthus reaction, particularly the varying predominance of neutrophils and mononuclear cells in lesions of different ages, fit with the histological observations in the biopsies of urticarial vasculitis lesions. The same holds for the frequently observed hemorrhage. Since these features are also seen in macules and papules of vasculitis, urticaria must be due to additional, probably more mast cell-related pathogenetic events. All of the factors that cause neutrophil secretion can also induce mast cells to release histamine and vasoactive arachidonate derivatives (see Fig. 8.3). One could postulate that in urticarial vasculitis, the vasoactive mediators predominate rather than the leukotactic and tissue destructive mediators of inflammation.

8.10.4 Other Pathogenic Factors

Several factors other than immune complexes must contribute to the development of urticarial vasculitis, particularly since immune complexes are not pathogenic under normal circumstances, unless histamine is injected (Braverman and Yen 1975). Devey et al. (1982) suggested that (1) the type of immune complex, (2) genetic factors, and (3) the sex of the individual are important for the development of the disease. In their experimental system, low affinity antibodies in immune complexes caused damage more easily than high affinity antibodies.

Certain strains of animals are also more susceptible to vasculitis than others, and female animals have ten times more free antibodies in the circulation than males (Devey et al. 1982).

In patients with hypocomplementemic urticarial vasculitis, an abnormal 7 S IgG-like C1q binding protein has been identified (Marder et al. 1978). This protein could result from (1) faulty synthesis of the Fc part of IgG or its alteration through factors in the circulation; (2) a small antigen that had reacted with both combining sites of a single IgG molecule, rendering the Fc portion available for binding; or (3) a complexing of IgG with a small antigen that has C1q binding properties (Marder et al. 1978).

As an alternative to the immune complex theory, complement abnormalities might be responsible for the vasculitis. Such abnormalities might be due to acquired or to intrinsic genetic defects. Opsonization by complement normally aids in the phagocytosis and elimination of immune complexes. Defects in the complement system or the phagocytic system could result in excessive levels of immune complexes which would activate the orchestration of pathogenic events, as depicted in Fig. 8.3.

These considerations are not entirely theoretical since patients with genetic defects of the C1r, C2, and C4 molecules tend to develop systemic lupus-like illnesses more frequently than the normal population. Excessive heparin and dextran sulfate can also cause complement consumption via C1 activation (Sissons et al. 1974) and may contribute to the disease.

9 Mastocytosis (Urticaria Pigmentosa)

9.1 Introduction

Mastocytosis first came to the attention of physicians at the end of the last century when the speckled brown pigmentation of the skin and the associated whealing after irritation was described (Nettleship 1869). Several years later, Unna observed a local proliferation of mast cells in the dermis underlying the brown spots (Unna 1887). The disease was called urticaria pigmentosa until the 1930ies when it became apparent that other organs than the skin could be involved, and the more general term mastocytosis was introduced at that time by Sézary (see Chapter 1, p. 3 for details).

Mastocytosis is a relatively rare disease, with an incidence of about one case in 1000–8000 dermatological outpatients (Sagher and Even-Paz 1967). At the department of dermatology of the University of Münster, 100 new cases were seen over the past 5 years (Table 9.1). About half of these patients had developed their disease before puberty, and in >90% of the latter, the diagnosis had been made at birth or during the first 6 months of life. The sex incidence is about equal, the symptomatology is low, particularly in children, and many adult patients have evidence of extracutaneous involvement.

Mastocytosis has been observed in all races, and it is found in many different types of mammals, particularly dogs (Cook 1969). The disease has been classified on the basis of many different criteria, including its highly variable clinical appearances. Table 9.2 shows a simple classification of mastocytosis, based on the extent of clinical involvement in different age groups and on prognostic criteria.

Table 9.1. Clinical data on 100 patients with cutaneous mastocytosis seen at the dermatology clinic, University of Münster, over 5 years.

Patient data	Juveniles (45)	Adults (55)
Age at onset (mean years)	0.3	31.1
♂/♀	1/1	1/1.6
Pruritus (%)	5.0	13.0
Diarrhea (%)	3.0	4.0
↑ MC, marrow (%)	n.d.	61.5

n.d., not done; MC, mast cells.

9.2 Cutaneous Mastocytosis

Solitary mastocytomas arise almost exclusively in childhood. They consist of up to 5–6 cm large, raised, pinkish or yellow papules or plaques that can be located anywhere on the body, with a preference for the hands and the wrists. The lesions regress in almost all instances within several years, and the chance of malignant transformation is extremely low (Johnson and Helwig 1961).

Disseminated cutaneous mastocytosis is the most frequent type of the disease (Sagher and Even-Paz 1967). In infants, it occurs mostly in form of multiple nodular lesions. Rare cases with large tumors have also been described (Bakos et al. 1972, Willemze et al.

Table 9.2. Classification of mast cell neoplasms, their relative frequency, and their prognosis.

Disease	Frequency	Spontaneous regression	Malignant transformation
I. Benign cutaneous mastocytosis			
1. solitary mastocytoma	11–15%	99%	0%
2. disseminated mastocytosis	85–89%		
juvenile	64%	80%	rare
adult	25%	rare	rare
II. Benign systemic mastocytosis	4.5–10%		
juvenile		yes	7%
adult		?	33%
III. Malignant mastocytosis	rare	no	(poor prognosis)

1980). The disseminated maculo-papular lesions represent the most frequent type of cutaneous mastocytosis (Fig. 9.1), particularly in the adult. Vesiculation and bulla formation, if present, occur on top of these lesions, mostly within the first years of life (Fig. 9.2). The tendency to blister formation disappears after the first year of life, or at the latest by age 3 (Robinson et al. 1962).

Other rare clinical manifestations of cutaneous mastocytosis are lichenoid, plaque-like, xanthelasmoid, haemorrhagic, and teleangiectatic or generalized erythrodermic changes of the skin. In rare cases, persistent skin lesions are absent, and the diagnosis is made on the basis of chronic urticaria and increased mast cell numbers on histological examination of the skin (Sahihi and Esterly 1972).

9.3 Systemic Mastocytosis

The incidence of benign systemic mastocytosis varies from 4.5 to 10% of the cases of mastocytosis in different series (Table 9.2), but may be much higher if thoroughly looked for through routine examinations of the bone marrow (see Table 9.1). Malignant mastocytosis is extremely rare and occurs much more frequently in adults than in children (Klaus and Winkelmann 1962, Caplan 1963, Sagher and Even-Paz 1967).

If systemic involvement is present, increased numbers of mast cells are found most frequently in the bone marrow (Webb et al. 1982). Enlargement of liver and spleen and X-ray changes of the skeleton may be noted in up to 70% of the cases, while lymphadenopathy is less frequent (28–46%) (Sagher and Even-Paz 1967). Changes in these organs do not necessarily imply a proliferation of mast cells. In the liver and the intestine, for example, one frequently finds only fibrotic changes of the reticuloendothelial system (Ammann and Spycher 1972, Rodermund et al. 1978).

X-ray changes may be present in form of single osteolytic lesions, particularly in the skull of children, while diffuse osteosclerotic changes are most frequent in adults. Increased numbers of mast cells have on rare occasions also been noted in the lungs, kidneys, the gastrointestinal tract, in striated muscles, the omentum, and in the central nervous system (Sagher and Even-Paz 1967).

9.4 Symptomatology

The majority of patients with mastocytosis come to the physician because they are disturbed by the pigmentary changes and the whealing on rubbing of their skin (Darier's sign) (Fig. 9.3). Less than 20% of the patients with only skin involvement complain of itching, and if present, this symptom is usually only of a mild degree and is rarely found in children (see Table 9.1). The frequency of pruritus and other symptoms is more frequent in patients with systemic involvement (Table 9.3). Flushing is relatively frequent, followed in frequency by gastro-intestinal disturbances such as nausea, vomiting, abdominal cramps, diarrhea, and peptic ulcers. Tachycardia, shock symptomatology, headache, and cardiovascular collapse may be observed after bouts of massive histamine release and may even result in death of the patient. Malaise, fever, and weight loss are signs of supervening malignancy. Local pain in bones and over joints, together with paresthesias, psychiatric disorders, and even convulsions are rare and are related to the mast cell-induced changes of the skeleton and the nervous system (Sagher and Even-Paz 1967).

9.5 Histology

The most frequent picture, particularly of the adult onset mastocytosis, is an increased number of spindle-shaped mast cells with long cytoplasmic processes, in a perivascular location or scattered throughout the upper corium (Fig. 9.4). Fibroblasts, lymphocytes, and occasional eosinophils may be seen in close apposition to the cells. In the nodular and plaque-type cutaneous lesions of childhood, cuboid mast cells with a smooth surface lie more closely together and have a nevoid appearance (Mihm et al. 1973, Ludatscher et al. 1977). Mast cells may be at very different stages of maturation (Drennan and Beare 1954). Even in diffuse cases of mastocytosis, mast cells have a normal appearance on electron microscopy and degranulate by extrusion of whole granules (Freeman 1967, Kolde et al. 1984).

In the bone marrow, either a focal (Fig. 9.5) or a diffuse proliferation of mast cells is observed. Bone marrow aspirates often yield false negative results because of the focal increase of mast cells, the sclerotic changes, or the adherence of mast cells to the connective tissue septa and the endosteum (Webb et al. 1982). Other possible changes in the marrow are myeloid hyperplasia with a shift to the left, a decrease of erythropoiesis, and a moderate to marked eosinophilia. Involvement of the marrow is rare in children (Rodermund et al. 1978).

For histological examination of tissue, special stains such as toluidine blue, methylene blue or Giemsa are

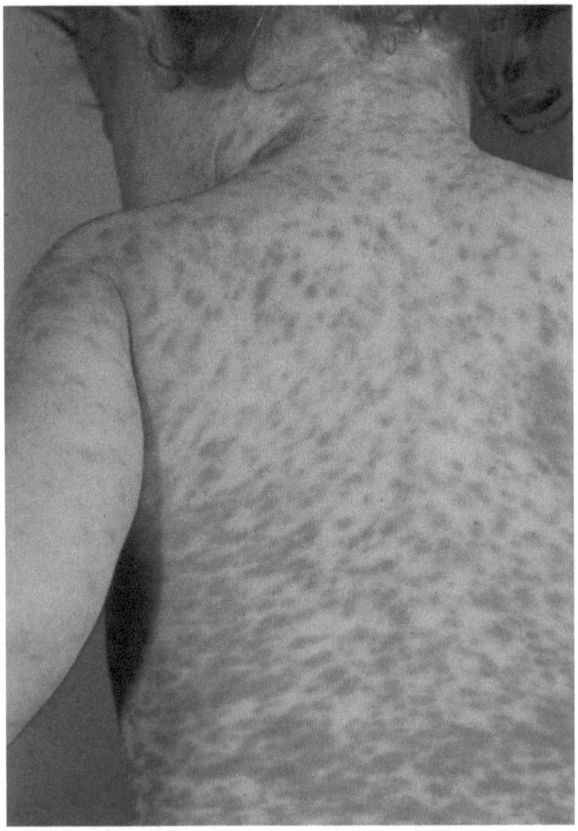

Fig. 9.1. Generalized maculopapular urticaria pigmentosa in a 9-month old girl. Note the intense erythema on the lateral back where the child's skin has been rubbed (+ Darier's sign).

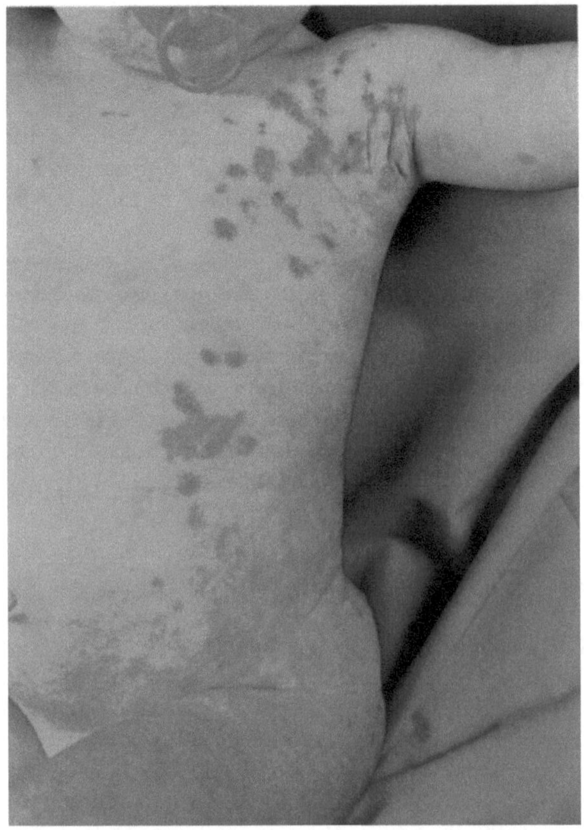

Fig. 9.2. Bullous lesions, many of which have ruptured, leaving eroded areas, in an 18-month old girl with mastocytosis. Note also the diffuse erythema and the thickening of the skin of the diaper area and the thighs. The child also suffers from seizures after massive histamine release.

necessary to recognize mast cells (Fig. 9.4, Fig. 9.5). Lennert (1962) believes that toluidine blue staining at higher pH is a sign for lower sulfatation and greater immaturity of the cells. Other possible signs for malignant transformation are a greater nuclear to cytoplasmic ratio, fewer cytoplasmic granules, an increase of atypical mitoses, and a greater cell and nuclear polymorphism with giant cells. Other authors

Fig. 9.3. Whealing and erythema of the skin after rubbing (Darrier's sign) in an adult patient with mastocytosis.

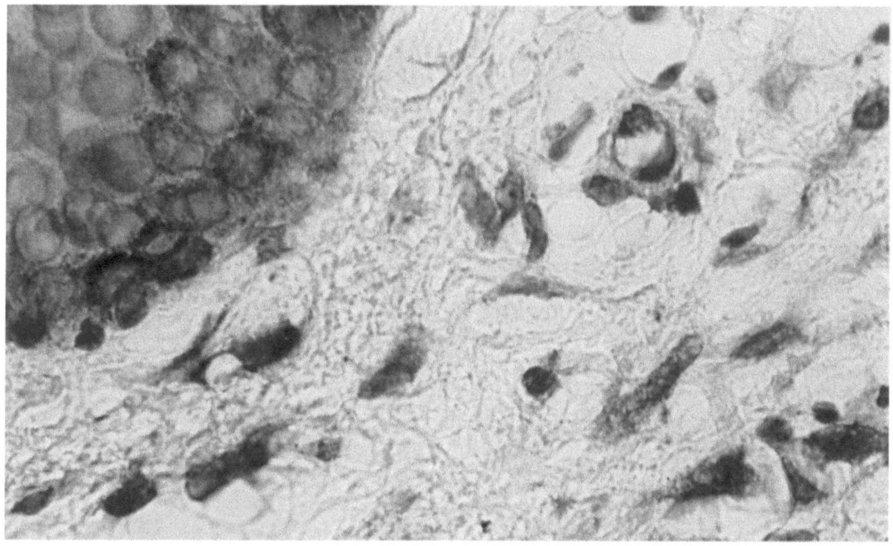

Fig. 9.4. Histological section of epidermis and upper dermis in an adult patient with mastocytosis. Note the purple discoloration of the mast cell granules in the dermis, due to their metachromatic staining characteristics. Toluidine blue stain, orig. magn. 400 ×.

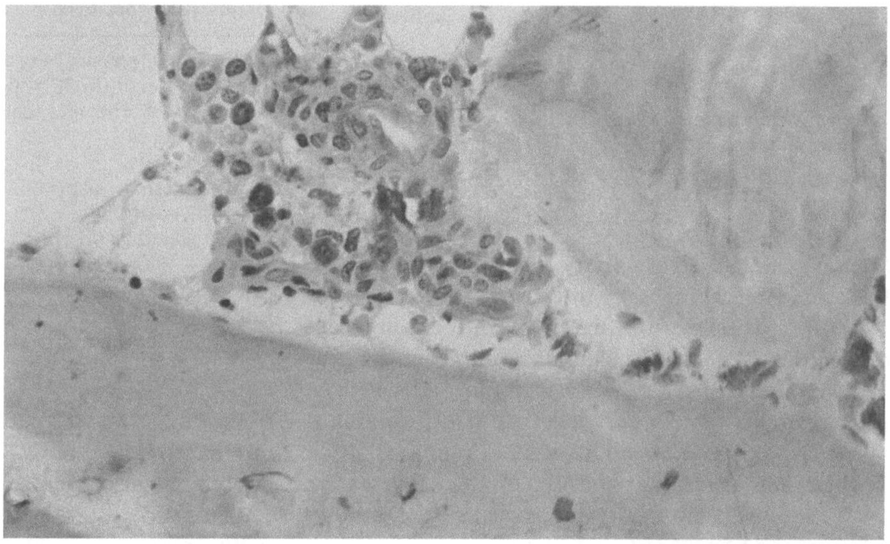

Fig. 9.5. Histology of the bone marrow in an adult patient with mastocytosis, demonstrating an increase of metachromatic mast cells (purple cells). Giemsa, orig. magn. 100 ×.

state that there are no such unequivocal criteria which help decide whether mastocytosis is benign or malignant, not even by electron microscopy (Desmons 1980).

Particularly in the adult form, it may at times be difficult to decide whether mast cell numbers are truly increased in the tissue. As a rule, 3–4 mast cells per high power field are suggestive if the diagnosis fits with the clinical picture, while 6 or more mast cells per high power field are highly suggestive. In cases of doubt, more than one biopsy from different locations should be performed to confirm the diagnosis (Lennert 1962).

Fig. 9.6. Test for dermographism in an adult patient with mastocytosis. The linear wheal has a beaded appearance due to more pronounced whealing at spots containing increased numbers of mast cells.

9.6 Laboratory Findings

Histamine levels are variably elevated in the skin, the serum, and the urine of patients with mastocytosis

Table 9.3. The frequency of symptoms of systemic mastocytosis.

Symptom	Frequency
Pruritus	41%
Flushing	36%
Nausea, vomiting, abdominal cramps	23%
Tachycardia	18%
Weakness, fatigue, malaise, fever	12%
Headache, dizziness	10%
Weight loss	10%
Peptic ulcer	4–7%
Respiratory symptomatology	rare
Bone pain	rare
Convulsions	rare

Table 9.4. Laboratory findings in mastocytosis.

Serum	Urine
↑ histamine	↑ hist. + metabolites
↑ alk. phosph. Ca, P	↑ PGD_2
↓ cholesterol	↑ hyaluronic acid + chondroitin sulfate
↓ prothrombin time	
↑ thromboxane B_2	
↓ 6 keto-$PGF_{1\alpha}$	

(Demis et al. 1961, Vella Briffa et al. 1983) (Table 9.4). Histamine metabolites in the urine are supposedly more closely related to the extent of proliferating mast cells in the tissue than is histamine itself (Granerus et al. 1983). Several other products of mast cells such as prostaglandin D_2, leukotrienes, and glycosaminoglycans may be elevated in skin, serum, or urine (Roberts et al. 1980, Ouwendijk et al. 1983, Czarnetzki et al. 1985). Elevation of serum alkaline phosphatase, calcium, and phosphorus and decreased serum cholesterol and prothrombin time may be secondary to hepatic and skeletal involvement (Sagher and Even-Paz 1967).

Hematological changes are generally a reflection of the replacement of the bone marrow by fibrotic connective tissue and are found exclusively in patients with systemic mastocytosis (Table 9.5). In these cases, signs which might indicate the development of leukemia should be watched for. Circulating tissue mast cells have been observed in up to 16% of patients with systemic mastocytosis, while an eosinophilia is seen only in 12% (Sagher and Even-Paz 1967).

Table 9.5. Changes in hematological parameters of patients with systemic mastocytosis.

Hematological abnormalities	Frequency
Anemia	42%
Leukemia	24%
Thrombocytopenia	21%
Coagulation defects	21%
Leukocytosis	18%
Leukopenia	13%
Eosinophilia	12%

9.7 Diagnosis

The more common types of cutaneous mastocytosis are readily recognized by the experienced physician because of their typical clinical appearance. Table 9.6 outlines the most important steps that should be taken in juvenile and adult patients in the sequence shown.

Table 9.6. Diagnosis of mastocytosis.

Diagnostic procedures	Juveniles	Adults
1. History + physical examination	↓	↓
2. Darier's sign (in 90% positive)	↓	↓
3. CBC, liver enzymes, calcium, phosphorus	↓	↓
4. Skin biopsy	↓	↓
5. Bone marrow aspirate + biopsy	—	↓
X-ray: skeleton, GI tract	⇣	⇣

The most important diagnostic procedures are shown with full arrows, optional procedures with dotted arrows. CBC, complete blood count; GI, gastrointestinal tract.

In 90% of the patients, the diagnosis can be confirmed by whealing and redness of the lesions after rubbing (Darier's sign, Fig. 9.3). About 50% of the patients also exhibit dermographic whealing in clinically normal skin (Demis et al. 1961, Hughes and Warin 1963) (Fig. 9.6).

To rule out systemic involvement, the patients or parents should be questioned about symptoms like gastrointestinal disturbances or flushing, and the physical examination should always include a palpation of liver, spleen, and peripheral lymphnodes. In all patients, an initial complete blood count should be performed and serum levels of alkaline phosphatase, calcium, and phosphorus should be measured.

A skin biopsy may be omitted in very small children with obviously benign disease. It is otherwise helpful to confirm the diagnosis and to rule out histological signs of malignant transformation. In adults, a bone marrow aspirate should be done routinely. Other tests like X-rays of the skeleton, a liver scintigram, and analysis of urinary histamine metabolites can be performed if clinically indicated or for scientific reasons.

9.8 Pathogenesis

The reason for the local or generalized proliferation of mast cells in mastocytosis is unknown. Recently, connective tissue mast cells have been shown to derive from the bone marrow (Kitamura et al. 1977). Our own in vitro studies have proven that mononuclear phagocytes of murine or human origin can be stimulated to transform into mast cells on exposure to fibroblast-derived conditioning factors (Czarnetzki et al. 1982 and 1984). Other groups have demonstrated that lymphocyte-derived conditioning factors can also stimulate mast cell differentiation (Thueson et al. 1979). Since fibroblasts and lymphocytes are frequently found in close apposition to cutaneous mast cells, factors from either cell type may stimulate the maturation of resident or immigrated precursor cells.

The reason for the increased production of mast cell stimulating factors may be diverse and may even include a genetic predisposition in 5% of these cases (Demis 1963, James and Eady 1981). This explains why no single common factor has so far been found at the beginning of mastocytosis, either during the pregnancy of mothers with affected infants or during the period before the appearance of the disease in adults.

Varying degrees of maturity of the mast cells and of the amount of mediators they contain may be a reason for differences in the symptomatology of the disease.

Table 9.7. Mast cell mediators explaining the clinical aspects of mastocytosis.

Mast cell mediator	Effect
1. histamine, LTC_4, LTD_4, (SRS), PGD_2, PAF	cutaneous whealing cardiovascular symptoms (flush, shock) GI and respiratory symptoms, pruritus, convulsions
2. glycosaminoglycans (heparin)	↑ CT turnover ↑ pigmentation ↓ cholesterol ↑ bleeding tendency (extremely rare) anti-inflammatory effect
3. LTB_4	↑ eosinophils in tissue
4. enzymes	↑ CT turnover ↑ kinin generation

LT, leukotrienes; PG, prostaglandin; PAF, platelet-activating factor; GI, gastrointestinal; CT, connective tissue.

Our current knowledge of the biological activity of mast cell mediators offers a basis for understanding practically all known symptoms of mastocytosis (see Table 9.7). The reactive, episodic changes in the skin and other organ systems can, for example, be caused by the intermittent release of histamine and other mast cell-derived lipid mediators like leukotrienes C_4 and D_4, PAF, and prostaglandin D_2. Heparin and other glycosaminoglycans which are stored in mast cell granules, can induce increased connective tissue turnover and hyperpigmentation (Sagher and Even-Paz 1967). Leukotriene B_4 and possibly also lymphocyte-derived factors can cause local accumulation of eosinophils, and mast cell enzymes can contribute to connective tissue turnover and kinin generation (see Chapter 2, p. 5 for details and references).

9.9 Prognosis

With a few exceptions, mastocytosis is a benign proliferative disease of mast cells (see Table 9.2). Dogs with mastocytosis have a normal or even prolonged lifespan (Cook 1969). In the childhood form, the stimulus for mast cell proliferation seems to be lost in the majority of cases, and cutaneous lesions rarely persist beyond puberty. In contrast, regression is a rare event if the disease begins after puberty, and even in children, the later the onset after birth, the less likely is regression (Klaus and Winkelmann 1962). Spontaneous regression may be observed even in systemic lesions (Robinson et al. 1962).

Of the adults with systemic disease, one-third may be expected to develop malignant mastocytosis or other malignancies of the reticuloendothelial system. The frequency is much lower in children with systemic diseases (Table 9.2) (Sagher and Even-Paz 1967).

Fatal complications in the absence of malignant disease may also occur because of cardiovascular shock after massive mast cell degranulation or due to peptic ulcers which are observed in 4–7% of patients with systemic mastocytosis (Sagher and Even-Paz 1967).

The latter should be looked for and treated appropriately. Parents and/or patients should be instructed to avoid factors or agents that cause sudden and extensive mast cell mediator release, or, if unavoidable, prophylactic treatment should be initiated (see Chapter 11.5, p. 148 for management and treatment).

10 Diagnosis

10.1 Introduction

The typical fleeting, pruritic urticarial lesion is so characteristic that it is readily recognized, even by inexperienced physicians and mostly also by the patient himself. The real diagnostic challenge lies in the recognition of the cause of this whealing reaction, particularly since this has important consequences for patient management (Chapter 11, p. 134).

In the preceding chapters, the diagnosis and differential diagnosis of each major category of urticaria has been discussed in detail, and the numerous clinical variants have been presented as well. The purpose of this chapter is to provide a flow-sheet-like guideline that should help the physician to group his patient's urticaria into one of the major diagnostic categories (Table 10.1). In addition, a detailed description of specific diagnostic tests is provided, and their relative value is discussed.

Hopefully, this chapter will help to make urticaria less of a vexing problem to both patient and physician. Like Dr. Watson with Sherlock Holmes, the patient should have the keen pleasure of following his doctor "in his professional investigations and in admiring the rapid deduction, as swift as intuitions, and yet always founded on a logical basis, with which he unravels the problems which were submitted to him" (Doyle 1901).

10.2 History

10.2.1 Clinical Appearance and Symptoms

Of all the diagnostic procedures for patients with urticaria, a carefully taken history represents the most important diagnostic step. At the first visit, the patient should be asked about the onset, the frequency, and the duration of the lesions. This will differentiate acute from chronic urticaria (Table 10.1).

The patient should then give a detailed description of the size, color, configuration, sensation, location, and duration of the individual wheals. These points will give first hints at a special type of urticaria. Reports on deeper tissue swellings would suggest the diagnosis of angioedema. More persistent urticarial lesions might be due to an underlying vasculitis. Macular or maculopapular, brown or red pigmentations indicate an urticaria pigmentosa.

An inquiry should be made about additional local or systemic symptoms. Some of them, such as shortness of breath, syncope, nausea, vomiting, and headache, are merely signs of massive mediator release. Flushing and edema of the face that spreads rapidly to the trunk, with associated itching of the scalp would, on the other hand, be suggestive of an aspirin-type intolerance reaction. Fever and arthralgias are seen only with familial cold urticaria, urticarial vasculitis, and pressure urticaria.

10.2.2 Potentially Provoking or Associated Factors

In contrast to chronic urticaria, the eliciting factor in acute urticaria is often evident. Specific foods, especially seafood, or drugs taken during an acute illness, can frequently be implicated. If the patient is unaware of such an association, he should be asked to relate or write down all that he has done during the 24 h preceding the onset of the urticaria. If this procedure provides no clues, it might be helpful to repeat it when another bout of acute urticaria occurs some weeks later.

In the initial phase, lesions due to light, cold, heat, pressure, or physical exertion might be viewed as an acute urticaria, but the distribution of the lesions, their configuration, and the time course of their appearance in relationship to certain stimuli will be helpful.

The diagnosis of chronic urticaria is much more problematic. Provoking factors, as noted above, are less readily evident. Patients will maintain that they have taken a type of food or drugs like laxatives, analgesics, or hormones for many years with impunity.

Important additional questions should inquire about a family history of similar illnesses since several types of urticaria are familial (see Table 5.2, p. 56), about smoking habits, occupation, recent travel, and past and present illnesses. In order not to miss any important points, it may be advisable to give the patient a checklist of drugs or diseases for which he might be taking medication and of odors and fumes which might provoke his symptoms (Speer et al. 1978, Table 10.2). Such lists should however not be a

Table 10.1. Important anamnestic features providing diagnostic clues for the different types of urticaria.

Question	Answer	Possible diagnosis	For further diagnostic procedures (Chapter)
1) Duration of disease	a) < 6 wks	acute urticaria	3 and 10
	b) > 6 wks	chronic urticaria	3 and 10
2) Size of lesions	a) pinpoint	1) aquagenic urticaria	5.11
		2) cholinergic urticaria	5.8
		3) solar urticaria	5.9
	b) giant, deep tissue swellings	1) angioedema	4.10
		2) pressure urticaria	5.6
3) Location of lesion	a) in areas exposed to sunlight	1) solar urticaria	5.9
		2) heat contact urticaria	5.10
	b) at pressure points	1) pressure urticaria	5.6
		2) dermographic urticaria	5.4
	c) at cold, exposed sites	cold urticaria	5.7
	d) at sites of vibration or friction	1) vibratory angioedema	5.5
		2) dermographic urticaria	5.4
	e) at site of exposure to chemicals	contact urticaria	6.8
	f) at sites of pigmented lesions	urticaria pigmentosa (mastocytosis)	9.7
4) Temporal appearance of lesions	a) delayed	1) pressure urticaria	5.6
		2) cholinergic urticaria	5.8
		3) cold urticaria	5.7
		4) heat contact urticaria	5.10
	b) rapid	most types of urticaria	
5) Duration of lesions	a) short (1/2–1 h)	1) dermographic urticaria	
		2) cholinergic urticaria	
		3) aquagenic urticaria	
		4) solar urticaria	5
		5) heat contact urticaria	
		6) cold urticaria	
		7) vibratory angioedema	
	b) prolonged (> 48 h)	1) urticaria vasculitis	8.7
		2) familial cold urticaria	5.7
6) Provoking factors	a) sunlight	solar urticaria	
	b) heat contact	heat contact urticaria	
	c) cold air	1) cold contact urticaria	
		2) familial cold urticaria	5
	d) cold water	1) cold contact urticaria	
		2) aquagenic urticaria	
	e) luke-warm water	aquagenic urticaria	
	f) physical exertion, stress	cholinergic urticaria	
	g) food – animal and plant proteins,	acute or chronic urticaria	3.7
	– preservatives, dyes	anaphylactoid reactions	7.6
	h) drugs (antibiotics, analgesics, laxatives, hormones)	ordinary urticaria	3.7
		(anaphylactoid reactions)	(7.6)
	i) acute or persistent viral illness (hepatitis B)	ordinary urticaria	3.7
	k) inhalants or contactants (smoking habits)	ordinary urticaria	3.7
	l) chronic illnesses	1) chronic urticaria	3.7
		2) urticaria vasculitis	8.7
	m) recent X-ray tests or surgical procedures	anaphylactoid reactions	7.6
	n) recent visits to tropical countries (parasitoses, insect bites)	1) acute or chronic urticaria	3.7
		2) papular urticaria	
7) Familial occurrence		several physical urticarias	Table 5.2
		hereditary angioedema	4.10
		aspirin intolerance syndrome	7.6
		atopy (cold and heat contact urticaria)	5.7 and 5.10

Table 10.2. Checklist for patients to determine possible causative factors in urticaria (after Speer et al. 1978).

Drugs	Diseases	Inhalants	Foods
antibiotics	acne	gasoline	alcohol
antihistamines	allergy	kerosene	milk
cold tablets	anemia	natural gas	eggs
cortisone	arthritis	paint, oil, thinners	fish
cough medications	asthma	paint remover	tomatoes
nasal decongestants	colds	tobacco smoke	strawberries
digitalis	colitis	trash fire	salads
diuretics	constipation	frying odors	mayonaise
douches	convulsions	leaf fire	tinned food
hormones	cough	lumber	citrus fruits
laxatives	depression	saw-sanding dust	
lozenges	diabetes	household cleaners	
mouth washes	diarrhea	polish	
muscle relaxants	epilepsy	bleaches, starch	
oral contraceptives	fungus infections	nail polish	
penicillin	gallbladder disorders	face powder	
rectal medications	glaucoma	deoderants	
reducing pills	gout	antiseptics	
sedatives	headache	alcohol	
sleeping pills	heart disease	witch hazel	
sulfa drugs	hemorrhoids	shaving lotion	
tetracyclines	high blood pressure	bubble bath	
thyroid hormones	indigestion	menthol or camphor	
tonics (quinine)	insomnia	Vick's vaporub	
tranquilizers	kidney disease	ammonia	
vaginal medications	menopause	chlorine	
"water pills"	menstrual disorders	pine odors	
vitamins	nervousness	moth balls	
	pinworms	lysol	
	sinus trouble	insect spray	
	stomach disorders	flowers	
	urinary infections	perfumes	
	vaginal infections	hair spray	
		newspaper ink	
		copying machines	
		carbon paper	
		adhesive tape	
		plastics	
		shoe polish	
		asphalt	
		food odors	

substitute for a thorough discussion of the specific provoking factors between patient and physician.

10.2.3 Physical Examination

Urticae and angioedema are usually present in patients with acute urticaria. These lesions should be examined for the typical clinical features of wheals and deep cutaneous edemas, and for their distribution. Dermographic wheals might be seen at sites of friction of tight clothing. The skin should also be inspected for pigment spots (mastocytosis), for signs of metabolic disorders, or for eczema.

A general physical examination should also include an inspection of the teeth, a palpation of the thyroid gland and the liver, and a cursory neurological check-up.

10.3 Laboratory Procedures

10.3.1 Screening Tests

Many authors suggest a battery of screening tests for the laboratory diagnosis of chronic idiopathic urticaria. This practice has been seriously challenged more recently since abnormal results are obtained in only 20.8% of the patients, and almost all of them were expected on the basis of a thorough history and physical examination (Kraig et al. 1980, see also

Table 10.3. Results of routine screening tests in two larger series of patients with (A) chronic (Kraig et al. 1980) and (B) acute and chronic urticaria (Stemmler and Lischka 1979). The number or percentage of patients who cleared their urticaria with therapy of the respective pathological findings are given in parentheses.

Lab results	%positive	
	A (100 patients)	B (75 patients)
Eosinophilia	2%	0%
↑ ESR (> 25 mm/h)	1%	–
Urinary abnormalities	3.5%	–
Stool + for parasites	0%	1%
Stool + for candida	–	9% (1% cleared)
+ ANA	1%	–
Cryoglobulins	3%	–
+ RA (> 1:10)	0%	–
↓ C3 and C4	1%	–
Sinusitis + tonsillitis	17%	15% (0% cleared)
Dental findings	16% (some cleared)	3% (1 patient cleared)

ESR, erythrocyte sedimentation rate;
ANA, antinuclear antibody;
RA, rheumatoid arthritis factor.

Chapter 3.6, p. 31). Exceptions were special investigations of the teeth for caries and of the sinuses for chronic inflammation (Table 10.3). In all other cases, laboratory tests are unnecessary and expensive and should be done only if they promise to help in confirming the suspected diagnosis or if they provide parameters by which one can better delineate the severity of the disease.

10.3.2 Specific Diagnostic Laboratory Tests

Certain types of urticaria and angioedema, once they are diagnosed on clinical grounds, can be confirmed by special laboratory tests. Table 10.4 lists tests that should be done when a specific type of urticaria is suspected. More details can also be obtained from the respective chapters that deal with these diseases.

10.3.3 Laboratory Tests for Diagnosis of IgE-Dependent Allergy (RAST and RIST)

Total IgE (radio-immunosorbent test, RIST) and the allergen-specific IgE (radio-allergosorbent test, RAST) can be measured in most hospital laboratories by a simple in vitro procedure (Fig. 10.1). Quantitation of the RAST is done on a scale of 0–4 or as %activity.

Since the first description of the RAST test by Wide et al. (1967), many technical modifications and simplifications of this technique have been published which have improved its accuracy and specificity (Adkinson 1980). The quantitation of total serum IgE levels generally offers no help in the diagnosis of the different causes of urticaria. The RAST test, on the other hand, provides an important diagnostic aid, particularly when skin tests cannot be performed due to ongoing skin disease or therapy. RAST determinations of specific circulating IgE are, however, of only limited value since they are semiquantitative and measure excess IgE and not the pathophysiologically more important IgE that is bound to mast cells and basophils. For this reason, RAST tests are often negative in patients with a weak or median degree of sensitization, even though IgE-dependent allergy is suggested by history, clinical aspects, skin tests, or oral provocation tests. Positive RAST tests in the presence of negative challenge tests are rare (5.7% for skin tests; 3% for inhalation tests) (Wüthrich and Kopper 1978). The correlation to disease is better with stronger and

Table 10.4. Laboratory tests required upon suspicion of a specific type of urticaria.

Suspected diagnosis	Laboratory test
1. Chronic urticaria due to	
a) thyroid disease	T_3, T_4, antimicrosomal thyroid antibody
b) systemic lupus erythematosus	ESR, ANA
c) viral infections	hepatitis B Ags
d) fungus infections	stool and vaginal smears for candida and trichomonas
e) bacterial infections	X-ray: chest, sinuses, teeth; urinalysis
f) parasitic infestations	stool for ova and parasites; blood count for eosinophilia, total IgE, chest X-ray
g) penicillin	RAST (or skin test)
2. Urticarial vasculitis	ESR, CH50, C1q, C4, C3, circulating immune complexes, histology of lesions, immunofluorescence of biopsy 3 h after histamine injection (1:10000, 0.1 ml intradermally) (see also Table 8.2)
3. Hereditary angioedema	C1 INH levels, CH50, C4, C1 (Tables 4.4 and 4.5)
4. Cold urticaria	syphilis serology, cryoglobulin, cryofibrinogens, cold hemolysins, serum electrophoresis, heterophile antibodies, ANA, leukocyte count
5. Pressure urticaria	ESR, leukocyte count
6. Solar urticaria	SLE and porphyria tests for differential diagnosis
7. Mastocytosis	skin biopsy, bone marrow biopsy

ANA, antinuclear antibodies.

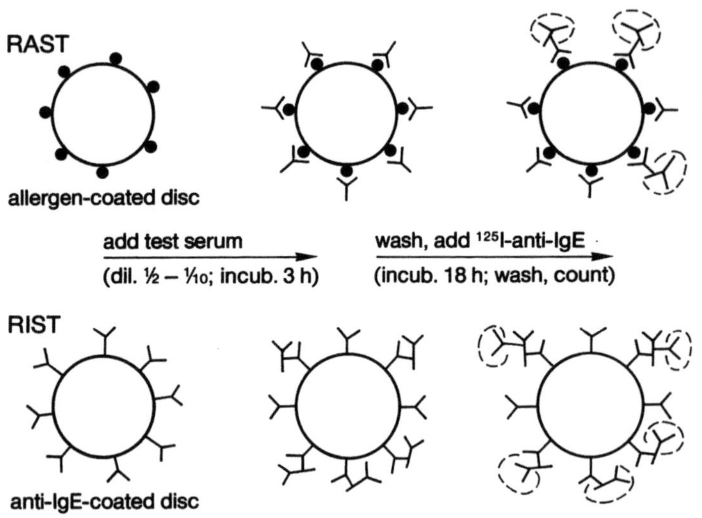

Fig. 10.1. Outline of in vitro measurement of allergen-specific serum IgE by the RAST (*r*adio*a*llergo*s*orbent) test and of total serum IgE by the RIST (*r*adio*i*mmuno*s*orbent) test.

purer allergens and with RAST classes 3–4. The superiority of the skin test over the RAST test holds also for bee sting hypersensitivity (Bar-Sela et al. 1983).

Since the RAST test is less sensitive, up to ten times more expensive than skin tests, and since it provides an answer in at most 2–3 days instead of 20 min, its indication is limited. Physicians should never yield to the temptation of using this test as a "search test" for the responsible antigen. They should also be cautioned against buying RAST tests for codeine, contrast media, or strawberries since IgE antibodies are not involved (Adkinson 1980).

Table 10.5 lists the three major indications for performing RAST tests. Difficulties in doing skin tests is the major reason. Besides the four points listed under this heading, some office physicians might also prefer to have RAST tests performed if they themselves and their helpers have little experience in performing skin tests and if they are not willing to deal with life-threatening anaphylactic reactions in some highly sensitive subjects. In rare instances, the RAST test will help to resolve discrepancies between the patient history and the results of skin tests. Finally, RAST tests are conventient to use as an objective measure of response in clinical studies, for testing and standardization of allergens, and for comparing data in multicenter trials. It should, however, be stressed that IgE-mediated allergy plays only a minor role in urticaria, particularly in the chronic type, and that in vivo tests via the cutaneous or oral route are of much greater diagnostic significance than the elegant RAST examinations.

Table 10.5. Indications for performance of RAST tests.

1. Skin tests are not possible or difficult to perform
   a) in babies and small children
   b) in patients with extensive skin disease (atopic eczema, erythroderma, ichthyosis)
   c) in patients with decreased cutaneous reactivity due to drugs or old age
   d) in patients with dermographic urticaria
2. Confirmation of allergy
   a) if there is a discrepancy between skin tests and patient history
   b) if bronchial provocation is not possible due to drug therapy or bad pulmonary function
   c) if skin testing is dangerous due to excessive reactivity
3. Research purposes
   a) control of desensitization therapy or of long-term allergen elimination
   b) standardization and testing of allergens
   c) epidemiological, multicenter studies

Other laboratory methods for testing IgE-dependent allergy will only be mentioned briefly since they are of little importance for routine diagnosis. Lichtenstein and Osler (1964) described a spectrofluorometric method for measuring histamine in extracts of leukocyte supernatants. Washed peripheral leucocytes were challenged in vitro with different antigens, and if the patient's basophils were sensitized with antigen-specific IgE, they released histamine into the supernatant. This test correlates well with RAST and skin test data and has been automated and simplified over the past two decades (Siraganian 1977, Diamant and Patkar 1982). It is nevertheless still too complicated for use during routine clinical diagnosis.

The basophil degranulation test (Shelley and Juhlin 1961, Hirsch and Zastrow 1972) is based on the same principle as the in vitro histamine release test, but it measures the number of basophils before and after antigen exposure of the cells by light microscopy. The test is less convenient and accurate than RAST and skin test techniques and offers no important additional information.

In vitro lymphocyte transformation tests which are a good measure of delayed type hypersensitivity reactions, are not used for the diagnosis of IgE-mediated immediate type allergy because they are, for example, positive in many patients who are treated with penicillin while only a few develop IgE-dependent allergies. Recently, these tests have been reevaluated for use in the diagnosis of food allergies (see Chapter 7.6.5, p. 104).

10.3.4 In Vivo Provocation Tests

In vivo allergy tests, in particular skin tests, have been in use in clinical medicine for more than a century and have proven to be superior to diagnostic laboratory tests up to this date. Their diagnostic value consists in the fact that the natural conditions which have caused anaphylactic or anaphylactoid reactions can be simulated. Furthermore, even non-IgE mediated reactions can be reproduced, for example during skin testing with mast cell liberators or during oral challenge with aspirin.

The skin is the most frequent organ used for testing, even for allergic reactions that have their primary clinical manifestation in other organs and their route of access along non-cutaneous epithelia. In a few instances, the skin is however not reliable for testing, and the oral, nasal, or tracheal routes have to be chosen instead. The procedures for nasal and pulmonary provocation tests are not discussed here since, even if urticaria is naturally elicited in rare instances by these means, the diagnosis is generally evident or can be established by other tests. Intramuscular provocation tests are done with an ongoing intravenous infusion, as during oral provocation tests (see Section 10.3.6, p. 131). Sublingual provocation tests should not be done since they are unreliable (position statement, American Academy of Allergy 1981).

Skin test procedures

Tests for mast cell-dependent urticarial reactions are performed by either of five methods: the open epicutaneous test, the "rub" test, the prick test, the scratch test, and the intradermal test.

Allergens, histamine liberators, and physical agents can be applied to intact skin. This is true also for the challenge tests for contact urticaria. In this instance, the technique of routine patch testing is used, except that readings are also taken at 30–45 min and at 6–8 h, and open patch tests are preferred (see Chapter 6.8.2, p. 95 for details). The tests for physical urticarias will be detailed below (10.3.5, p. 130).

Most allergens and chemicals do not readily cross the epidermal barrier, and their penetration is therefore enhanced by mechanical injury to the skin. The least invasive means of this kind which is used in highly sensitive subjects, is the "rub" test (Gronemeyer and Debelic 1967). The test is executed by rubbing the allergen with a firm object into the skin of the forearm. Penetration of the allergen occurs principally along the hair follicles, resulting in a follicular pattern of the early whealing reaction. The test can be evaluated after 20 min; it is 10000 times less sensitive than the intradermal tests.

The prick and scratch tests are also relatively insensitive (100 times less than the intradermal test) but are safe to use in highly reactive subjects. They are widely used because of the simplicity of the testing technique, the speed of performance, the low level of discomfort to the patient, and the good correlation to clinical disease (Nelson 1983). They are however far more variable than the intracutaneous tests (Voorhorst and van Krieken 1973a).

For prick testing, a drop of the extract is placed on the skin, and a sharp instrument is passed through the drop at a 45° angle. The skin is thus lifted, creating a small break in the epidermis. Alternately, a lancet with a tiny tip that barely penetrates the epidermis, is touched to the skin at a 90° angle, leaving no bleeding point (Fig. 10.2). Approximately 3 µl of the test solution are introduced intradermally by this technique (Nelson 1983). In the scratch test, a superficial abrasion is made with a knife, a needle, or a lancet (Fig. 10.3), and the extract is then applied to the skin. In the intradermal test, 20 µl of a solution is injected into the skin with a 30 gauge needle and a 0.1 ml syringe. Slow injection will cause less discomfort to the patient.

The needle or lancet can be wiped off with a wet sponge between each prick or scratch and can then be reused without causing significant false positive results. This procedure is also faster than changing the needle between each test. A disposable needle must of course be used for each patient in order to avoid transfer of infectious diseases. The drop of the test solution can be wiped off from the skin after testing without changing the size of the reaction (Nelson 1983).

All these tests are usually performed on the lower or upper arm since the extremity can be tied off easily in case of strong reactions. They can also be applied to the back, but during intradermal testing, it is advisable to know the reactivity of the patient, for example by first doing a prick test. On the back, the test sites should be about 5 cm apart from each other to prevent test reactions from influencing each other (Voorhorst and van Krieken 1973b). A negative control, consisting

Table 10.6. Contraindications to skin testing.

Severe systemic disease (pneumonia, cardiac insufficiency)
First 4 months of pregnancy
Thrombocytopenia
Intrinsic clotting defects (not coumarin therapy)
Acute allergic symptoms
Impetigo
Generalized skin disease

of the test solution without an antigen, and a positive control of histamine (0.01%), compound 48/80 0.01%, or codeine should also be included in the test battery.

A normal histamine wheal at the recommended test concentration should be about 6 mm in diameter in the prick test and 12–16 mm in the intracutaneous test. The other test reactions are evaluated semiquantitatively in relation to the histamine wheal. Similar reactions are called 3+, twice the reaction size 4+, one-half the histamine reaction 2+, and very small wheals 1+. For better quantitation, wheals can also be measured with a planimeter. The product of two diameters at right angles yields equally good results (Nelson 1983). Readings should also be taken at 6–8 h so as not to miss late cutaneous reactions.

Skin tests are an extremely valuable diagnostic tool which is widely used by physicians throughout the world. If done properly and if interpreted adequately, the tests provide important information about the cause of urticaria. There are only a few situations in which they cannot be used. These are listed in Table 10.6, and the reasons are generally obvious. Many authors suggest not testing children below the age of 8, although reliable data were recently reported by others (Ménardo et al. 1985).

Modulating factors on skin test reactivity

The intensity of skin test reactions depends on a number of factors (Table 10.7): the amount of allergen injected, the degree of sensitivity of the cutaneous mast cells which is closely related to allergen-specific IgE on the mast cells, the state of releasability of the mast cells, and finally, the reactivity of the cutaneous target tissue to mast cell-derived pharmacological mediators.

The sensitivity of the test also varies with the body region, the forearm being more sensitive close to the anticubital fossa than at the wrist, and on the ulnar side more than on the radial side. The back is again more sensitive than the forearm, and more so in the upper and midregion than close to the belt line. Maximal size reactions occur from 7–11 pm, smallest ones at 7 am (Lee et al. 1977). At birth, less so during childhood, and again after 50 years of age, the reactivity is low, while it is maximal during the third decade. Women have weakest reactions during days 20 to 1 of a 28-day menstrual cycle. Finally, the depth of intradermal injection will also cause variations in the whealing response.

The size of skin reactions will be augmented in patients who have dermographic urticaria and erythroderma, or who receive β-agonist treatment (Shereff et al. 1973). Patients with ichthyosis have smaller reactions, and in atopic eczema, the flare reaction is smaller and the maximal size of the wheal is reached already at 8–10 min (Voorhorst and van Krieken 1973b). Effective anti-allergic immunotherapy will also result in smaller skin reactions.

One should always make sure that patients do not take drugs that might influence their skin test reactivity. The size of the histamine control injection is a good gauge as to whether suppressive factors are operative or not. Antihistamines directed against the H1 receptor are potent inhibitors of the allergen-induced whealing response. Galant et al. (1972) found significant suppression of scratch test reactions to allergens up to 1 week after stopping treatment with these drugs. Cook et al. (1973) found the mean recovery of skin test reactions after a 3-day treatment period with diphenhydramine to be 1.9 days, with chlorpheniramine 2.5 days, and with hydroxyzine 4.3 days. Tranquilizers, tricyclic antidepressants, and neuroleptics with antihistamine activity also cause a depression of wheal and flare reactions.

The effect of steroids is less striking. Several larger, well controlled studies have shown no effect on wheal size in patients treated with oral prednisone for 1 week at a dose of up to 40 mg (Nyfors and Heegaard 1968,

Table 10.7. Factors influencing size of skin test reactions.

Amount of allergen
Responsiveness of mast cells
Responsiveness of target tissue
Depth of injection
Body region (↑ on upper back)
Time of day (↑ in the evening)
Menstrual cycle (↑ prior to menstruation)
Age (↑ in 3rd decade)
Associated diseases (↑ with dermographic urticaria and erythroderma, ↓ with ichthyosis and atopic eczema)
Immunotherapy (↓)
Refractory state of the skin (after recent urtication at that site)
H1 antihistamines (↓)
Corticosteroids (↓ with long, high-dose therapy)
Sympathomimetic drugs (↓)

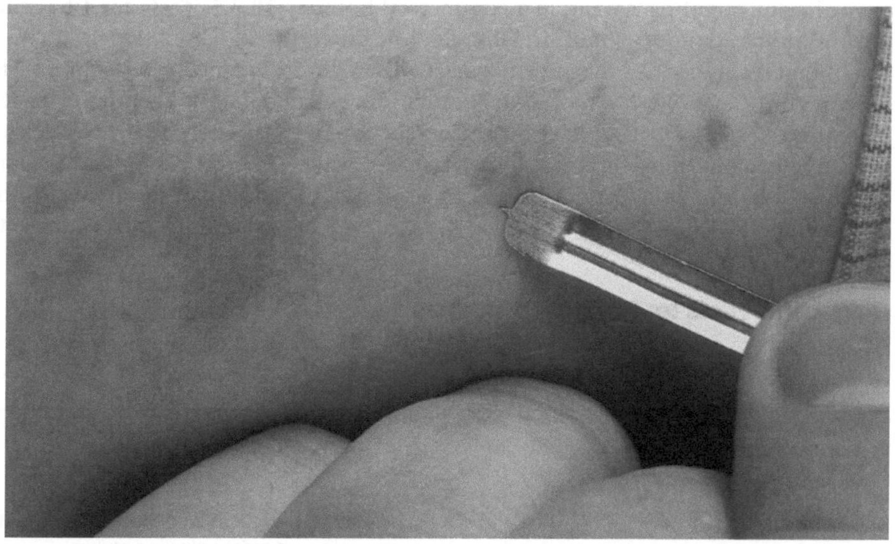

Fig. 10.2. The prick test technique. A drop of test substance is placed on intact skin and the skin is pricked through this drop with a lancet. A positive reaction to walnut is shown on the left.

Galant et al. 1973, Slott and Zweiman 1974). There are however no data in the literature on the effect of high dose, long-term therapy.

Sympathomimetic drugs should be stopped 1 day before testing. Many other antiallergic drugs, like H2 antagonists, disodium cromoglycate, aspirin, and theophylline, have no effect on the wheal and flare reaction (reviewed in Merget and Schultze-Werninghaus 1983).

False positive skin tests occur in 2–8% of normal patients who are tested with pollen extracts and in 5% with house dust. Since this unexpected reactivity can be passively transferred, it must be due to subclinical allergy. False positive tests might also be due to cross-reactions between allergens, due to similarity of the antigenic structure (e.g., birch and hazel pollens), or to the choice of test sites too close to each other or to the histamine control. Histamine in venoms or foods (Doeglas and Nater 1968), a direct liberating action of a chemical (e.g., codeine), or a toxic concentration of the solution should also be considered when unexpected positive reactions are observed.

Skin tests can also be false negative. Allergen extracts are more stable when they are most concentrated. Dilutions, if kept for too long, will deteriorate with storage. Allergen extracts used for prick testing can have 50% glycerin added for stabilization, but even 6% glycerin will cause a high incidence of false positive reactions on intradermal testing. Fruit and vegetable antigens are particularly unstable (Nelson 1981). Different allergens are released at different rates from native material during the extraction procedure. It is therefore also possible that the most relevant antigen for the patient is lacking or is present at only low concentrations in the commercial extract. Also, the antigen present in the patient's own

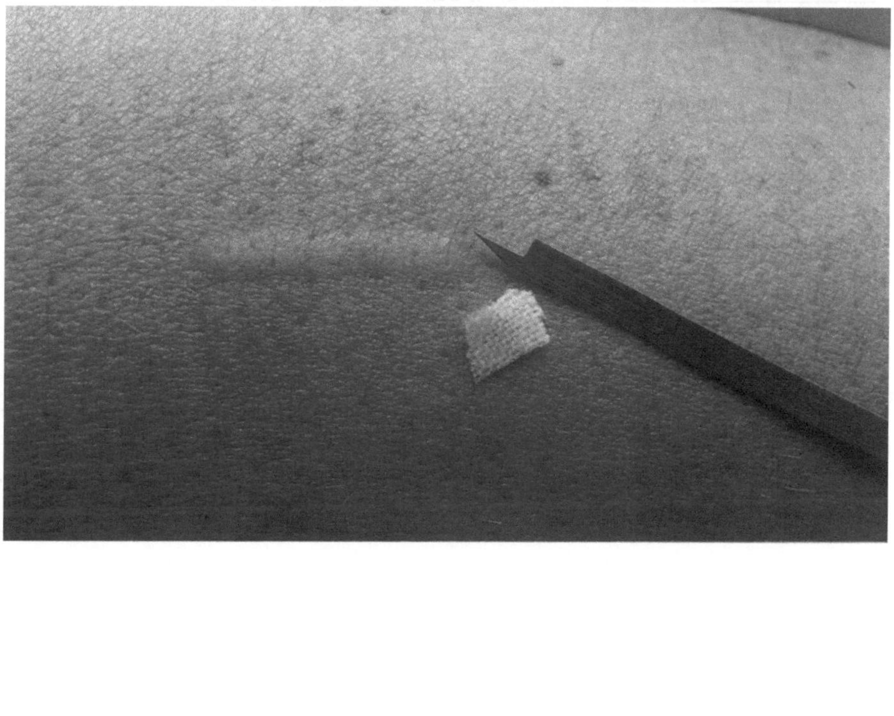

Fig. 10.3. The scratch test technique. A superficial scratch is performed with a lancet, and a small piece of linen soaked with the test material is briefly applied to the scratch. A positive histamine wheal is demonstrated.

environment might be lacking in a commercial house dust or animal dander extract. Finally, false negative tests might result because the patient's mast cells are in a refractory state due to recent degranulation and mediator release. After a massive urticarial reaction to bee stings or penicillin, it is generally advisable to wait 2–3 weeks before skin testing is done (Nelson 1983, Wortmann 1984).

10.3.5 Tests for Physical Urticarias

Diagnostic tests for physical urticarias are described in detail in Chapter 5, p. 55.

Figure 10.4 provides a flow sheet that can be used for recording the test data of a patient in response to different mechanical, thermal, and radiant energy stimuli. Details of these tests and their evaluation are

Diagnostic Tests for Physical Urticarias

Name: Date:

Date of birth: Time:

1) Dermographic Urticaria — **Test Site:** upper back

erythema after min, h.

edema after min, h.

itch after min, h.

application of firm scratch with a safety pin or a stylus

2) Delayed Pressure Urticaria — **Test Site:** back, (weights on a rod or thigh, with weights applied to a strap)

weights	whealing: immediate	4 h	6 h	8 h
900 g 5 min				
900 g 10 min				
1800 g 5 min				
1800 g 10 min				

3) Heat Contact Urticaria — **Test Site:** arm

whealing and erythema: immediate: / delayed (2–4 h): / temperature:

bath at 37–41° C, 3–10 min, if negative, higher temperature

4) Cholinergic (Heat reflex) Urticaria — **Test Site:** arm

pinpoint wheals and erythema:

(bath at 37–41° C, 3–10 min; if negative, higher temperature)

5) Cold Urticaria — **Result**

		Result: immediate	8 h	24 h
a) ice bag or ice cube, 3–5 min, lower arm				
b) arm bath, 5–10 min	10° C			
	21° C			
c) cold room (4° C) until shivering (5–10 min)				

6) Solar Urticaria — **Test Method:** Expose 1 cm^2 areas of skin on the back for increasing time periods

	whealing: up to 2 h	24 h	48 h
solar simulator			
solar simulator + glass			
visible light (projector)			

Diagnosis: Remarks:

Fig. 10.4. Flow sheet to record test reactions in patients suspected of suffering from physical urticaria.

given under the specific headings in Chapter 5, p. 55. Tests for rare types of physical urticaria, like aquagenic urticaria and vibratory angioedema, are not listed in Fig. 10.4, but are described in Chapter 5, p. 64 and p. 87.

10.3.6 Oral Challenge Tests

Agents that cause urticaria after oral intake are either foods and drinks or drugs. Oral provocation tests are indicated when the diagnosis is unclear from the history and when skin tests are irrelevant, as applies for agents that cause intolerance reactions (see Chapter 7, p. 96). They are also performed to find drugs that can be taken with impunity. As oral challenge tests are not without risk, they should be conducted under the supervision of a physician and be replaced by other diagnostic means whenever possible, including diet elimination tests.

A detailed description of oral challenge tests is given in Chapter 7.6.4 p. 102. Patients must be free of symptoms at the time of challenge, increasing doses should be given, and an intravenous infusion should be in place when there is a history of severe reactions. At the University of Münster, this is done on a routine basis to also reduce the level of anxiety and anticipation of the patient.

Oral challenge tests can also be done for diverse food stuffs. If the tests are not done on an open basis, the foods are hidden in an oblate. Oral provocation tests are very useful when skin tests are negative despite a suggestive history, or when commercial skin test solutions are not available. We have given patients oblates containing boiled potatoes, tomatoes, and diverse spices, and have obtained some valuable diagnostic information by these means.

10.4 Diagnosis by Avoidance

10.4.1 Social Habits and Environmental Factors

The importance of habits and environmental factors in the elicitation and maintenance of chronic urticaria is most evident in patients who are relieved of their urticaria only after a short hospital stay. A history of improvement during weekends, while on vacation, or after changing work or home might indicate that factors at work or home are involved. In this way, inhalants, contactants, or stress factors which cause or contribute to the urticaria might be identified (see Chapter 3.7, p. 32). The frequency of improvement with hospitalization alone is however relatively low.

There are a few cases on record where cigarettes have caused chronic urticaria (see Chapter 3.7.12, p. 40). Patients should therefore be firmly advised to stop smoking and, if that is impossible, to switch to another brand, preferably one without menthol.

10.4.2 Drugs

Patients often take a sizable number of different drugs and do not even consider agents like laxatives as belonging to this category. To determine which drugs might cause the urticaria, the optimal procedure is to stop all of them, possibly for several weeks, depending on their half-life in the body. If that cannot be done without the patient developing serious medical problems, only those drugs that can be easily dispensed with should be eliminated, and others should be replaced by chemically different agents. Such a decision should be made after consultation and in agreement with the family physician or the specialist. Some drugs are more apt than others to cause urticaria, for example antibiotics, diuretics, and hypotensive agents; digitalis preparations are rarely implicated. A temporal relationship to the start of drug therapy and the urticaria is also at times helpful, particularly if therapy was instituted after the urticaria had begun. The coloring of the tablets should also be examined since they and similar non-therapeutic additives might also be responsible for the urticaria.

10.4.3 Diet

The most radical procedure for obtaining clarity on the role of food in urticaria is a potato, rice, and water diet. This can be followed for at most 10 or 12 days with a highly motivated patient, preferably in the hospital.

An answer can often be arrived at by simpler methods, before such extreme steps are taken. The patient can be provided with a diet plan that avoids food colorings and preservatives, which he should follow for a minimum of 2 weeks. An example of which foods should be taken or avoided is given in Table 10.8. If the patient clears within a few weeks, the responsible agent can then be identified by oral provocation tests. The patient should also keep a diary of his symptoms so that possible additional contributing factors can be identified in his diet or daily life.

If urticaria occurs only in bouts and not on a daily basis, an elimination diet might be considered. One way to do this is to eat only one single, simple foodstuff at one meal and wait until the next meal to see if it has provoked the urticaria. Water, cane sugar, and non-

Table 10.8. Foods allowed or prohibited during a diet free of preservatives and food colorings.

Category	Allowed	Prohibited
General		all preserved food in cans, tins or tubes, prefabricated meals or sauces in tins or boxes, Indian and Chinese food
Meats	fresh meat, fish, crustaceans, poultry	sausage, cold cuts, canned meat
Milk and fats	fresh milk, cream, cottage cheese, butter (non-colored), oil	condensed milk, ultra-heated milk, magarine, fats for frying, yoghurt (esp. with fruits), mayonaise, salad dressings
Bread and cereals	flour, potatoes, meal, farina, rice, oat meal	pre-packaged bread, cakes with baking powder
Vegetables	leeks, beans, carrots, cabbage, cauliflower, brussel sprouts, fresh potatoes	peas, rhubarb, tomatoes, paprika, cucumber, tomato paste and ketchup, French fries
Fruits	pears	apples; fruits with stones: peaches, apricots, plums; berries: raspberries, strawberries, gooseberries, blackberries, loganberries, cranberries; bananas, grapes, melons, citrus fruits
Beverages	tea, coffee, carbonated water, milk	soft drinks, tonic water, juices, beer, wine, hard liquor
Miscellaneous	sugar, honey, artificial sweeteners, home-made marmelade without salicylate, vinegar (not wine vinegar), spices (not cinnemon), nuts, fresh mushrooms	chocolate, candy, ice cream, wine vinegar, almonds, mints, mouth washes, pudding, tooth pastes with added preservatives, sweat sauces, gelatins

iodized salts can be taken throughout the test period. Rice, oatmeal, beef, beets, milk, and bread are tested first at successive meals and can be eaten from then on if they have caused no reactions. If urticaria develops after one type of food, it is not eaten for 1 week and is then retested. No new food should be tested until the urticaria has completely subsided. Keeping a careful diary is again very important during this approach.

Table 10.9. Sequentially build-up diet, ending with big challenging meal (Illig 1977).

Step I:	*Milk and eggs*: cheese, yoghurt, cottage cheese, milk, eggs, butter, salt, onions. No fruits.
Step II:	*Carbohydrates*: bread, baked goods, pudding, honey, marmelade, fruit juices, tomatoes, celery, fresh fruit.
Step III:	*Meat and sausages*: bacon, beef, pork, chicken. No canned sausages or meat.
Step IV:	*Fish and crustaceans*: tomatoes, canned fish, cooked or boiled fresh fish, herring (also pickled), sardines.
Step V:	*Big meal*: normal breakfast and supper. At noontime oxtail soup, shrimp with mayonaise, meat with sauce, potato dumplings, sauerkraut, whipped cream with fruit, red or white wine, coffee.

Illig (1977) suggested a method which allows the patient, after being free of symptoms on a potato-rice diet, to eat only certain types of food sequentially at 1–2 day intervals (Table 10.9). A big, challenging meal is consumed on the last day. This can provide an answer as to which type of food is involved within 10 days. Preferably, this "search diet" should be done in the hospital, in close cooperation with a dietitian. Individual components of foods to which the patient has reacted can then be tested separately.

When food allergy is suspected in early childhood, infants under 3 months of age should receive a milk substitute only. From 3–6 months, rice cereal can be added to the milk substitute, and from 6 months to 2 years, applesauce, pears, carrots, lamb, rice, and a colorless vitamin supplement are added in a gradual sequence. Older children and adults can also follow this diagnostic diet. The persistence of symptoms under this regimen indicates that the urticaria is not caused by food. When symptoms subside, additional foods can be added gradually, again keeping a diet diary (Metcalfe 1984). Omitted foods should be reinstituted with extreme care. David (1984) reported recently that four of eight children with atopic eczema developed severe anaphylactic shock under such circumstances.

10.5 Diagnosis by Therapy

If an underlying disease or alteration is discovered in the course of the diagnostic procedures, proof that it causes the urticaria should be obtained by trying to eliminate the underlying cause. This applies to infectious agents, exemplified by chronic bacterial infections of teeth or sinuses, by fungal infections with candida, or by parasites like scabies (see Chapter 3.7.11, p. 38). Hormonal defects, particularly thyroid disease (Chapter 3.7.13, p. 41) and chronic inflammatory disease should be treated appropriately (Chapter 3.7.13, p. 41). An urticaria due to malignancies may clear with chemical or surgical treatment. The positive yield is however only modest.

11 Therapy

11.1 Basic Therapeutic Considerations

For the treatment of urticaria, a vast armamentarium of therapeutic modalities has become available in the past few decades, particularly at the level of pharmacological modulation of the disease. Each of these tools is, however, most effective if it is chosen on the basis of as accurate a diagnosis as possible. Failure of therapy is mostly found among the group of patients for whom the cause of urticaria cannot be properly identified.

Figure 11.1 outlines the three major pathological events at which the treatment of urticaria is aimed. A cure can only be expected with therapy that is directed against the initiating event of the disease. Therapy that is aimed at the activity of the effector cells, in almost all instances the basophils and mast cells, and at the target tissue, primarily the cutaneous vessels, is accomplished almost exclusively through drugs. In this situation, symptoms are alleviated only as long as the pharmacological modulation is in effect.

Our greatest handicap in the treatment of urticaria is our present limited knowledge. It is entirely unclear why certain persons develop an IgE-mediated allergy. Furthermore, the vast majority of urticarias are not even IgE-dependent, and in these cases, the reason for the development of the disease is even more of a mystery. Hyposensitization which is aimed at modulation of the IgE-dependent immune apparatus, is cumbersome, dangerous, and can be applied to only a very small group of patients. In all those cases where the stimulus can be identified, patients are relieved of their symptoms by removing or avoiding the eliciting cause.

One additional approach to improve the clinical situation is to instruct patients to avoid aggravating factors. This applies mostly to agents that modulate the releasability of mast cells and basophils or the

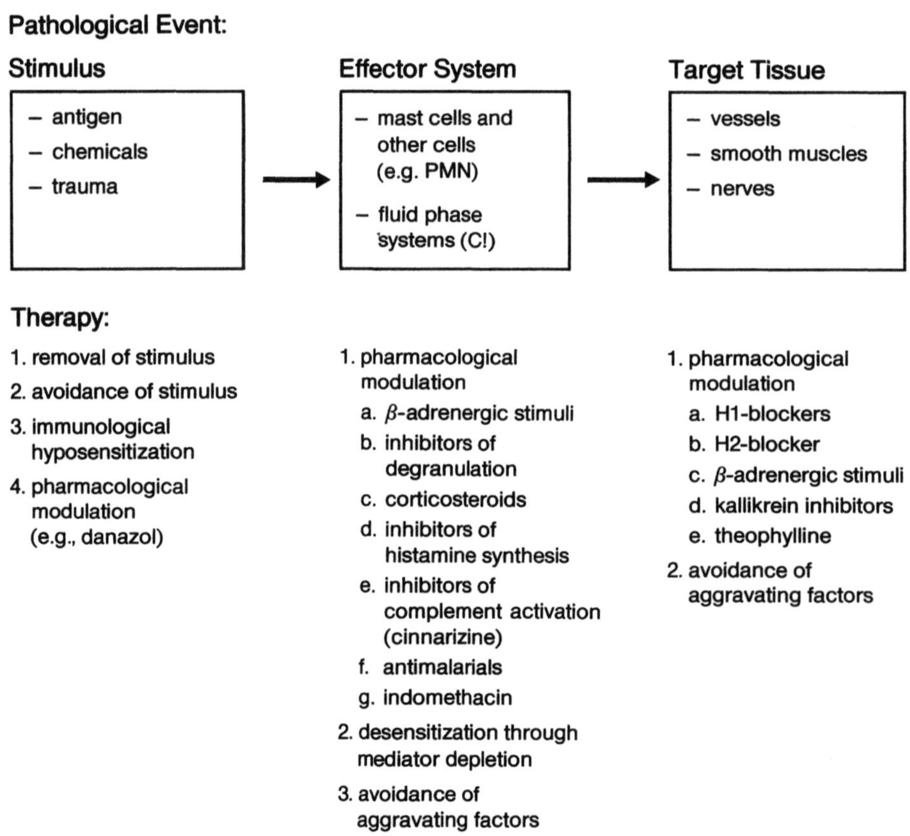

Fig. 11.1. The major aspects of the development of urticaria and angioedema and possible therapeutic measures.

responsiveness of the cutaneous vasculature. Examples are alcohol, aspirin, heat, exertion, and emotional stress.

The vast majority of patients with urticaria have to be treated with drugs. Failures in this category are primarily due to the choice of an inappropriate drug for the respective condition, too low a dose, or loss of patient compliance by not giving proper instruction about the drug's mode of action and use in the patient's specific life situation. For example, many patients are afraid to take antihistamines regularly because of the general widespread fear of taking drugs in the population. Physicians often also fail to reinsure patients that in many instances, the bothersome symptoms of tiredness will disappear after about a week of regular consumption of the drugs.

In the following two parts of this chapter, the pharmacology or the mode of action of the most important therapeutic principles will be discussed primarily in relation to their use in urticaria, and thereafter, the therapy for the major disease categories of the urticarias will be dealt with (Sections 11.3–11.7, p. 142–152).

11.2 Specific Therapeutic Modalities

11.2.1 Antihistamines

Basic pharmacology

Histamine antagonists act by occupying the pharmacological receptor sites at their different target tissues (Fig. 2.10, p. 15). Histamine can attach to cells by either one of its ends (H1 or H2, see Fig. 2.9, p. 14). The more common H1 receptors, first described by Ash and Schild (1966), are located on smooth muscles and vessels and are responsible for the histamine-induced contraction of vascular, bronchial, and intestinal smooth muscles, and for increased vascular permeability. The first histamine antagonists discovered by Staub and Bovet (1937) were directed against these pharmacological activities of histamine. Once drugs became available with low enough toxicity for clinical use (Halpern 1942), a large number of new compounds with a similar spectrum of activities flooded the market and keep doing so even today.

All these H1 receptor antagonists, or H1 blockers, inhibit the basic features of the whealing reaction: (1) the edema due to the effect of histamine on vascular permeability, (2) the flare and the itch which are caused by the action of histamine on the nerve endings, and (3) together with H2 blockers, the histamine-induced vasodilatation and less so also the vasoconstriction of small vessels. Effects of H1 blockers on the central nervous system and the local anesthetic and anticholinergic activities explain some of the undesirable side effects of the drugs.

H2 receptors were discovered only in 1972 (Black et al.), and clinically useful antagonists have only recently appeared on the market. Their therapeutic effect in urticaria is still controversial (see below and Section 11.3.3, p. 144). H2 receptors are located on the gastric mucosa, on leukocytes, and as observed by Commens and Greaves (1978), also on cutaneous blood vessels (see Fig. 2.10, p. 15).

For most antihistamines, the onset of action is observed 1/2–1 h after ingestion, a maximum is reached after 1–3 h, and a loss of 50% of the therapeutic effect after 5–7 h. The delay of action is not due to the absorption through the gastrointestinal tract, but to the time needed to attach to the tissue receptor sites. Antihistamines can also be given by subcutaneous, intramuscular, or intravenous routes, but even then the maximal action is reached only after 2–3 h.

Antihistamines such as diphenhydramine leave the circulation very rapidly, reaching maximal levels in the lung, with progressively lower concentrations in spleen, kidney, brain, lung, and skin. Most of the drug is excreted in the urine 24 h later. The duration of action of other antihistamines, such as promethazine and hydroxyzine, lasts for several days.

Pharmacological tolerance to the action of antihistamines does not develop after many months of therapy, although fluctuations in the severity of the disease might suggest that.

Antihistamines often also have antiserotonin, antiacetylcholine, and tranquilizing effects, and newer compounds also inhibit the release and effect of mediators of inflammation other than histamine (see below).

Side effects

H1-type antihistamines belong to the most innocuous therapeutic agents presently available. The list of their potential side effects is nevertheless long (Table 11.1), and the severity of these side effects varies depending on the individual patient and the specific chemical structure of the compound.

Antihistamines have side effects most frequently on the central nervous system. They include sedation, dizziness, tinnitus, lassitude, incoordination, fatigue, blurred vision, diplopia, euphoria, nervousness, insomnia, and tremors. More rarely, patients experience weakness, incoordiantion, and twitching of the skeletal muscles, or gastrointestinal symptoms like anorexia, dryness of the mouth, nausea, vomiting, con-

Table 11.1. Side effects of H1-type antihistamines.

Target organ	Side effects
Central nervous system	sedation, fatigue, nervousness, lassitude, euphoria, insomnia, temors intoxication: convulsions
Eye	blurred vision, diplopia
Ear	tinnitus, dizziness
Muscle	weakness, incoordination, twitching
Gastrointestinal tract	anorexia, dryness of the mouth, nausea, vomiting, diarrhea, constipation, epigastric pain
Immune system	urticaria, maculopapular exanthems, light sensitivity (promethazine, tripolidine), contact allergy, leukopenia, agranulocytosis
Reproductive system	teratogenicity in laboratory animals with cyclizine and meclizine, male impotence at high dosage

stipation, diarrhea, and epigastric pain. Some of these side effects can be explained by the atropine-like effects of antihistamines. The CNS symptoms often disappear after 1 week. Some newer antihistamines are claimed not to cross the blood-brain barrier (e.g. terfenadine), and patients receiving them do not complain about tiredness or dizziness. In rare instances, antihistamines have been observed to cause urticaria; but this is mostly due to intolerance reactions to the colored coating of the capsules. Light sensitivity can be observed during therapy with promethazine and tripolidine, and local application of antihistamines might lead to contact or photocontact allergy. Because of the generalized nature of most types of urticaria and the fact that the drugs must be given to prevent the action of histamine rather than treat existing lesions, local antihistamines are rarely used to treat urticaria and should not be either.

Development of leukopenia and agranulocytosis has been attributed to therapy with antihistamines, but these events, even though they must be mentioned, have never caused serious concern because of their extremely low incidence (Goodman and Gilman 1980).

An overdosage of antihistamines due to accidental poisoning results in convulsions and can lead to death. Large therapeutic doses may also trigger convulsions in epileptic patients.

Teratogenicity in laboratory animals has been observed with cyclizine, chlorcyclizine and meclizine. Antihistamines have been used in the past during the first trimester of pregnancy for vomiting because of their relative safety, but drug companies have become more cautious in recommending these agents in the light of negative past experiences with apparently safe drugs during periods of fetal development (Goodman and Gilman 1980).

Antihistamines with anticholinergic activity are contraindicated in patients with glaucoma, during urinary retention, renal insufficiency, and during monoaminoxidase therapy. Patients should also be warned of the potentiating effect of H1 blockers when consumed with alcohol or centrally depressing drugs.

H2 antagonists were expected to cause far more side effects than H1 antagonists, due to their broad spectrum of activities, also on the immune system (see Fig. 2.10, p. 15). Since the first clinically acceptable H2 blocker, cimetidine, became available several years ago, these fears have not been substantiated, although many more years of clinical experience are necessary before firm conclusions can be reached about the drug. Major, rare side effects which should be mentoined are mental confusion, particularly in elderly patients and in those with renal and hepatic dysfunction, a weak antiandrogen action which can result in a reduction of sperm count after long-term therapy, gynecomastia, galactorrhea, prolongation of the prothrombin time in patients on oral anticoagulants (reviewed in Domschke and Domschke 1980), and rarely bone marrow suppression (Chang and Morrison 1979). Headache, dizziness, fatigue, muscle

Table 11.2. Responsiveness of cutaneous and pulmonary tissue to different types of drugs (from Hutchcroft et al. 1979, Altounyan 1980, Harvey and Schocket 1980, Smith et al. 1980).

Tissue reaction	Inhibitors					
	H1 Blocker	H2 Blocker	H1 + H2 Blocker	Steroids	DSCG	β-2 Stimulants
Histamine response	+	−	++	+/−	−	++
Immediate, antigen-induced response	+	−	++	−	++	++
late, antigen-induced response	−	−	++	++	++	+/−

−, no effect; +, moderate; ++, strong effect; DSCG, disodiumcromoglycate.

pain, constipation, diarrhea, and skin rashes are other, minor side effects (Goodman and Gilman 1980). Ranitidine, a newer H2 blocker, has in contrast to cimetidine no effect on plasma hormone levels or on the P450-dependent mono-oxygenase activity (information of the manufacturer).

Clinical effect

The effectiveness of H1 blockers on the experimentally induced wheal and erythema reaction, also on reverse type passive anaphylaxis reactions, has been repeatedly proven in numerous studies (see Table 11.2). H1 antagonists also inhibit the itch in urticaria, but they fail to do so in eczema or psoriasis, unless the H1 blockers are also good centrally acting sedatives (Krause and Shuster 1983). Illig and Paul (1978) observed that pruritus and reflex erythema is almost always suppressed by H1 blockers, but that the wheal is influenced less, and the central erythema not at all.

Even though H2 blockers act on histamine receptors on blood vessels, most studies show that they have little effect of their own on the histamine-induced response, unless they are combined with H1 blockers (see Table 11.2). Kaliner et al. (1982) showed however that H2 blockers were useful in inhibiting anaphylactoid reactions to intravenous histamine.

Numerous, carefully designed clinical studies have proven the efficacy of H1 blockers in the treatment of acute and chronic urticaria. However, even in the very early studies, it became apparent that a small percentage of patients were unresponsive. Curtis and Brechner Owens (1945) observed disappearance of the urticarial lesions in 11 of their 18 patients on treatment with diphenhydramine. Three were improved, and four patients needed variable doses to control their urticaria. Minor side effects of drowsiness and muscle aching were observed in two, and dizziness and weakness in one. Most older studies agree with these authors that about one-third of urticaria patients respond poorly or not at all to H1 blockers alone (Warin and Champion 1974).

In more recent studies, it could be clearly demonstrated that patients who fail to improve with ordinary antihistamines, respond to more potent antihistamines at a high dosage (e.g. hydroxyzine, 25 mg three or four times daily) or on combination therapy (see Section 11.3.3, p. 144 and Harvey et al. 1981). Newer drugs which do not cross the blood-brain barrier should be tried, but a certain percentage of patients will fail on this treatment as well (Cerio and Lessof 1984). No side effects were observed in the 24 patients treated with terfenadine by the latter authors, whereas Gibson et al. (1984) found that 7 of his 20 patients noted tiredness on a similar drug, compared to three patients who did so on placebo.

The lack of any effect of H2 blockers alone on histamine or antigen-induced wheals (Table 11.2) is striking, but was confirmed by most authors who studied the effect of cimetidine in patients with urticaria. Exceptions are a report by Kaiser et al. (1980) who noted that 9 of 10 patients with chronic urticaria improved on cimetidine (900 mg daily) after they had failed to respond to H1 blockers. Farnam et al. (1984) reported on one unique patient with urticaria and angioedema who had been well controlled for 3 years on cimetidine. When this patient was studied by the group, his wheals responded better to cimetidine than to chlorpheniramine, but a combination of both drugs was even more effective.

The synergistic effect of a combination of H1 and H2 blockers was observed by all groups who studied the immediate wheal reaction (Table 11.2). The suppression of the late reaction was unexpected since this reaction is thought to be mediated by mediators other than histamine (see Chapter 2.1, p. 5). One possible explanation would be that the histamine-independent late wheal can only develop as a consequence of the histamine-dependent immediate wheal, and effective suppression of the latter would curb the mechanisms that initiate late wheal production. This agrees with the observations on delayed wheals in cold urticaria (Chapter 5.7.10, p. 75).

Clinically, the combination of H1 and H2 blockers did not prove as successful as expected from the experimental models. Commens and Greaves (1978), in a study of 19 patients with chronic urticaria on a combination therapy of chlorpheniramine and cimetidine, found no improvement over chlorpheniramine treatment alone, even though both regimens were better than placebo. More recently, Cook and Shuster (1983b) confirmed these findings on 20 patients with chronic urticaria who were treated with the same drugs.

This stands in contrast to a study by Phanuphak et al. (1978) on eight patients with chronic urticaria who had failed to respond to H1 blockers, ephedrine and corticosteroids. Fifty percent of the patients improved on a combination therapy of cyproheptadine (16 mg daily) and cimetidine (1200 mg daily) within 4–5 days, with a maximal therapeutic effect by 7–10 days. These authors concluded that a combination with the more effective H1 blocker hydroxyzine might be even more effective, and studies by Monroe et al. (1981) and by Harvey et al. (1981) proved that they were right. The first group treated 18 patients with treatment refractory chronic urticaria by a combination of hydroxyzine (60 mg/day) and cimetidine (1200 mg/day), and the latter group used even 75 mg hydroxyzine daily. Compared to combinations of hydroxyzine with other H1 blockers or terbutaline, addition of cimetidine was most effective, both by the patient's choice and on the basis of skin test reactions to histamine or compound 48/80. These authors speculate that the negative combination studies by the British authors are due to incomplete H1 blockade which would impair recognition of the H2 effects on the skin.

11.2.2 Beta-Adrenergic Agonists

Epinephrine is the drug of first choice to relieve symptoms of acute hypersensitivity reactions to drugs, sera, other allergens, and to non-IgE mediated reactions. Its high effectiveness in counteracting histamine- induced whealing (see Table 11.2) is due to a direct action on peripheral vessels, causing constriction of the precapillary arterioles and the subcapillary venules of the skin. This peripheral vasoconstriction is also important in counteracting anaphylactic shock. Another reason for its effectiveness in the treatment of shock is its ability to increase cardiac action by enhancing coronary flow and the activity of the cardiac pacemaker and the conducting tissue. In the pulmonary system, epinephrine causes bronchodilatation, increases the vital capacity by relieving the congestion of the bronchial mucosa and by constricting the pulmonary vessels, and inhibits additional antigen-induced mediator release by raising intracellular cAMP levels. The net effect is an effective alleviation of the bronchospastic symptoms that may accompany acute urticaria and shock and an interruption of stimulus-induced mediator release.

Other effects of epinephrine are an increased blood flow through the skeletal muscles, as part of the "fight or fly" reaction. Reactions such as fear, anxiety, tenseness, restlessness, throbbing headache, tremor, weakness, dizziness, pallor, respiratory difficulties, and palpitations are part of an exaggerated pharmacological effect of the drug. Serious side effects like cerebral hemorrhage and cardiac arrhythmias are especially seen after intravenous use (Goodman and Gilman 1980).

Epinephrine also causes neutrophilia and lymphocytosis. These reactions are probably due to a stimulation of the endothelial cell β-receptors, resulting in an increase of intracellular cAMP and a decreased leukocyte adherence to the vessel walls (Boxer et al. 1980). This reversal of margination of the leukocyte pool is probably not important in the therapy of anaphylactic reactions.

Since the drug is destroyed in the gastrointestinal tract, it should be given by other routes, e.g., in form of sprays, solutions, sublingual tablets, or suppositories via the oral, respiratory, or rectal mucosae. It is also incorporated into ointments. The most common form of administration is via subcutaneous injection, at a dosage of 0.1 to maximally 0.5 ml of a 1 : 1000 dilution (= 0.1 – 0.5 mg). The intravenous route is very rarely chosen, usually in extreme emergencies. The drug is then infused in diluted form and very slowly, at a dosage of maximally 0.25 mg. Intracardiac injection is rarely practiced nowadays. Epinephrine is rapidly eliminated in the body via enzymatic destruction in the liver through monoamine oxidases or catechol-O-methyltransferase. It is excreted in the urine in its inactive form. Suspension of the drug in an oily emulsion helps to retard its action. Ephedrine and other drugs related to epinephrine are used for long-term therapy for allergic disorders (Goodman and Gilman 1980).

Epinephrine rapidly relieves itching, urticaria, swelling of the mucosae, bronchospasms, and shock and should always be at hand during skin testing for immediate-type reactions. Beta-agonists are widely employed in the treatment of bronchial asthma, but have been used only rarely in the treatment of chronic urticaria. This may be due to the fact that antihistamines which work only poorly in bronchial asthma, are highly effective in urticaria without causing the bothersome side effects of the beta-agonists.

Spangler et al. (1980) studied the effect of terbutaline (2.5 mg three times daily) in 18 patients with chronic idiopathic urticaria. They observed no statistically significant difference between verum and placebo in their double-blind, crossover study. Nevertheless, 53% of the patients on terbutaline versus 12% on placebo noted smaller wheals. Two patients reported experiencing severe tremors while taking terbutaline.

Using the same drug and dosage, Kennes et al. (1977) found terbutaline more effective than antihistamines in 16 patients with chronic urticaria. The effect was less good in five patients with cholinergic and three patients with pressure urticaria. Only one patient noted palpitations while on terbutaline.

Combinations of terbutaline and H1 blockers were studied by Harvey et al. (1981) and by Saihan and Littlewood (1983) in patients with treatment-resistant chronic urticaria. Only two of the 19 patients of the first group chose a combination of hydroxyzine and terbutaline over other combinations, while one patient of the latter study responded to terbutaline alone and nine of eleven to a combination of terbutaline and ketotifen.

11.2.3 Corticosteroids

The indications for the use of corticosteroids in acute and chronic urticaria is far more limited than those for antihistamines and beta-adrenergic drugs. This is primarily due to the fact that corticosteroids have no striking effect on the immediate urticarial reaction (see Table 11.2). They are instead excellent inhibitors of the more general inflammatory response. This explains their suppression of late whealing reactions (Table 11.2) which are due to mediators other than histamine and which involve cellular infiltrates.

Corticosteroids, when incubated with mast cells or basophils, have no effect on mediator release unless they are preincubated with the cells for 16–24 h (Daëron et al. 1982, Schleimer et al. 1982). Histamine release from mast cells and basophils is controlled by phospholipase A_2-mediated events (Hirata et al. 1979), and corticosteroids have a potent inhibitory effect on phospholipase A_2. This inhibition is due to the synthesis of an inhibitory glycoprotein in cells. This protein has recently been identified and named lipomodulin, macrocortin, or lipocortin (Hirata 1981, Hirata et al. 1982).

The RNA-dependent synthesis of this inhibitory protein which is induced through corticosteroid receptors on cells, explains most of the anti-inflammatory action of corticosteroids (see Table 11.3). It also makes apparent why the onset of action of steroids is delayed and why these drugs are therefore not useful in combatting acute symptoms of anaphylactic shock.

As discussed in Chapter 2.3, p. 13, phospholipase A_2 controls the production of important mediators of inflammation, such as platelet activating factor (PAF), prostaglandins, and leukotrienes (Fig. 2.11, p. 18). Corticosteroids also increase the activities of prostaglandin-metabolizing enzymes (Moore and Hoult 1980). The inhibition of the synthesis and activity of these mediators and of histamine secretion from cells explains the reduction of edema, redness, and pain after administration of corticosteroids.

Table 11.3. Anti-inflammatory effects of glucocorticosteroids.

A. Phospholipase A_2- and lipomodulin-mediated effects
1. suppression of synthesis and secretion of
   a) prostaglandins
   b) leukotrienes
   c) platelet-activating factor
2. inhibition of histamine release
3. inhibition of IgE synthesis
4. inhibition of lymphocyte mitogenesis

B. Unknown mechanisms
1. decreased chemotaxis
2. decreased phagocytosis
3. decreased lysosomal enzyme secretion
4. decreased chemiluminescence, O_2 and H_2O_2 production
5. lymphopenia, eosinopenia, monocytopenia

Phospholipase A_2-dependent events also control lymphocyte mitogenesis (Hirata et al. 1980), the distribution and metabolism of T- and B-lymphocytes, and the secretion of lymphokines, but they affect antibody synthesis only at very high doses (Claman 1975). Ishizaka (1984) showed in a series of elegant studies that macrocortin is identical to glycosylation inhibiting factor from lymphocytes which, together with macrophages, suppresses IgE formation. The significance of this controlling system in human disease needs to be further explored.

Although the precise mechanisms by which corticosteroids induce lymphopenia, monocytopenia, and eosinopenia are not clear, these drugs suppress many of the inflammatory activities of these cells and of neutrophils. This inhibition is not mediated through inhibition of DNA, RNA, or protein synthesis alone, but also through a decrease of phagocytosis, chemotaxis, and enzyme secretion of the cells (Ignarro 1977, Werb 1978, Gee et al. 1980). Corticosteroids also induce a decrease of chemiluminescence and of O_2- and H_2O_2 production, without affecting the bactericidal capacity of neutrophils (Shea and Morse 1978, Levine et al. 1981).

The broad range of action of the corticosteroids is responsible for the well-known and feared number of side effects which become apparent only during long-term, high-dose use. For this reason, their use in the treatment of chronic urticaria should be avoided. They may be used in rapidly decreasing doses in severe cases of acute urticaria where they help to suppress the acute symptomatology. Steroids are usually also infused during the treatment of anaphylactic shock. It should always be kept in mind, however, that these drugs work only after several hours. They are therefore not indicated in the treatment of acute, life-threatening symptoms.

11.2.4 Inhibitors of Mast Cell Secretion

Several years ago, the first antiasthmatic drug was discovered which had the unique ability to inhibit mast cell-dependent histamine release (reviewed by Altounyan 1980). Disodiumcromoglycate inhibits both immediate and late pulmonary reactions to antigen challenge (Table 11.2), but it has no effect on basophils at all. According to recent findings, the drug induces the phosphorylation of a protein with a molecular weight of 78 kd. Within seconds, this protein can switch off the anti-IgE- or compound 48/80-induced mast cell secretion. Other cromo-compounds work via the same mechanism. This phosphorylation switch-off is not activated by compounds that inhibit histamine release via elevation of cAMP, such as beta-agonists or phosphodiesterase inhibitors like theophylline (Wells and Mann 1983).

Disodiumcromoglycate does not readily enter cells since it is very hydrophilic, less than 1% of the drug being absorbed via the oral route. The drug also inhibits the release of mediators other than histamine, such as neutrophil chemotactic factor, from mast cells (Orr et al. 1980).

Because of its poor intestinal absorption, the drug is primarily useful when applied locally, as is possible with sprays or aerosols for the lungs or the nose, or in capsules for intestinal allergy. The drug has been shown to be effective in the treatment of food allergy by Finn and Cohen (1978) and Vaz et al. (1978), although Harries et al. (1978) and Thormann et al. (1980) saw no effect in 3 and 15 patients, respectively, with chronic urticaria due to food additives and analgesics. In mastocytosis, the drug is excellent for the control of gastrointestinal symptoms, whereas its effect on cutaneous symptomatology has a slow onset and is not as good as that of ordinary H1 blockers (Soter et al. 1979, Czarnetzki and Behrendt 1981).

Recently, a few other inhibitors of mast cell secretion have become available. They promise to be superior to disodiumcromoglycate, for they are absorbed via the oral route, and most of them also work on basophils (quercetin, doxantrazole, ketotifen) (Middleton 1981, Wahn and Müller 1983). Fields et al. (1984) have rated the relative potency of inhibition of histamine release as follows: azelastine > ketotifen > theophylline > disodiumcromoglycate. Azelastine, ketotifen, and oxatomide are also H1 blockers, ketotifen and oxatomide have anti-SRS effects, and oxatomide has anti-serotonin activities (Demaubeuge et al. 1982, Wang et al. 1984).

Clinical studies with these latter drugs appear promising. Oxatomide acts rapidly in patients with chronic urticaria, is reasonably effective, and causes only moderate tiredness (Verhaegen and De Cree 1980, Peremans 1981, Demaubeuge et al. 1982). Ketotifen works very well in controlling the cutaneous symptoms of patients with mastocytosis and dermographic urticaria, less so those of patients with cholinergic urticaria (Czarnetzki 1983, Cap et al. 1985). In combination with terbutaline, it yielded good results in 8 of 12 patients with chronic urticaria and in one patient each with dermographic and cold urticaria (Saihan 1981).

11.2.5 Kallikrein Inhibitors

Since kinins seem to be involved in the pathogenesis of certain types of urticaria, it was reasonable to test the effect of kallikrein inhibitors in urticaria patients, once such agents became available.

Juhlin and Michaelsson (1969) treated six patients with intravenous infusions of Trasylol, a commercial kallikrein inhibitor. This substance has a molecular weight of 6500 d and is purified from lungs and parotid glands of cattle. The urticae of the treated patients disappeared within 24 h, but reappeared within 5–90 days. Side effects included hypersalivation, flushing, perspiration, orthostatic hypotension, worsening of the urticaria in one patient, and anaphylactic shock in one of two patients with hereditary angioedema. The authors did not treat any more patients after the latter incident.

Berova et al. (1974) treated 52 patients with various forms of urticaria with 100,000 antikallikrein units of Trasylol intravenously on alternate days. They observed excellent results in 44% and improvement in 37% of their patients. The failures were usually among the patients with acute urticaria. Significant side effects were not recorded.

Treatment with Trasylol has nevertheless not become established for the treatment of urticaria, probably because of its route of administration and its potential side effects.

11.2.6 Mast Cell Mediator Depletion

Many decades ago, attempts were made to treat urticaria via depletion of mast cell mediators, based on the observation that patients have a refractory period after massive attacks of urticaria. This approach is still practiced for several physical urticarias, and if kept up by the patient, yields excellent results.

The same approach has been taken by developing drugs that inhibit the synthesis of histamine. Tritoqualin, an inhibitor of histidine decarboxylase, has been on the market for several years. In our experience, it is not very effective in the treatment of urticaria.

11.2.7 Miscellaneous Therapeutic Agents

Cinnarizine, an antihistamine and inhibitor of complement activation, has been tried in 35 patients with chronic urticaria and yielded good results with practically no side effects (Valsecchi et al. 1977). In a double-blind crossover trial, cinnarizine proved to be as effective as dexchlorpheniramine, compared to placebo, but was better tolerated (Kalimo and Jansen 1980).

Injections or oral solutions of calcium have been used for many decades to treat urticaria, particularly in central European countries. A sound scientific basis for this treatment cannot be found in the literature. We were unable to show any effect of intravenous calcium on the formation of resorption of experimental wheals of histamine, compound 48/80, or concanavalin A in ten allergic individuals and ten controls, compared to intravenous normal saline. Pruritus was not affected either (Pokropp and Czarnetzki 1983).

Since corticosteroids inhibit the formation of arachidonate metabolites, indomethacin was studied in 24 patients with chronic urticaria. The drug had no clinical effect on whealing or pruritus (Zachariae et al. 1969). Aspirin had also no effect on histamine wheals or immediate and delayed antigen-induced wheals (Smith et al. 1980).

Indomethacin and aspirin are primarily prostaglandin synthetase inhibitors. Studies with benoxaprofen which also inhibits the lipoxygenase (see Fig. 2.11, p. 18) and therefore the synthesis of leukotrienes, have shown reduction of SRS and histamine release in guinea pig and human lung (Boot et al. 1982). However, the drug has numerous serious side effects (Hindson et al. 1982) and is no longer marketed. Other, less toxic lipoxygenase inhibitors would be interesting to investigate in urticaria.

Antimalarials, such as dapsone, are used in the treatment of allergic vasculitis and have been tried with the urticarial vasculitis syndrome (see Chapter 11.6, p. 148). They can inhibit phospholipase A, the myeloperoxidase-peroxide-halide system, and the chemiluminescence of neutrophils (Mallorga et al. 1980, Webster et al. 1984). Not much else is known about their possible mechanism of action in the suppression of acute inflammation and allergy.

Casale et al. (1984) recently reported an interesting observation in patients who were treated with dopamine for hypotension. The drug depressed the histamine wheal and the penicillin-induced wheal in allergic patients, but had no effect on wheals induced by morphine, compound 48/80, ragweed, or mold antigens. This drug might provide a tool for probing the role of histamine in urticarial reactions and be useful in the therapy of certain subtypes of urticaria.

11.2.8 Hyposensitization

This type of treatment, also termed desensitization or "immunotherapy" by allergists, is aimed at downmodulating the basic immunological responsiveness of an individual to a specific allergen. Its use in urticaria is limited to the small group of patients with IgE-dependent disease who cannot avoid the eliciting agent or whose urticaria is associated with potentially life-threatening symptoms.

Hyposensitization in urticaria patients is practiced most frequently with bee and wasp sting allergic patients. In rare instances, patients with urticaria due to inhalant allergy or drug allergy (penicillin, insulin, isoniazid, diphenylhydantoin) are also treated in this fashion.

Hyposensitization against bees and wasps is done with the natural, commercially available venoms. Lichtenstein et al. (1979) described an ambulatory therapy regimen at weekly intervals until twice the dose of an insect sting is reached. Some patients may even need higher doses for protection and for monthly maintenance therapy (Ménardo et al. 1984). Müller (1981) and Glowania and Schulz (1981) described hyposensitization in hospitalized patients, with initially 4, then 3 daily doses until maintenance therapy levels were reached, usually by day 5. At our hospital, up to 8 daily injections are given. The most frequent side effects are local erythema and swelling at the site of subcutaneous injection on the lateral upper arm (Fig. 11.2). Systemic reactions, generally not life threatening, occur in 1 of 100 injections during these procedures. A tourniquet for tying off the arm after an

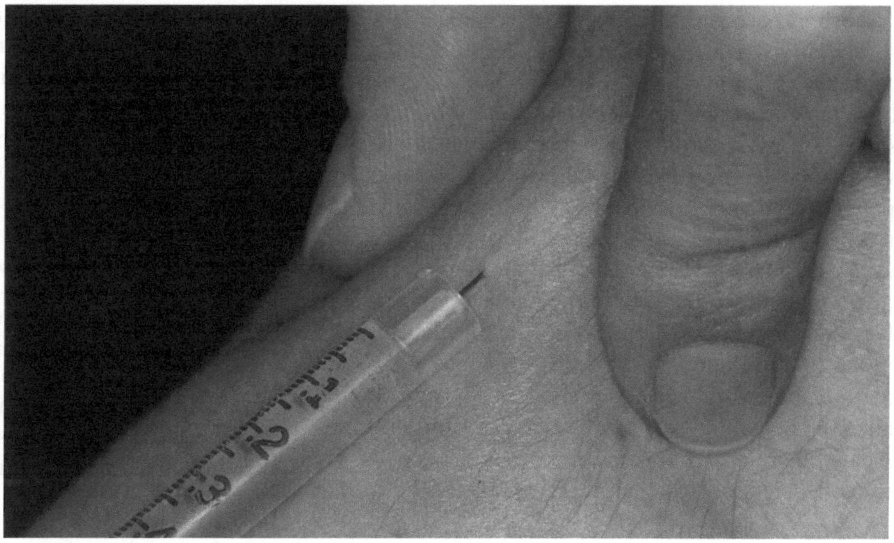

Fig. 11.2. Technique of subcutaneous injection. The outer aspect of the upper arm during immunological hyposensitization of a patient with bee venom allergy.

Table 11.4. Antigen preparations in clinical use for hyposensitization (1–3) and under experimental study to improve the effectiveness of hyposensitization (4–8) (from Norman 1980, Ishizaka 1984, Wüthrich 1984).

1. Aqueous extracts
2. Alum precipitated pyridine extracts
3. L-Tyrosine absorbed, glutaraldehyde, or formaldehyde treated extracts
4. Alum absorbed, urea denatured extracts
5. Ovalbumin-polyethylene glycol substituted allergens
6. Copolymerization with D-glutamic acid or D-lysine
7. Dinitrophenyl conjugates of polyvinyl alcohol
8. Anti-idiotype antibodies

injection and emergency drugs should be available during immunotherapy, and the patient should be observed by medical personnel for 30 min after each injection. The effectiveness of this treatment is good, and the end point of therapy is thought to be an undetectable level of specific IgE (Urbanek et al. 1984).

Inhalant allergy is not an important cause of urticaria, and the indication for hyposensitization, the technique for its execution, its efficacy, its side effects, and its theoretical basis have recently been thoroughly reviewed (Norman 1980, Wüthrich 1984). Since patients are usually allergic to several allergens, and since the extracts contain mixtures of antigens, the results of immunotherapy for inhalant allergy are not as good as with insect venom therapy. Treatment is always done on an outpatient basis. Instead of aqueous extracts, chemically modified allergens with a depot action are frequently used (Table 11.4). In recent years, a number of attempts have been made to make treatment with allergens more effective by chemically modifying the allergens (Table 11.4). Their clinical usefulness in humans is, however, still uncertain.

Rush hyposensitization can be accomplished within 4–24 h in patients who urgently need a drug, for example, in patients with bacterial endocarditis who have a penicillin allergy. Parker (1975), who has used such therapy without major incidents in 24 patients with skin test positive penicillin allergy, started his patients on a very low dose (1000 units or less) via the relatively safe oral route and added increasing doses every 20–30 min. He switched to parenteral administration when 50,000 units of penicillin were reached. Naclerio et al. (1983) described a schedule that initially involved parenteral administration for 4 days and maintenance oral doses thereafter in one highly allergic, penicillin-sensitive patient. A similar treatment schedule can be used for other drugs that are urgently needed. However, it should always be kept in mind that these procedures are very dangerous and that the patients need careful, constant supervision.

The mechanisms that induce tolerance to allergens through rapidly increasing doses of the allergens are not known. Careful immunologic monitoring has shown several changes in the patients' immune system: a gradual increase of IgG, particularly of IgG_4, a decrease of antigen-induced in vitro histamine release from basophils, decreased in vitro lymphocyte responsiveness to the specific allergen, an increase of IgE-specific suppressor T-cells, and after some weeks, a decrease of specific IgE. None of these changes are consistently observed in all individuals who undergo hyposensitization; therefore, other, as yet unknown mechanisms must be operative (Norman 1980, Ishizaka 1984).

11.3 Treatment of Acute and Chronic Urticaria

11.3.1 Acute Urticaria

Treatment of acute urticaria, with no associated pulmonary or cardiovascular symptoms, is not a major challenge to the physician (Table 11.5). He must identify the cause and remove or stop further contact with the eliciting agent, if possible. Induction of vomiting was practiced in former times in food allergy but is probably of little help since in most cases, the food or drug has passed already into the intestines.

Reassurance of the patient is the next important measure. He should be instructed to contact the treating physician or a nearby hospital in case of respiratory difficulties and signs of vascular collapse, and he should be told that his urticaria might last for several weeks since it often takes that long for certain drugs to be eliminated from the body.

Local treatment of the existing wheals is not necessary, but one can prescribe a shaking lotion to alleviate the itch. This gives the patient reassurance that something is being done for his skin. The use of topical steroids is not indicated, unless the so-called papular urticaria due to insect stings or localized contact urticaria are present.

Table 11.5. Treatment of acute urticaria and angioedema.

Removal or reduced absorption of eliciting agent
Patient reassurance and instruction to report at once to the physician if breathing difficulties should occur
Antihistamines (H1-antagonists)
Corticosteroids in severe cases
Topical lotions, if desired or otherwise indicated

Antihistamines of the H1 type should be prescribed for the entire period of persistence of lesions. Each physician will have certain antihistamine preparations with which he is most familiar and his patients are most satisfied. In general, it is preferable to prescribe newer antihistamines with little or no depressing effect on the central nervous system (terfenadine, ketotifen). A drug with more sedating qualities and a longer acting antihistamine such as hydroxyzine may be desirable for the night. The dosage should be adjusted according to the severity of the urticaria and the patient's discomfort.

In severe, acute urticaria which is bothersome to the patient in his daily work and where the eliciting agent is evident, symptoms can be alleviated by intramuscular or oral corticosteroids. One can start with 60–80 mg of prednisone daily, decreasing the dose rapidly every other day for the following 10 to 14 days. This treatment has the disadvantage that it delays the time until diagnostic skin tests can be performed. Precautions which are necessary for long-term steroid therapy, such as treatment with antacids, tuberculostatic agents, and drugs against osteoporosis, are not necessary in this situation.

11.3.2 Anaphylaxis

The cardinal rule for the treatment of acute anaphylaxis is reduction of the absorption or increased elimination of the offending agent (Table 11.6). Epinephrine is the mainstay of therapy, and its primary use is mandatory to reduce local resorption, to decrease peripheral vasodilation and bronchospasm, to increase cardiac output, and to decrease further release of cellular mediators. Maintenance of a patent vein, fluid replacement, and open airways are important additional measures. Antihistamines and corticosteroids are infused to counteract the effect of additionally released histamine and to reduce the late systemic effects of anaphylaxis. In case of severe bronchospasms, aminophylline is infused intravenously. Resuscitation measures may have to be taken in case of severe cardiovascular collapse. Lidocaine (1–1.5 mg/kg body wt.) should be infused to strengthen cardiac output and prevent arrhythmias; sodium bicarbonate (1–1.5 mg/kg) should be given at regular intervals to combat acidosis; and plasma expanders, such as hydroxyethyl starch, should replace the dextrose infusion.

There are patients who suffer from recurrent anaphylaxis due to insect stings, food, or unknown cause (Bacal et al. 1978, Lieberman and Taylor 1979). These patients and their families should be taught the use of subcutaneous epinephrine and be instructed to go to an emergency room as soon as possible. If the episodes are more frequent, regular treatment with antihistamines and ephedrine should be instituted, and if episodes are very frequent and severe, prednisone should be given regularly, starting at 50 mg daily and tapering to the lowest dose possible, with a switch to alternate day therapy to minimize side effects. Precautions against gastric ulcers, worsening of osteoporosis, diabetes, and reactivation of tuberculosis should be taken as indicated.

In patients with previous reactions to contrast media who need another X-ray examination, oral prednisone (50 mg) should be given 13, 7, and 1 h before the procedure. Diphenhydramine (50 mg) or another H1 blocker should be given in addition 1 h before, and, to further reduce the incidence of serious reactions, ephedrine can also be added 1 h before the examination (Greenberger et al. 1984). A combination of an H2 blocker (cimetidine) with the H1 blocker has also been effective (Myers and Bloom 1981). Such a preventive regimen can also be instituted in patients who have a positive history of previous incidents

Table 11.6. Treatment of acute anaphylaxis (modified from Katz 1975).

I. General measures
   1. Eliminate or reduce absorption of the offending material (tourniquet proximal to site of challenge for several minutes; application of ice; local, subcutaneous injection of epinephrine (0.2 ml of a 1:1000 dilution) to decrease absorption; see II.1)
   2. Start an intravenous infusion with 5% dextrose in water
   3. Place patient in supine position and clear airways
   4. Maintain observation for at least 30 to 60 min after patient is stabilized
   5. Have resuscitation equipment available
   6. Observe vital signs

II. Respiratory distress
   1. Inject aqueous epinephrine (0.3 to 0.5 ml, 1:1000 dilution) subcutaneously; repeat in 15 min, if necessary
   2. Give H1-antihistamines (e.g. diphenhydramine, 2 mg/kg) i.v. or i.m. and cimetidine (200 mg) i.v.
   3. Maintain airways (intubation), and make a tracheotomy (surgically or with a large bore needle) for severe laryngeal edema
   4. Infuse aminophylline (5–10 mg/kg) in 1000 ml 5% dextrose in water over 1 h for bronchospasm
   5. Infuse hydrocortisone (300–1000 mg) by direct push and 7 mg/kg/24 h via the infusion (or dexamethasone, up to 20 mg/kg), to reduce the late effects of generalized reactions

III. Cardiovascular collapse
   1. Infuse aqueous epinephrine i.v. (0.5 to 1.0 ml, diluted 1:10000) (5–10 ml), slowly; watch heart rate!
   2. Give antihistamines and corticosteroid, as in II.2 and II.5

Table 11.7. Treatment of chronic urticaria.

Avoid the eliciting agents (e.g., foods, drugs) and stimulants
Treat potential causes (e.g., infections, metabolic alterations)
Give H1-antihistamines or an inhibitor of mast cell degranulation or complement activation on a maintenance basis
If there is no response, try a combination of
H1 and H2 blockers
an H1 blocker and an inhibitor of degranulation
an H1 blocker and a beta-agonist

during anesthesia or surgery but in whom the exact cause cannot be ascertained. The same holds for patients with mastocytosis who react more readily to histamine liberators used during anesthesia. None of these measures are helpful in patients with hereditary or acquired C1-deficiency angioedema (see Chapter 11.7, p. 149).

11.3.3 **Chronic Urticaria** (Table 11.7)

The treatment discussed here applies to chronic idiopathic urticaria, urticaria due to intolerance reactions, and urticaria due to causes other than physical agents, vasculitis, and mastocytosis.

As in acute urticaria, the cardinal rule for therapy is the elimination or avoidance of the noxious agents (Table 11.7). This might involve such esoteric approaches as treating an urticaria due to surgically implanted tantalum staples with disulfiram chelation therapy (Werman and Rietschel 1981). Even if the cause is not known, 55–57% of patients will be cured or improved if they keep an additive-free diet, according to the guidelines given in Table 10.8 (Gibson and Clancy 1980, Verschave et al. 1983). Aspirin desensitization which has improved asthma and rhinosinusitis in patients with these afflictions and has also "cross-desensitized" them to indomethacin and other non-steroidal anti-inflammatory agents (Pleskow et al. 1982, Lumry et al. 1983, Stevenson et al. 1984) has not yet been tried in chronic urticaria and aspirin intolerance.

Antihistamines should be given to patients on a maintenance basis, and patients should be reassured that this is a relatively safe therapy. Drugs with little central depressant action should be given preference, and the timing of treatment should be adjusted to the rhythm of worsening of the urticarial lesions. Thus, some patients might need treatment only at night. Patients should also be informed that they must expect a worsening of their symptoms with aggravating factors such as alcohol or viral infections.

Illig and Paul (1978) maintain that in treatment failures, antihistamines are often not given at a sufficient dose or that the patients reduce the dosage on their own. They consider retard H1 preparations which are given by some physicians at night (Warin and Champion 1974) unnecessary since antihistamines are excreted anyway very slowly.

If an ordinary antihistamine (e.g. diphenhydramine, chlorpheniramine) is not helpful, a more potent antihistamine such as hydroxyzine may be instituted in addition, particularly at night (Harvey et al. 1981). One should, however, be cautious of the long-term use of hydroxyzine because it can cause a psychological dependence and can have hallucinogenic effects. An oral inhibitor of mast cell degranulation with H1 activity, such as ketotifen or oxatomide, may also be tried as an alternative or in combination with a classical H1 blocker.

In patients who fail on these regimens, a combination of H1 and H2 blockers or H1 and β-agonists can be tried. Although the results of such regimens are good (see Sections 11.2.1, p. 135 and 11.2.2, p. 138), more long-term experience is necessary to prove their safety and effectiveness.

11.4 The Physical Urticarias

In general, the principles of treatment, as outlined for chronic urticaria (Table 11.7), apply also to the physical urticarias. Since this group differs, however, in its responsiveness to drugs, and since some types of physical urticaria do not respond to antihistamines at all, the major types of the physical urticarias are dealt with separately.

11.4.1 **Dermographic Urticaria** (Table 11.8)

In many instances, patients with this affliction require no treatment at all because the symptoms are mild and the disease disappears again after a certain time. Exposure of the skin to wind and sun to cause "hardening" of the skin, and vigorous rubbing at regular intervals to cause mediator depletion, are helpful conservative measures. Rare patients whose dermographic urticaria is due to penicillin should avoid taking this drug.

Doeglas (1975) observed four spontaneous remissions among his 25 patients with this condition, and 16 of 22 were well controlled with H1 blockers. Illig and Paul (1978) observed no response to antihistamines in 5 of 9 patients, and Marcussen (1950) in 8 of 38. Marcussen observed that addition of sedatives and psychotherapy yielded excellent results in his patients.

The need for a sedative action and the better H1 blocking activity may explain why hydroxyzine was found to be superior to other H1 blockers for the treatment of dermographic urticaria (Matthews et al. 1973, Breathnach et al. 1983). A combination of either chlorpheniramine or hydroxyzine with cimetidine was found to be even better (Matthews et al. 1979, Kaur et al. 1981, Breathnach et al., 1983, Cook and Shuster 1983a). We observed excellent control of symptoms with ketotifen in more than 95% of our patients and would prefer this treatment to combined H1 and H2 blockers because of the lower side effects (Cap et al. 1985). Newer agents with similar properties as ketotifen such as oxatomide should also be tried in this condition.

11.4.2 Cholinergic Urticaria

Since cholinergic urticaria (Table 11.8) has a well-defined refractory period in most patients, deliberate provocation of the condition through regular hot baths or exercise can ensure freedom of symptoms for certain time periods. Such a regular desensitization program might also cause a reduction in general symptomatology. Antihistamines should be taken by patients with severe symptoms to prevent serious systemic reactions. Avoidance of situations that elicit the urticarial reaction and psychotherapy may also be recommended. A spontaneous remission can be expected in a small percentage of patients (3 of 17 in the series of Doeglas 1975).

The effectiveness of antihistamines is variable. Illig and Paul (1978) found that all of their 13 patients responded to oral H1 blockers, and only 1 of 5 failed on parenteral antihistamine therapy. Doeglas (1975) observed good control in 4 of 5 patients on H1 blockers and in 10 of 15 on hydroxyzine. The latter drug was suggested to be particularly helpful in cholinergic urticaria because of its anticholinergic activity. Moore Robinson and Warin (1968) found, in a double-blind study, that 8 of 14 patients were better while on hydroxyzine (25 mg three times daily), only 4 of 14 were improved on brompheniramine (4 mg three times daily), and two patients observed no difference between the two types of therapy. We have tried ketotifen in a double-blind crossover study in patients with cholinergic urticaria and have observed a good response in slighly less than 70% of the patients. Obviously, a search for a convincingly effective therapy in this condition is still warranted. Trials with a combination therapy of different drugs have not been published to date.

11.4.3 Cold Urticaria (Table 11.8)

Once an underlying cause of cold urticaria is excluded through routine diagnosis (see Section 5.7.6, p. 71), patients should be given a course of penicillin i.m., daily or every other day, at a total dose of 10–12 million units. From 25%–50% of the patients are cured or improved with this treatment (Liebeskind and Schwarze 1974, Doeglas 1975, Haustein and Kirchhoff 1984). The drug has to be given parenterally, and care should be taken not to give this treatment to patients who are allergic to penicillin. The mechanism of action is not known.

Table 11.8. Treatment of special types of urticaria.

Condition	Treatment
Dermographic urticaria	1. desensitization (rubbing, shower) 2. H1 blockers (hydroxyzine, ketotifen) 3. if not effective, combine with H2 blockers
Cholinergic urticaria	1. desensitization (hot baths, exercise) 2. H1 blockers (hydroxyzine) 3. ketotifen
Cold urticaria	1. penicillin i.m., 10–12 million units 2. desensitization (cold baths) 3. orally effective inhibitors of mast cell degranulation (ketotifen, oxatomide) 4. cyproheptadine
Solar urticaria	1. desensitization (UV-A, PUVA or sunlight) 2. sunscreens: 280–320 nm: p-aminobenzoic acid 320–400 nm: benzophenones, titanium oxide, zinc oxide 400–500 nm: titanium oxide, zinc oxide 3. H1 blockers or antimalarials
Heat urticaria	1. desensitization (hot baths) 2. H1 blockers 3. H1+H2 blockers 4. chloroquine
Pressure urticaria	1. avoidance 2. corticosteroids
Mastocytosis	1. avoidance of degranulating agents 2. symptomatic treatment of a) gastrointestinal symptoms: disodiumcromoglycate cimetidine b) blistering: disodiumcromoglycate c) pruritus: H1 blockers, ketotifen d) flush: nifedipine; combined H1, H2, and prostaglandin antagonists e) cosmetic problems: PUVA
Urticarial vasculitis syndrome	1. dapsone or hydroxychloroquine 2. corticosteroids, alone or combined with 1. 3. cyclophosphamide 4. indomethacin 5. plasma exchange

Desensitization by depletion of mast cell mediators through gradually increased exposure to the cold was already practiced in the thirties (Horton et al. 1936). One recommended method is to immerse the body for 5 min at hourly intervals into cold water. This is usually tolerated without development of wheals, within 4–5 h. Maintenance treatment is done with cold showers every 12–24 h (Leigh et al. 1974).

A more cautious method of desensitization is done by starting to submerge one forearm in 15° C water for 5 min at hourly intervals until no more urticarial swelling develops, usually after the 4th or 5th treatment. The interval is then extended to every 2 h and, when no more urticaria occurs, to 4, 6, 8, 12, and 24 h intervals. The same procedure is repeated with each limb, then the face, and finally the trunk (Bentley-Phillips et al. 1976).

A third possibility of desensitization is to have the patient take 15-min baths twice daily, starting about 5° C above his threshold temperature, with exposures at gradually lower degrees to the point where the patient can tolerate the temperatures that normally produce his urticaria.

Side effects of cold desensitization are frequent headaches, flushing, and feeling of faintness during all these procedures. Because of the danger of syncope, the patient should be under careful supervision and be told of the potential danger of this treatment. While the results are excellent if the patient is highly motivated and willing to keep up the procedure at home, there is rarely a person who is compulsive enough to maintain desensitization over months and years. The hardening effect is lost within 5 days without treatment. The patient should be aware of this to prevent major reactions if he has not taken his therapy for a few days.

The response of cold urticaria to H1 blockers is only variably effective. Doeglas (1975) observed good control in 7 of 11 patients. Wanderer et al. (1977) compared cyproheptadine (4 mg three times daily) to chlorpheniramine (4 mg three times daily) and placebo. They observed significant improvement only in the eight patients on cyproheptadine. Cyproheptadine is a powerful H1 blocker with antiserotonin and weak anticholinergic properties. Side effects are a moderate central depression, weight gain, stimulation of growth in children, and confusion and ataxia at higher doses (Goodman and Gilman 1980). The good response to cyproheptadine was confirmed by Sigler et al. (1980) in six patients, while Haustein and Kirchhoff (1984) observed a response in only 20 %, and weight gain and tiredness in all his patients.

Neittaanmäki et al. (1984) studied doxepin (30 mg daily), an H1 and H2 blocker with anticholinergic effects at high doses, comparing it with cinnarizine (30 mg daily), an inhibitor of complement activation, and hydroxyzine (40 mg daily). They found all three drugs to be equally effective, compared to placebo. Doxepin caused less tiredness, but patients complained of dryness of the mouth.

Studies with inhibitors of mast cell degranulation offer new perspectives in the treatment of cold urticaria. Haustein and Kirchhoff (1984) observed no therapeutic effect in three patients with oral disodium-cromoglycate, probably because of bad absorption of the drug via the oral route. In nine patients with cold contact and two with cold reflex urticaria, there was good control of itching and whealing with ketotifen (2 mg daily), and only two patients observed slight initial sedation. Sauer and Steigleder (1983) found that oxatomide (60 mg daily), another orally effective inhibitor of mast cell degranulation, was superior to ketotifen, even though both drugs caused decreased histamine levels in the venous effluent on cold exposure and a good control of symptoms in the four patients studied.

Kobza-Black et al. (1981) treated six patients with oral prednisone (20–25 mg for 1–5 days), recording decrease of venous histamine release and of pruritus, but not of edema and redness. This treatment is therefore obviously no alternative to that with inhibitors of mast cell degranulation, also in view of the side effects of corticosteroids.

11.4.4 **Solar Urticaria** (Table 11.8)

As with other types of physical urticaria, improvement of solar urticaria can be obtained by controlled, gradually increasing exposure to natural sunlight or to artificial light sources. Tolerance can be produced by hourly exposure of individual body regions to fluorescent lamps, achieving tolerance with 2–5 exposures (Fig. 11.3). The intervals of irradiation are then increased to 3, 6, 12, and 24 h, and tolerance is maintained by irradiation at these intervals (Ramsay 1977). Initiation of tolerance with UV-A, which does not readily cause erythema and sunburn, is preferable and also helps patients to tolerate the UV-B of natural sunlight (Keahey et al. 1984). The desensitization procedure can be accelerated by oral methoxsalen (0.6 mg/kg) 2 h before a UV-A irradiation, starting at 80 % of the minimal dose to induce urticaria. Treatments are given 3x a week, with an increase of 5×10^3 J/m^2 at each session (Parrish et al. 1982). As the refractory state lasts only 48–72 h, most authors have the patient continue treatment during the sunny season by exposure to the noontime sun, starting with 15 min and increasing the time by 5–10 min each time until noon sunlight is tolerated for 2 h (Keahey et al. 1984). Most patients respond well to this treatment, although there are occasional failures (Bernhard et al. 1984).

The mechanisms of this rapidly achieved and equally quickly lost tolerance to light cannot be due to slowly developing processes, such as epidermal hyperkeratosis, hyperplasia, or increased melanin pigmentation in response to irradiation. While it can readily be shown that mast cells fail to degranulate on exposure to radiant light in tolerant skin, the cells still degranulate in response to codeine, and the tissue reacts normally to histamine, so that the tolerance must be very specific for radiant energy (Horio 1978, Bernhard et al. 1984, Keahey et al. 1984).

In patients who cannot undergo desensitization, topical sunscreens and drugs should be prescribed. In recent years, very good sunscreen preparations have appeared on the market. A particular sunscreen should be chosen on the basis of the eliciting spectrum for each individual patient (see Table 11.8).

Topical sunscreens alone yield good to fair protection in about 50% of the patients (Ravits et al. 1982). Various forms of drug therapy must therefore be used in addition. Chlorpheniramine gives only slight improvement of light tolerance (Michell et al. 1980, Parrish et al. 1982), whereas hydroxyzine was considered effective by Ratanen and Suhonen (1980). Several other authors have found H1 blockers to be good (Baart de la Faille et al. 1975), variable (Ravits et al. 1982), or ineffective (Willis and Epstein 1974, Hasei and Ichihashi 1982). H2 blockers, indomethacin, and β-carotene are not helpful (Kobza et al. 1973, Horio and Minami 1977, Michell et al. 1980, Wennersten 1980, Parrish et al. 1982). Chloroquine (250 mg orally twice daily) suppressed symptoms within 3 weeks in two patients who were unresponsive to antihistamines. Control could be maintained on 250 mg every 5 days (Willis and Eppstein 1974). Others could not confirm this improvement by antimalarials in their patients (Ratanen and Suhonen 1980). Risks of long-term treatment with antimalarials should be considered when starting patients on this therapy, and trials with modern antihistamines and blockers of mast cell degranulation should be tried instead. Moderate improvement was seen in one of our patients on ketotifen (unpublished observation).

Fig. 11.3. Effect of hardening through UV-A (long wavelength) therapy in a patient with solar urticaria. The irradiated, tanned skin no longer urticates on challenge with UV light, whereas the unirradiated skin (lower half) does.

11.4.5 Heat Contact Urticaria (Table 11.8)

As this rare condition is based on several different pathomechanisms (see Chapter 5.10.10, p. 85), it is not uniformly responsive to one type of therapy. Desensitization by increasing exposure to hot water was found helpful by some (Duke 1924, Doeglas 1975, Leigh and Ramsay 1975, Atkins and Zweiman 1981), but not by others (de Moragas et al. 1973, Daman et al. 1978, Johansson et al. 1984). A successful procedure is to take hot baths, 4 × daily for two days, and once daily thereafter (Atkins and Zweiman 1981). Another method is to start with a 1 min exposure of one limb every hour, and to gradually increase the time of immersion to 5 min, at increasing intervals of 3, 6, and 12 h, followed by exposure of the other limbs, then the lower, and finally the upper trunk. Total tolerance should be reached in this fashion by 10 days (Leigh and Ramsay 1975).

Many authors have not even attempted this cumbersome and potentially dangerous procedure, but have tried their patients on drug therapy instead. H1 blockers were rated good to helpful by some (Michaelsson and Ros 1971, Greaves et al. 1974, Wise et al. 1978, Grant et al. 1981, Johansson et al. 1984), and ineffective by others (Willis and Epstein 1974, Starr et al. 1980, Atkins and Zweiman 1981). Wüthrich (1979) observed a partial effect with ketotifen and a good response with the retard H1 blocker dexchlorpheniramine maleate, at 2 × 2 tablets daily. H1 plus H2 blockers as well as chloroquine were ineffective, according to Starr et al. (1980), although they gave good therapeutic responses in the hands of

Irwin et al. (1984) and Willis and Epstein (1974). Oral disodiumcromoglycate was not helpful either (Atkins and Zweiman 1981). Obviously, patients with this rare condition should be subjected to a number of treatment regimens to find the one that they respond to best.

11.4.6 Pressure Urticaria (Table 11.8)

Among the physical urticarias, pressure urticaria is the type most resistant to treatment. Oral or intravenous antihistamines of various types are not effective (Doeglas 1975, Illig and Paul 1978). Doeglas (1975) observed relief in three of eight patients with prednisone, in one of seven patients with tranexamic acid, and in one with chloroquine. Sussman et al. (1982) claim that aspirin ameliorates pressure urticaria, but more than 90% of their patients had chronic urticaria, and the authors did not specify which symptoms were improved. In my own experience, aspirin was useless in pressure urticaria. Pilot therapies with oral disodiumcromoglycate, danazol, ketotifen, cimetidine, indomethacin, propanolol, lipopolysaccharide injections, and combinations of these drugs also had no influence on the disease. The only effective agents were corticosteroids (unpublished observations).

Davis et al. (1984) claimed that their ten patients with documented delayed pressure urticaria developed delayed skin tests to compound 48/80 and multiple food antigens. Fasting and elimination of the foods that were positive on testing cleared the disease in each instance. Although several of our patients had delayed skin reactions to foods, inhalant allergens, and even to normal saline, none of them lost their symptoms while on a diet that lacked the suspected agents.

Avoidance of situations that provoke the lesions, and treatment of painful lesions with analgesics and corticosteroids are therefore the only means to treat pressure urticaria.

11.5 Mastocytosis (Table 11.8)

Since the majority of patients with mastocytosis have the limited, benign form of the disease and are free of symptoms, one should avoid excessive diagnostic procedures and unnecessary treatment, particularly in small children. The patient or the parents should be educated about the disease and informed that mast cell degranulating stimuli should be avoided.

Until now, no therapeutic agent has been found that can induce regression of benign or malignant mastocytosis. Antihistamines with H1 receptor specificity are excellent drugs to reduce the symptoms of pruritus, shock, and flushing. H2 antagonists have been used successfully for the treatment of peptic ulcers (Johnson et al. 1980), and combinations of H1 and H2 antagonists have yielded good control of blistering (Fenske et al. 1985), but dinatriumcromoglycate is safer in this situation (see below and Section 11.2.4). The chronic use of a combination of H1, H2, and prostaglandin antagonists has been advocated to prevent severe flushing and shock (Roberts et al. 1982). Aspirin should, however, be given carefully in such cases and only at gradually increasing doses because it can also act as a histamine liberator in intolerant patients.

Disodiumcromoglycate is an excellent drug for controlling gastrointestinal symptomatology. As it is absorbed to <1%, it is only moderately effective for the treatment of other symptoms such as pruritus (Soter et al. 1979, Czarnetzki and Behrendt 1981, Businco et al. 1984). It is also reported to be useful in the control of cutaneous blistering in very small children (40–100 mg/day) (Evans and Vickers 1981, Welch et al. 1983). Ketotifen, an orally effective inhibitor of mast cell degranulation, is more effective than cromolyn in controlling the cutaneous, but not the gastrointestinal symptoms (Czarnetzki 1983). Nifedipine (30 mg daily), an organic calcium channel blocker, has suppressed urtication and flushing in a young adult woman (Fairley et al. 1984).

Psoralen plus UV-A (PUVA) treatment yields excellent cosmetic results, causes some of the lesions to disappear, reduces itching, and decreases histamine and leukotriene contents of the skin (Christophers et al. 1978, Vella Briffa et al. 1983, Czarnetzki et al. 1985). Total mast cell numbers do not decrease, but the cells translocate to lower regions of the dermis (Kolde et al. 1984). Symptoms, skin lesions, and all morphological and biochemical changes revert however to pretreatment levels after discontinuation of treatment (Vella Briffa et al. 1983; Czarnetzki et al. 1985). Thus, this transient improvement does not justify the use of a potentially harmful (carcinogenic) therapy. Acute shock should be treated as outlined in Section 11.3.2, p. 143 and Table 11.6.

Corticosteroids, X-rays, and cytostatic drugs have been used in an attempt to control the symptoms or the progression of mastocytosis, particularly in patients with the malignant variety of the disease. All these modalities are useless for the long-term management of the disease, but they may be instituted judiciously for palliative reasons. Fifty percent of the patients with malignant mastocytosis die within 2 years of the diagnosis.

Because of the almost universally benign nature of mastocytosis, management of the patients should concentrate on the diagnostic delineation of the extent of the disease, on treatment and prevention of symptomatology, and above all on the education and the reassuring guidance of the patient and his relatives by the physician.

11.6 Urticarial Vasculitis Syndrome

(Table 11.8)

There is almost no uniformly effective therapeutic agent for this condition, as would be expected from the broad spectrum of potential clinical manifestations that are part of the syndrome. Whereas H1 and H2 blockers are ineffective (O'Loughlin et al. 1978, Lopez et al. 1984), dapsone and hydroxychloroquine are the most effective agents. Lesions cleared within 48 h and a gradual improvement of complement abnormalities within the following 3 months was observed in patients with SLE, urticaria, and neutrophilic vasculitis who received 100 mg daily (Matthews et al. 1978, Ruzicka and Goerz 1981, Jones et al. 1983). A combination of this treatment with prednisone (20 mg daily) also yielded good results (Highet 1980). Hydroxychloroquine (200 mg daily) resulted in remission of the hypocomplementemic urticarial vasculitis in four patients, and a fifth patient also responded but had to stop treatment because of therapy-dependent diplopia. Two of the patients eventually developed systemic lupus erythematosus despite the good initial therapeutic response (Gurd and Zuraw 1984). O'Loughlin et al. (1978) noted good control in 4 of their 12 patients on chloroquine. A good response of joint symptoms and a partial response of the urticaria were achieved with chloroquine (400 mg daily) in one patient (Lopez et al. 1984), and Van der Horst and Bronsveld (1981) observed a response with chloroquine (600 mg daily) and prednisone (40 mg daily).

Corticosteroids alone in a dosage of up to 30 mg of prednisone daily have been found to be ineffective (Soter 1977), although symptoms can be controlled, with lower doses (G. Goerz, personal communication). Lopez et al. (1984) noted a partial improvement, with persistence of arthralgias and urticaria, on 40 mg daily. The urticaria was suppressed with 30 mg daily in one patient of Ruzicka and Goerz (1981), and Callen and Kalbfleisch (1982) could control the vasculitis in seven of their nine patients. Hintner and Tappeiner (1979) suppressed the disease with steroids, but stopped treatment because of side effects.

Cytotoxic drugs, alone or in combination with steroids, are an additional potential mode of treatment (McDuffie et al. 1973, Sissons et al. 1974). Hintner and Tappeiner (1979) induced remission with cyclophosphamide which lasted for 5 months. Ruzicka and Goerz (1981) however obtained no response with prednisone (10 mg) and azathioprine (100 mg daily). Treatment failure was also noted by Lopez et al. (1984) with azathioprine (100 mg daily).

Millns et al. (1980) made the exciting observation that indomethacin (2 × 25 mg–4 × 50 mg daily) induced a complete remission within 17 days in six of their ten patients with urticarial vasculitis, angioedema, arthralgias, abdominal pain, and low grade fever. Three additional patients had a partial response. Eight patients had a recurrence of lesions within 48 h after discontinuation of therapy. Gastrointestinal irritation was the only side effect. We have not seen such a therapeutic benefit with indomethacin in any of our patients, nor have Jones et al. (1983) and Lopez et al. (1984). Nevertheless, it seems worthwhile to try this treatment in patients before initiating therapy with agents that have a much higher risk of side effects.

Finally, it should be mentioned that plasma exchange was found to yield good results by Jones et al. (1983). Wherever the facilities are available, this relatively innocuous treatment modality is also worth a trial.

11.7 Hereditary Angioedema

11.7.1 Danazol

The observation that attacks of hereditary angioedema can be prevented by treatment with methyltestosterone (Spaulding 1960) paved the way for one of the most significant and satisfying advances in the treatment of this condition. Davis (1974) tested androgens with less severe virilizing effects, fluoxymesterone for men and oxymetholone for women. These good therapeutic results were confirmed by Rosse et al. (1976) and by Sheffer et al. (1979). C1INH and C4 levels rose during treatment, and side effects were less marked with these synthetic androgens.

The most satisfying therapeutic results with relatively few side effects were obtained in a series of studies with danazol. The drug is a 2,3-isoxazol derivative of 17-alpha-ethynyl testosterone. Its main mechanism of action was initially thought to relate to a suppression of the pituitary-ovarian axis by inhibiting the output of gonadotropins from the pituitary gland. This effect is seen primarily in hypogonadic patients. The drug's more important effects in normals are due to the inhibition of enzymes that control sex steroid synthesis and to the competitive binding of sex steroids to their cytoplasmic receptors in the target tissue (Madanes and Farber 1982, Table 11.9). Other actions

Table 11.9. Therapeutic effects and undesirable responses caused by danazol (from Hosea and Frank 1980, Madanes and Farber 1982).

A. Pharmacological effects of danazol
  1. enzymatic inhibition of sex steroid synthesis
  2. competitive inhibition of binding of sex hormones to their cytoplasmic receptors
  3. decreased thyroxin binding globulin, pregnancy zone protein, sex hormone binding protein
  4. increased serum prealbumin, haptoglobin, transferrin, antithrombin III, prothrombin, plasminogen, α_1-antitrypsin
  5. increase of C1 INH levels
  6. increase of C2 and C4 levels

B. Clinical uses of danazol
  1. prevention of attacks of angioedema due to C1INH deficiency
  2. treatment of endometriosis and cystic disease of the breast

C. Undesirable side effects of danazol
  1. weight gain (38–100% of patients)
  2. menometrorrhagia (34%)
  3. myalgias, muscle cramps (28–30%)
  4. headache (22%)
  5. mild alopecia (17%)
  6. amenorrhea (16%)
  7. episodes of anxiety and tremor (16%)
  8. elevated serum transaminases (14%)
  9. decreased libido (5–14%)
  10. microscopic hematuria (13%)
  11. hot flashes (12–17%)
  12. deepening of the voice (7–10%)
  13. hirsuitism, acne, seborrhea (8–30%)
  14. nausea (4%)

of the drug include increases in various serum proteins, the increase of C1INH and C4 being the basis for its therapeutic use in hereditary and acquired angioedema. The increase of other serum factors which interact with the Hageman-factor dependent inflammatory processes (see Fig. 4.2, p. 51; Table 11.9) may add to the beneficial effect of the drug.

Gelfand et al. (1976) provided convincing evidence that danazol prevents attacks of angioedema in a double-blind study, with nine patients as subjects. A rise in serum C1INH and C4 was noted after only 3–4 days of treatment. A number of changes in serum hormone binding proteins and in other serum proteins were noted as well (Table 11.9, reviewed in Madanes and Farber 1982).

The therapeutic benefit of danazol in the treatment of hereditary angioedema has been confirmed in a number of studies with both men and women (Lagrue et al. 1978, Pitts et al. 1978, Hintner et al. 1979, Hosea and Frank 1980). The drug also improved the clinical and laboratory alterations in a patient with acquired angioedema due to rectal carcinoma (Cohen et al. 1978) and in patients due to inactive or albumin-bound C1INH (Gadek et al. 1979, Kövary et al. 1981). It does not work in ordinary urticaria and angioedema. Tappeiner et al. (1979) reported on the successful treatment of an 5-year-old boy with severe hereditary angioedema. Initially, 400 mg daily were given and then a maintenance dose of 200 mg daily for 1 year. No side effects were observed.

At 600 mg daily, danazol causes a reversion of serum complement to normal levels in practically all patients (Lagrue et al. 1978). Since the virilizing side effects correlate with dosage and duration of therapy, it is very important to find the minimal dose which will prevent attacks in each individual patient through downward titration. There is no correlation between body weight or area and the therapeutic effect. Lagrue et al. (1978) maintained their patients at 200 mg daily with good clinical effects, even though the biological effects were barely detectable. Hosea and Frank (1980) could maintain 50% of their 69 patients on a maintenance dose of 300 mg daily. At this minimal dose, C1INH levels were 71% and C4 levels were 36% below normal.

Although the drug has a low incidence of side effects, and the therapeutic levels are not high enough to suppress ovulation, masculinization of minor degree develops in 10% of patients at doses of more than 300 mg daily and with longer therapy. These changes are more obvious and their incidence is higher in females (Table 11.9). Menometrorrhagia can be treated with combinations of estrogens and progesterons without increasing the frequency of attacks. Severe headaches develop mostly in patients who suffer from them anyway, but they may be a reason to discontinue therapy. Episodes of anxiety and tremor are very infrequent and last at most for 30–60 min. Microscopic hematuria clears on reduction of the dose (Hosea and Frank 1980).

Signs of liver damage, such as increased size (38%), elevated serum transaminases (31%), and increased conjugated bilirubin (8%), occur mostly in females and on long-term therapy, according to a study of Cicardi et al. (1983). Histology showed slight cholestasis, intralobular necrosis, hepatitis, and steatosis in four of their patients, and examination of ultrastructure revealed scattered giant mitochondria and intracanalicular biliary pigment in nine patients. No evidence for hepatic tumors was detected. It is suggested that treatment be restricted to severe cases (with more than two attacks per month) and that the minimal effective dose should be established for each patient. The authors are aware of the fact that most patients refuse to stop therapy with danazol because it is so highly effective.

11.7.2 Plasmin Inhibitors

Although not quite as effective as danazol, these drugs offer an alternative mode of prophylactic treatment for patients with hereditary angioedema, particularly for young children or pregnant women (Rosen and Austen 1976). Epsilon-aminocaproic acid (EACA) was ineffective during an acute attack (Landerman et al. 1962), but prevented attacks at a dose of 6 g daily (Lundh et al. 1968, Champion and Lachmann 1969). This therapeutic effect was confirmed in four of five patients during a double-blind study (Frank et al. 1972). The drug was also useful during prophylaxis of oral surgery (Pence et al. 1974) and for the treatment of children (Gwynn 1974).

Tranexamic acid, a cyclized EACA derivative, has fewer side effects than its parent compound. Sheffer et al. (1971) treated 12 patients with the drug. Seven obtained good, four only moderate, and one no improvement. Blohmé (1972) also observed good suppression of attacks in three of five patients, and Zachariae et al. (1975) found the same results in all their eight patients while normal urticaria and non-hereditary angioedema patients were not affected. Agostini et al. (1978) evaluated 16 patients who had been treated for 8 to 34 months. Four patients did not respond, and therapy was stopped after 2 months. The other 12 patients were well controlled on a treatment regimen of 2–3 g daily for adults and 1.5 g for children. Brackertz (1974) used suramin to maintain the therapeutic response of patients who had originally responded to tranexamic acid.

Both drugs reduce C1 activation in vitro, but do not change C1INH, C3, C4, or C2 levels during therapy (Frank et al. 1976). Although thrombosis, myonecrosis, with increased serum creatininphosphokinase and aldolase, retinal changes, urticaria, and tumorigenesis in animals (tranexamic acid) have been reported (Frank et al. 1976), tranexamic acid causes only few and no severe side effects in humans. Nausea, headache, slight diarrhea, dyspepsia, dysmenorrhea, and superficial venous thrombosis have been observed in less than 10% of the patients. Changes in the liver or alterations of blood fibrinolytic activity were not observed either (Blohmé 1972, Agostini et al. 1978).

11.7.3 Replacement Therapy with Fresh Frozen Plasma and C1INH

The only effective therapy during acute attacks of angioedema is the infusion of fresh plasma or of purified C1INH. The latter has recently become available commercially (Behring AG, Marburg, FRG). Pickering et al. (1969) and later Cohen and Peterson (1972) transfused fresh frozen plasma during acute attacks and observed a rapid subjective relief, with a decrease of symptoms shortly thereafter. After infusion of 1 liter, there was only a slight, transient increase of C1 and C1INH. Jaffe et al. (1975) treated six patients with 500 ml one day prior to surgical procedures and saw no complications, except for slight symptoms in three patients 5–8 days after the procedure. Potential problems with this treatment are the transmission of viral diseases and allergic or pseudoallergic transfusion reactions.

Only a few reports are available as yet on the use of C1INH injections. Schulz (1974) treated three patients during ten attacks and observed relief within 1–2 h, with a gradual resolution of the attacks by 24 h. In moderately severe attacks, 3000 units of lyophilized C1INH, corresponding to about 500 ml of pooled plasma, are dissolved in 10 ml and injected slowly intravenously.

While C1INH cannot influence existing lesions, it can stop their further progression, thus allowing for their resolution. It also suppresses the development of new lesions. C1INH should therefore not be given when an attack is about to resolve. Its use in mild attacks should also be weighed against the potential danger of inducing antibody formation. Commercial C1INH has been widely used in the Federal Republic of Germany and elsewhere during the past few years, without major adverse reactions (Agostini et al. 1980, Opferkuch et al. 1980, Bork et al. 1984). It can also be used for short-term prophylaxis before surgery. Gadek et al. (1980) used their own semipurified C1INH with similar good results, also in patients with abdominal pain and laryngeal edema.

11.7.4 Practical Clinical Guidelines

Table 11.10 summarizes the agents that should be used in different clinical situations in hereditary angioedema.

It is extremely important to note that drugs which are used to treat ordinary urticaria, angioedema, and shock are not effective in angioedema due to hereditary or acquired C1INH deficiency with angioedema.

The use of fresh frozen plasma, and better even of C1INH preparations, should therefore be instituted early, particularly if swellings are present in the region of the head and of the lungs or kidneys in order to prevent progression of the already existing swellings and the development of new ones. Children and adults receive 3,000 units of C1INH, dissolved in 10 ml, by slow intravenous injection. The dosage can be increased to 6,000 or even 12,000 units if there is worsening or no improvement after 30–60 min. If

Table 11.10. Treatment of various clinical situations in hereditary or acquired angioedema due to C1INH deficiency.

A. Acute attacks
1. analgesics or narcotics for pain
2. C1INH (3000 units in 10 ml) slowly i.v.; repeat by 15–30 min, if no improvement or worsening, up to a total of 12000 units
3. if 2. not available, fresh frozen plasma (500 ml); repeat if necessary
4. intubation or tracheostomy, if indicated

Note: epinephrine, steroids, and antihistamines are ineffective

B. Short-term prophylaxis
1. danazol (600 mg daily), 1–10 days before surgery,
2. or EACA, (6 g daily), 2–3 days before surgery,
3. or C1INH (3000–6000 units) i.v., shortly before surgery,
4. or fresh plasma (500 ml) i.v., 1 day before surgery

C. Long-term prophylaxis
1. danazol; start at 600 mg daily; reduce to 200–300 mg daily, if possible,
2. or EACA (6 g daily),
3. or tranexamic acid (2–3 g daily); 1.5 g for children

EACA, epsilon-aminocaproic acid.

C1INH is not available, fresh frozen plasma should be given instead, starting with 500 ml. In case of severe breathing difficulties due to laryngeal swelling, a tracheostomy or, if still possible, intubation is recommended. Analgesics or narcotics can be given for severe pain. Patients should choose a physician's office or treatment center close to their home where C1INH is kept for them. They should take C1INH along when they travel. Some patients report improvement of acute symptoms of their angioedema by adjunctive treatment with diazepam (Opferkuch, personal communication).

For short-term prophylaxis before surgical procedures, it is most convenient, inexpensive, and safe to give danazol. The effectiveness of this treatment has been discussed (11.7.1, p. 149). Alternative measures are listed in Table 11.10.

For long-term prophylaxis, treatment with danazol can be given at the lowest possible dose that will suppress attacks. Possible side effects should be discussed with the patient, and basic laboratory data should be obtained, prior to and at regular intervals during treatment, particularly with regard to liver function (see Table 11.9 and Section 11.7.1, p. 149). Prophylactic treatment should be withheld from pregnant women and also from children, unless urgently indicated in the latter case. EACA or tranexamic acid can be tried in severe cases instead (see Table 11.10 and Section 11.7.2, p. 150).

References

Chapter 1 (History of Urticaria)

Bovet D, Staub A (1937) Action protectrice des éthers phénoliques au cours de l'intoxication histaminique. C r Séan Soc Biol 124:547–549

Dale HH, Laidlaw PP (1910) The physiological action of β-imidazolethylamine. J Physiol (London) 41:318–344

Donaldson VH, Evans RR (1963) A biochemical abnormality in hereditary angioneurotic edema. Am J Med 35:37–44

Dukor P, Kallos P, Schlumberger HD, West GB (1980) PAR. Pseudoallergic reaction. Genetic agents and anaphylactoid reactions. Karger, Basel

Ehrlich P (1879) Beiträge zur Kenntnis der granulierten Bindegewebsmastzellen und der eosinophilen Leukozyten. Arch J Anat Physiol 3:166–169

Eppinger H (1913) Über eine eigentümliche Hautkrankheit, hervorgerufen durch Ergamin. Wien Med Wschr 63:1413–1416

Fox GH (1883) The treatment of urticaria. J Cutan Ven Dis 1:197–202

Gilchrist TC (1908) Some experimental observations on the histopathology of urticaria factitia. J Cutan Dis 26:122–123

Ishizaka K, Ishizaka T, Hornbrook MM (1966) Physicochemical properties of reaginic antibody. V. Correlation of reaginic activity with E globulin antibody. J Immunol 97:840–853

Johnsson SGO, Bennich H (1967) Immunological studies of an atypical (myeloma) immunoglobulin. Immunology 13:381–394

Lewis Th (1927) The blood vessels of the human skin and their responses. Shaw, London

Nettleship E (1869) Rare forms of urticaria. Br Med J 2:323–324

Osler W (1888) Hereditary angioneurotic edema. Am J Med Sci 95:362–367

Prausnitz K, Küstner H (1921) Studien über die Überempfindlichkeit. Zbl Bakt 86:160–169

Quincke H (1882) Über akutes umschriebenes Hautödem. Mschr Prakt Dermatol 1:160–169

Riley JF, West GB (1953) Presence of histamine in tissue mast cells. J Physiol (London) 120:528–537

Rook A (1974) The historial background. In: Warin RP, Champion RH (eds) Urticaria. Saunders, London-Philadelphia-Toronto, pp 1–9

Sagher F, Even-Paz Z (1967) Mastocytosis and the mast cell. History. Karger, Basel-New York, pp 4–7

Schadewaldt H (1981 a) Geschichte der Allergie. Urtikaria. Dustri, Dr Karl Feistle, München-Deisenhofen, Vol 3, pp 45–176

Schadewaldt H (1981 b) Geschichte der Allergie. Quincke Ödem. Dustri, Dr. Karl Feistle, München-Deisenhofen, Vol 3, pp 177–218

Schadewaldt H (1981 c) Geschichte der Allergie. Physikalische Allergie. Dustri, Dr. Karl Feistle, München-Deisenhofen, Vol. 4, pp 50–53

Spaulding WB (1960) Methyltestosterone therapy for hereditary episodic edema (hereditary angioneurotic edema). Ann Int Med 53:739–745

Swingle WW, Pfiffner JJ (1930) Experiments with active extract of suprarenal cortex. Anat Rec 44:225–226

Török L (1928) Urticaria. In: Jadasson J (ed) Handbuch der Haut- und Geschlechtskrankheiten. Springer, Berlin, Vol 6, pp 145–215

Unna PG (1887) Beiträge zur Anatomie und Pathogenese der Urtikaria simplex und pigmentosa. MH Prakt Dermatol 6:EH I

Windaus A, Vogt W (1907) Synthese des Imidazoläthylamins. Chem Berichte 40:3691

Chapter 2 (Basic Mechanisms)

Archer CB, Page CP, Paul W, Morley J, Macdonald DM (1984) Inflammatory characteristics of platelet activating factor (PAF-acether) in human skin. Br J Dermatol 110:45–50

Arthur R, Shelley W (1955) The role of proteolytic enzymes in the production of pruritus in man. J Invest Dermatol 25:341–346

Atkins FM, Metcalfe DD (1983) Degradation of the heparin matrix of mast cell granules by cultured fibroblasts. J Immunol 131:1420–1425

Atkins PC, Norman M, Weiner H, Zweiman B (1977) Release of neutrophil chemotactic activity during immediate hypersensitivity reactions in humans. Ann Int Med 86:415–418

Benveniste J, Vargaftig BB (1983) Platelet-activating factor: An ether lipid with biological activity. In: Mangold HK, Paltauf F (eds) Ether Lipids. Academic Press, New York, pp 355–376

Bienenstock J, Befus AD, Pearce F, Denburg J, Goodacre R (1982) Mast cell heterogeneity: derivation and function, with emphasis on the intestine. J Allergy Clin Immunol 70:407–412

Bisgaard H, Kristensen J, Sondergaard J (1982) The effect of leukotriene C_4 and D_4 on cutaneous blood flow in humans. Prostaglandins 23:797–801

Borgeat P, Samuelsson B (1979) Transformation of arachidonic acid by rabbit polymorphonuclear leukocytes. Formation of a novel dihydroxyeicosatetraenoic acid. J Biol Chem 254:2643–2646

Boswell RN, Austen KF, Goetzl EJ (1978) Intermediate molecular weight eosinophil chemotactic factors in rat peritoneal mast cells: Immunologic release, granule association, and demonstration of structural heterogeneity. J Immunol 126:15–20

Busse WW, Swenson CA, Borden EC, Treuhaft MW, Dick EC (1983) Effect of influenza A virus on leukocyte histamine release. J Allergy Clin Immunol 71:382–388

Camp RDR, Coutts AA, Greaves MW, Kay AB, Walport MJ (1983) Responses of human skin to intradermal injection of leukotrienes C_4, D_4 and B_4. Br J Pharmac 80:497–502

Casale TB, Bowman S, Kaliner M (1984) Induction of human cutaneous mast cell degranulation by opiates and endogenous opioid peptides: Evidence for opiate and nonopiate receptor participation. J Allergy Clin Immunol 73:775–781

Center DM (1983) Identification of rat mast cell-derived chemoattractant factors for lymphocytes. J Allergy Clin Immunol 71:29–35

Center DM, Cruikshank WW, Berman JS, Beer DJ (1983) Functional characteristics of histamine receptor-bearing mononuclear cells. I. Selective production of lymphocyte chemoattractant lymphokines with histamine used as a ligand. J Immunol 131:1854–1859

Chi EY, Henderson WR, Klebanoff SJ (1982) Phospholipase A_2-induced rat mast cell secretion. Role of arachidonic acid metabolism. Lab Invest 47:579–585

Chi EY, Ignacio E, Lagunoff D (1978) Mast cell granule formation in the beige mouse. J Histochem Cytochem 26:131–137

Clark RAF, Gallin JI, Kaplan AP (1975) The selective eosinophil chemotactic activity of histamine. J Exp Med 142:1462–1476

Cohen S, Ward PA (1971) In vitro and in vivo activity of a lymphocyte and immune complex-dependent chemotactic factor for eosinophils. J Exp Med 133:133–146

Colley DG (1973) Eosinophils and immune mechanisms I. Eosinophil stimulation promoter (ESP): A lymphokine induced by specific antigen or phytohemagglutinin. J Immunol 110:1419–1423

Crunkhorn P, Willis AL (1971) Cutaneous reactions to intradermal prostaglandins. B J Pharmacol 41:49–56

Curtain C, Looney FD, Smelstorius JA (1981) Glycosphingolipid clustering and mast cell degranulation. Int Archs Allergy appl Immun 65:34–41

Czarnetzki BM (1982) Release of mediators from purified rat mast cells during phagocytosis. Scand J Immunol 15:581–586

Czarnetzki BM (1983) Increased monocyte chemotaxis towards leukotriene B_4 and platelet activating factor in psoriasis and atopic eczema. Clin Exp Immunol 54:486–492

Czarnetzki BM, Benveniste J (1981) Effect of synthetic PAF-acether on human neutrophil leukocytes. I. Analysis of the in vitro migration of human neutrophils. Chem Phys Lip 29:317–326

Czarnetzki BM, Figdor CG, Kolde G, Vroom T, Aalberse R, deVries JE (1984b) Development of human connective tissue mast cells from purified blood monocytes. Immunol 51:549–554

Czarnetzki BM, Grabbe J (1983) Biological and chemical characterization of eosinophil chemotactic factors from human leukocytes. Agents Actions 12 suppl:204–216

Czarnetzki BM, Kern F, Lichtenstein LM (1976) Defective release of eosinophil chemotactic factor from peripheral leukocytes in patients with chronic urticaria. J Invest Derm 67:276–278

Czarnetzki BM, König W, Lichtenstein LM (1975) Antigen-induced eosinophil chemotactic factor (ECF) release by human leukocytes. Inflammation 1:201–215

Czarnetzki BM, Meentken J, Rosenbach T, Pokropp A (1984a) Clinical, pharmacological and immunological aspects of delayed pressure urticaria. Brit J Dermatol 111:315–324

Czarnetzki BM, Panneck W, Frosch PJ (1980) Inhibitory effect of heparin on leukocyte chemotactic factors. Clin Exp Immunol 39:526–531

Czarnetzki BM, Pawelzik B (1983) The effect of eosinophil chemotactic factors on the in vitro eosinopoiesis in the guinea pig. Blut 47:287–296

Czarnetzki BM, Rosenbach T (1984) Analysis of the neutrophil and eosinophil chemotactic activity of leukotriene B_4 and its oxidation products. J Invest Dermatol 82:414 (abstract)

Czarnetzki BM, Rosenbach T, Kolde G, Frosch PJ (1985) Phototherapy of urticaria pigmentosa: Clinical response and changes of cutaneous reactivity, histamine and chemotactic leukotrienes. Arch Derm Res 277:105–113

Daëron M, Voisin GA (1979) Mast cell membrane antigens and Fc receptors in anaphylaxis. I. Products of the major histocompatibility complex involved in alloantibody-induced mast cell activation. Immunology 38:447–458

Dahlén SE, Björk J, Hedqvist P, Arfors KE, Hammarström S, Lindgren J-A, Samuelsson B (1981) Leukotrienes promote plasma leakage and leukocyte adhesion in postcapillary venules: In vivo effects with relevance to the acute inflammatory response. Proc Natl Acad Sci 78:3887–3891

de Shazo RD, Levinson AI, Dvorak HF, Davis RW (1979) The late phase skin reaction: Evidence for activation of the coagulation system in an IgE-dependent reaction in man. J Immunol 122:692–698

Doeglas HMG, Bleumink E (1975) Protease inhibitors in plasma of patients with chronic urticaria. Arch Dermatol 111:979–985

Dolovich J, Denberg J, Kwee YN, Belda T, Blajchman J, Hargreave FE (1983) Does non-immunologic mast cell mediator release/activation elicit a late cutaneous response? Ann Allergy 50:241–244

Dorsch W, Ring J, Weber P-C, Strasser T (1985) Detection of immunoreactive leukotrienes LTC_4/D_4 in skin blister fluid after allergen testing in patients with late cutaneous reactions (LCR). Arch Derm Res, in press

Douglas WW (1980) Histamine and 5-hydroxytryptamine (serotonin) and their antagonists. In: Goodman LS, Gilman A (eds) The pharmacological basis of therapeutics. MacMillan, New York, pp 609–649

Drobis JD, Siraganian RP (1976) Histamine release from cultured human basophils: lack of histamine resynthesis after antigenic release. J Immunol 117:1049–1059

Du JT, Foegh M, Maddox Y, Ramwell PW (1983) Human peritoneal macrophages synthesize leukotrienes B_4 and C_4. Biochim Biophys Acta 753:159–163

Dvorak AM, Galli SJ, Morgan EM, Galli AS, Hammond ME, Dvorak HF (1982) Anaphylactic degranulation of guinea pig basophilic leukocytes. II. Evidence for regranulation of mature basophils during recovery from degranulation in vitro. Lab Invest 46:461–475

Dvorak HF, Hammond ME (1978) Cutaneous basophil hypersensitivity. In: Bach M (ed) Immediate hypersensitivity. Marcel Dekker, New York, pp 659–686

Dyer J, Warren K, Merlin S, Metcalfe DD, Kaliner MA (1982) Measurement of plasma histamine: description of an improved method and normal values. J Allergy Clin Immunol 70:82–87

Eady RAJ, Cowen T, Marshall TF, Plummer V, Greaves MW (1979) Mast cell population density, blood vessel density and histamine content in normal human skin. Brit J Dermatol 100:623–633

Ezeamuzie IC, Assem ESK (1984) Modulation of the effect of histamine releasing lymphokine on human basophils. Agents Actions 14:501–505

Feldberg W, Kellaway CH (1938) Liberation of histamine

and formation of a lecithin-like substance by cobra venom. J Physiol 94:186–226

Feltkamp-Vroom TM (1977) Mast cells in atopic and non-atopic subjects. Scand J Resp Dis 58:8–12

Findlay SR, Kagey-Sobotka A, Lichtenstein LM (1984) In vitro basophil histamine release induced by mannitol in a patient with a mannitol-induced anaphylactoid reaction. J Allergy Clin Immunol 73:578–583

Foreman JC (1984) Mast cells and the action of flavonoids. J Allergy Clin Immunol 73:769–774

Forni M, Klatt EC, Shaw ST, Taylor CR, Lukes RJ, Meyer PR (1983) Immunohistochemical characterization of reactive and neoplastic mast cells. Am J Clin Pathol 80:660–665

Garcia Leme J (1978) Bradykinin System. In: Vane JR, Ferreira SH (eds) Inflammation. Springer-Verlag, Berlin, pp 464–522

Ginsburg H, Nir I, Hammel I, Eren R, Weissman B-A, Naot Y (1978) Differentiation and activity of mast cells following immunization in cultures of lymph node cells. Immunology 35:485–502

Gleich GJ (1982) The late phase of the immunoglobulin E-mediated reaction: a link between anaphylaxis and common allergic disease? J Allergy Clin Immunol 70:160–169

Goetzl EJ (1980) Mediators of immediate hypersensitivity derived from arachidonic acid. N Engl J Med 303:822–825

Goetzl EJ, Austen KF (1975) Purification and synthesis of eosinophilotactic tetrapeptides of human lung: Identification as eosinophil chemotactic factor of anaphylaxis. Proc Natl Acad Sci USA 72:4123–4127

Gorski JP, Hugli TE, Müller-Eberhard HJ (1979) C4a: The third anaphylatoxin of the human complement system. Proc Natl Acad Sci 76:5299–5302

Grabbe J, Czarnetzki BM, Mardin M (1982) Chemotactic leukotrienes in psoriasis. Lancet II:1464

Grosman N (1982) Histamine release from human basophils and isolated rat mast cells induced by ketobemidone, pethidine and the spasmolytic A 29. Acta pharmacol et toxicol 50:78–80

Hadding U (1981) Das Komplementsystem und seine Rolle bei der Entzündung. Hautarzt 32 (Suppl V): pp 104–115

Haddy FJ (1960) Effect of histamine on small and large vessel pressures in the dog foreleg. Am J Physiol 198:161–168

Hagermark O, Strandberg K (1977) Pruritogenic activity of prostaglandin E_2. Acta Derm Venereol 57:37–43

Ham EA, Soderman DD, Zanetti ME, Dougherty HW, McCauley E, Kaehl FA (1983) Inhibition by prostaglandins of leukotriene B_4 release from activated neutrophils. Proc Natl Acad Sci 80:4349–4353

Hanahoe THP (1984) Mechanism of histamine release from rat isolated peritoneal mast cells by dextran: the role of immunoglobulin E. Agents Actions 14:468–474

Henderson WR, Kaliner M (1979) Mast cell granule peroxidase: Location, secretion, and SRS-A inactivation. J Immunol 122:1322–1328

Henderson WR, Klebanoff SJ (1983) Leukotriene B_4, C_4, D_4 and E_4 inactivation by hydroxyl radicals. Biochem Biophys Res Comm 110:266–272

Higgs GA, Moncada S (1983) Interactions of arachidonate products with other pain mediators. In: Bonica JJ (ed) Advances in Pain Research and Therapy. Raven Press, New York, pp 617–626

Hübscher T (1975) Role of the eosinophil in the allergic reactions. I. EDI – An eosinophil-derived inhibitor of histamine release. J Immunol 114:1379–1388

Ida S, Hooks JJ, Siraganian RP, Notkins AL (1977) Enhancement of IgE-mediated histamine release from human basophils by viruses: role of interferon. J Exp Med 145:892–906

Ida S, Hooks JJ, Siraganian RP, Notkins AL (1980) Enhancement of IgE-mediated histamine release from human basophils by immune-specific lymphokines. Clin Exp Immunol 41:380–387

Igarashi R, Sudo S, Morohashi M, Takeuchi S, Sato Y (1982) Immunofluorescence studies on Clq in mast cells. Acta dermatovener 62:27–30

Ishizaka K, Ishizaka T (1967) Identification of γE antibodies as a carrier of reaginic activity. J Immunol 99:1187–1198

Ishizaka K, Tomioka H, Ishizaka T (1970) Mechanisms of passive sensitization. I. Presence of IgE and IgG molecules on human leukocytes. J Immunol 105:1459–1467

Ishizaka T (1982) Biochemical analysis of triggering signals induced by bridging of IgE receptors. Federation Proc 14:17–21

Ishizaka T, Stark AR, Ishizaka K (1979) Demonstration of Fcγ receptors on human basophil granulocytes. J Immunol 123:578–583

Jacques LB (1979) Heparin: An old drug with a new paradigm. Science 206:528–533

James MP, Kennedy AR, Eady RA (1982) A microscopic study of inflammatory reactions in human skin induced by histamine and compound 48/80. J Invest Dermatol 78:406–413

Juan H, Sametz W (1980) Histamine-induced release of arachidonic acid and of prostaglandins in the peripheral vascular bed. Arch Pharmacol 314:183–190

Juhlin L, Michaelsson G (1969) Cutaneous reaction to kallikrein, bradykinin and histamine in healthy subjects and in patients with urticaria. Acta Derm Venereol 49:26–36

Kaliner MM (1984) Hypotheses on the contribution of late-phase allergic responses to the understanding and treatment of allergic diseases. J Allergy Clin Immunol 73:311–315

Kaliner M, Shelhamer JH, Ottesen EA (1982) Effects of infused histamine: correlation of plasma histamine levels and symptoms. J Allergy Clin Immunol 69:283–289

Kaplan AP, Gray L, Shaff RE, Horakova Z, Beaven MA (1975) In vivo studies of mediator release in cold urticaria and cholinergic urticaria. J Allergy Clin Immunol 55:394–402

Kaplan AP, Horakova Z, Katz SI (1978) Assessment of tissue fluid histamine levels in patients with urticaria. J Allergy Clin Immunol 61:350–354

Kennerly DA, Sullivan TJ, Sylwester P, Parker CW (1979) Diacylglycerol metabolism in mast cells: A potential role in membrane fusion and arachidonic acid release. J Exp Med 150:1039–1044

Kern F, Lichtenstein LM (1976) Defective histamine release in chronic urticaria. J Clin Invest 57:1369–1377

Kindblom L-G (1982) Factor VIII related antigen and mast cells. Acta Path Microbiol Immunol Scand 90:437–439

Kitamura Y, Shimada M, Hatanaka K, Miyano Y (1977) Development of mast cells from grafted bone marrow cells in irradiated mice. Nature 268:442–443

Klickstein LB, Shapleigh C, Goetzl EJ (1980) Lipoxygenation of arachidonic acid as a source of polymorphonuclear leukocyte chemotactic factors in synovial fluid and tissue in rheumatoid arthritis and spondyloarthritis. J Clin Invest 66:1166–1170

Komiyama A, Spicer SS (1975) Acid phosphatase demonstrated ultrastructurally in mast cell granules altered by pinocytosis. Lab Invest 32:485–491

Kraeuterkops S, Tsakalos ND, Theoharides TC, Askenase PW (1982) Mast cell secretion of serotonin and histamine induced by parathyroid hormone (PTH). Fed Proc 41:376 (abstract)

Krüger PG, Aas P, Onarheim J, Helle KB (1982) Neurotensin-induced release of histamine from rat mast cells in vitro. Acta Physiol Scand 114:467–469

Kurose M, Saeki K (1981) Histamine release induced by neurotensin from rat peritoneal mast cells. Eur J Pharmacol 76:129–136

Lagunoff D, Martin T, Read G (1983) Agents that release histamine from mast cells. Ann Rev Pharmacol Toxicol 23:331–351

Laurell AB, Martensen U, Sjoholm AG (1977) Studies of C1 subcomponents in chronic urticaria and angioedema. Int Arch Allergy Appl Immunol 54:434–442

Lemanske RF, Guthman DA, Kaliner M (1983) The biologic activity of mast cell granules. VII. The effect of anti-neutrophil antibody-induced neutropenia on rat cutaneous late phase reactions. J Immunol 131:929–933

Levy DA (1974) Histamine and serotonin. In: Weissman G (ed) Mediators of inflammation. Plenum Press, New York, pp 141–162

Lewis T (1927) Blood vessels of the human skin and their responses. Shaw, London

Lichtenstein LM, Gillespie E (1973) Inhibition of histamine release by histamine is controlled by H_2 receptor. Nature 244:287–288

Lichtenstein LM, Margolis S (1968) Histamine release in vitro: inhibition by catecholamines and methylxanthines. Science 161:902–903

Lieberman P, Rice MC, Mallette JE jr (1977) Studies of urticaria and acute serum sickness with the C1q precipitin test. Arch Intern Med 137:440–442

Lomax P, Green MD (1981) Histaminergic neurons in the hypothalamic thermoregulatory pathways. Fed Proc 40:2741–2745

MacGlashan DW jr, Schleimer RP, Peters SP, Schulman ES, Adams GK, Sobotka AK, Newball HH, Lichtenstein LM (1983) Comparative studies of human basophils and mast cells. Fed Proc 42:2504–2509

Marder RJ, Rent R, Choi EYC, Gewurz H (1976) C1q deficiency associated with urticarial like lesions and cutaneous vasculitis. Amer J Med 61:560–565

Marom Z, Casale TB (1983) Mast cells and their mediators. Ann Allergy 50:367–370

Marquardt DL, Parker CW, Sullivan TJ (1978) Potentiation of mast cell mediator release by adenosine. J Immunol 120:871–878

Mathison DA, Arroyave CM, Bhat KN, Hurewitz DS, Marnell DJ (1977) Hypocomplementemia in chronic idiopathic urticaria. Ann Int Med 86:534–538

Mayrhofer G, Bazin H (1981) Nature of the thymus dependency of mucosal mast cells. III. Mucosal mast cells in nude mice and nude rats, in B rats and in a child with the Di George Syndrome. Int Arch Allergy Appl Immunol 64:320–331

Melewicz FM, Spiegelberg HL (1980) Fc receptors for IgE on a subpopulation of human peripheral blood monocytes. J Immunol 125:1026–1031

Mellblom L, Enerbäck L (1979) Protein content, dry mass and chemical composition of individual mast cells related to body growth. Histochemistry 63:129–143

Mensing H, Czarnetzki BM (1984) Leukotriene B_4 induces in vitro fibroblast chemotaxis. J Invest Dermatol 82:9–12

Metcalfe DD (1983) Effector cell heterogeneity in immediate hypersensitivity reactions. Clin Rev Allergy 1:311–325

Metcalfe DD, Kaliner M, Donlon MA (1981) The mast cell. CRC Crit Rev Immunol 3:23–74

Metzger H, Goetze A, Kanellopoulos J, Holowka D, Fewtrell C (1982) Structure of the high-affinity mast cell receptor for IgE. Fed Proc 41:8–11

Morishima T (1970) 5-Hydroxytryptamine (serotonin) and 5-hydroxytryptophane in mast cells in human mastocytosis. Tohoku J Exp Med 102:121–126

Mossmann H, Schmitz B, Lauer W, Stauffer U, Gehrung M, Günther E, Hammer DK (1979) Relationship between histocompatibility antigens, other surface determinants and the IgE receptor on rat mast cells. Eur J Immunol 9:219–224

Murphy MF, Haarstad VB, Hahn FB (1974) Molecular orbital studies of the mast cell zinc-histamine storage complex. Int J Quantum Chem 1:149–157

Murphy RC, Hammarström S, Samuelsson B (1979) Leukotriene C: A slow-reacting substance from murine mastocytoma cells. Proc Natl Acad Sci USA 76:4275–4279

Nair MPN, Schwartz SA (1983) Effect of histamine and histamine antagonists on natural and antibody-dependent cellular cytotoxicity of human lymphocytes in vitro. Cell Immunol 81:45–60

Natbony SF, Phillips ME, Elias JM, Godfrey HP, Kaplan AP (1983) Histologic studies of chronic idiopathic urticaria. J Allergy Clin Immunol 71:177–183

Nials AT, Vordey CJ, Skidmore IF (1983) The release of histamine from mast cells by chymotrypsin. Int Arch Allergy Appl Immunol 70:83–87

Nicholson A, Fearon DT, Austen KF (1978) Complement. In: Vane JR, Ferreira SH (eds) Inflammation. Springer Verlag, Berlin, pp 425–463

Oehling A, Neffen H, Subira ML, Sanz ML (1979) Humoral and cellular immunity in chronic urticaria. Allergol Immunopathol 7:351–356

Oertel HL, Kaliner M (1981) The biologic activity of mast cell granules. III. Purification of inflammatory factors of anaphylaxis (IF-A) responsible for causing late-phase reactions. J Immunol 127:1398–1402

Omini C, Folco GC, Vigano T, Rossoni G, Brunelli G, Berti I (1981) Leukotriene-C_4 induces generation of PGI_2 and TXA_2 in guinea-pig in vivo. Pharm Res Com 13:633–640

Orenstein NS, Galli SJ, Dvorak AM, Silbert JE, Dvorak HF (1978) Sulfated glycosaminoglycans of guinea pig basophilic leukocytes. J Immunol 121:586–592

Orning L, Hammarström S, Samuelsson B (1980) Leukotriene D: a slow reacting substance from rat basophilic leukemia cells. Proc Natl Acad Sci 77:2014–2017

Padawer J (1974) Mast cells: Extended lifespan and lack of granule turnover under normal in vivo conditions. Exp Mol Pathol 20:269–280

Padawer J (1979) Mast-cell structure: Implications for normal physiology and degranulation. In: Pepys J, Edwards AM (eds) The mast cell. Pitman Medical Publ Co, Tunbridge Wells, pp 1–8

Parker CW (1982) The chemical nature of slow-reacting substances. In: Weissmann G (ed) Advances in Inflammation Research. Raven Press, New York, Vol 4, pp 1–24

Parker CW, Huber MM, Hoffman MK, Falkenhein SF (1979) Characteristization of the two major species of slow reacting substance from rat basophilic leukemia cells as glutathionyl thioesters of eicosatetraenoic acids oxygenated at the 5 position. Evidence that peroxy groups are present and important for spasmogenic activity. Prostaglandins 18:673–686

Parker CW, Schechtel T, Falkenheim SF, Huber MM (1983) Induction of IgE receptors on human lymphocytes. Imm Comm 12:1–10

Perelmutter L (1984) IgG_4: Non-IgE mediated atopic disease. Ann Allergy 52:64–68

Perez HD, Goldstein IM (1981) Regulation of the biological activity of C5-derived peptides. In: Weissmann G (ed) Advances in Inflammation Research, Raven Press, New York, Vol 1, pp 1–19

Peters SP, Siegel MI, Kagey-Sobotka A, Lichtenstein LM (1981) Lipoxygenase products modulate histamine release in human basophils. Nature 292:455–457

Pinckard RN, McManus LM, Hanahan DJ (1982) Chemistry and biology of acetyl glyceryl ether phosphorylcholine (platelet-activating factor) In: Weissmann G (ed) Advances in Inflammation Research, Raven Press, New York, Vol 4, pp 147–180

Plaut M, Lichtenstein LM (1978) Histamine, 5-hydroxytryptamine, SRS-A: Discussion of type I hypersensitivity (anaphylaxis). In: Vane JR, Ferreira SH (eds) Inflammation. Springer-Verlag, Berlin, pp 345–373

Pokropp A, Czarnetzki BM (1983) Untersuchungen zur Wirkung von intravenösem Kalzium auf experimentelle Quaddel- und Erythembildung. Allergologie 6:82–83

Poothullil J, Umemoto L, Dolovich J, Hargreave FE, Day RP (1976) Inhibition by prednisone of late cutaneous allergic responses induced by antiserum to human IgE. J Allergy Clin Immunol 57:164–167

Regal JF, Pickering RJ (1981) C5a-induced tracheal contraction: Effect of an SRS-A antagonist and inhibitors of arachidonate metabolism. J Immunol 126:313–316

Renner H, Foreman JC, Jordan CC, Oehme P (1982) Histamine release from mast cells by substance P and substance P sequences. Pharmazie 37:12

Rivkin J, Becker EL (1972) Possible implication of cyclic 3′5′-adenosine monophosphate in the chemotaxis of rabbit polymorphonuclear leukocytes (PMNs). Fed Proc 31:657 (abstract)

Rocklin RE, Breard J, Gupta S, Good RA, Melman KL (1980) Characterization of the human blood lymphocytes that produce a histamine-induced suppressor factor (HSF). Cell Immunol 51:226–237

Rola-Pleszczynski M, Borgeat P, Sirois P (1982) Leukotriene B_4 induces human suppressor lymphocytes. Biochem Biophys Res Com 108:1531–1537

Rola-Pleszczynski M, Gagnon L, Sirois P (1983) Leukotriene B_4 augments human natural cytotoxic cell activity. Biochem Biophys Res Com 113:531–537

Ruzicka T, Simmet T, Peskar BA, Braun-Falco O (1984) Leukotrienes in skin of atopic dermatitis. Lancet I:222–223

Samuelsson B, Borgeat P, Hammarström S, Murphy RC (1979) Introduction of a nomenclature: leukotrienes. Prostaglandins 17:785–787

Sandberg AL (1981) Complement. In: Oppenheim JJ, Rosenstreich DL, Potter M (eds) Cellular functions in immunity and inflammation. Edward Arnold Publ Ltd, London, pp 373–396

Sasai J, Ichihashi M (1975) Histochemical demonstration of hyaluronic acid in human dermal mast cells. Tokohu J Exp Med 116:285–293

Schwartz A, Sutton SL, Askenase PW, Gershon RK (1981) Histamine inhibition of concanavalin A-induced suppressor T-cell activation. Cell Immunol 60:426–439

Schwartz LB, Austen KF (1980) Enzymes of the mast cell granule. J Invest Dermatol 74:349–353

Sedgwick JD, Holt PG, Turner KJ (1981) Production of a histamine-releasing lymphokine by antigen- or mitogen-stimulated human peripheral T cells. Clin Exp Immunol 45:409–418

Sher A, Hein A, Moser G, Caulfield JP (1979) Complement receptors promote the phagocytosis of bacteria by rat peritoneal mast cells. Lab Invest 41:490–499

Simson JAV, Hintz DS, Munster AM, Spicer SS (1977) Immunocytochemical evidence for antibody binding to mast cell granules. Exp Mol Pathol 26:85–91

Siraganian RP, Hook WA (1977) Mechanism of histamine release by formyl methionine-containing peptides. J Immunol 119:2078–2083

Siraganian RP, McGivney A, Barsumian EL, Crews FT, Hirata F, Axelrod J (1982) Variants of the rat basophilic leukemia cell line for the study of histamine release. Fed Proc 41:30–34

Skurkovich S, Skurkovich B, Bellanti JA, Banerjee DK (1983) Interferon increases IgE binding to basophils. Ann Allergy 50:305–308

Slott RI, Zweiman B (1974) A controlled study of the effect of corticosteroids on immediate skin test reactivity. J Allergy Clin Immunol 54:229–234

Sondergaard J, Greaves MW (1971) Prostaglandin E_2: Effect on human cutaneous vasculature and skin histamine. Br J Dermatol 84:424–428

Sosman J, Busse W (1976) Reduced H_2 receptor response of granulocytes of asthmatic patients. J Allergy Clin Immunol 57:222 (abstract)

Soter NA, Lewis RA, Corey EJ, Austen KF (1983) Local effects of synthetic leukotrienes (LTC_4, LTD_4, LTE_4 and LTB_4) in human skin. J Invest Dermatol 80:115–119

Stanworth DR (1980) Oligopeptide-induced release of histamine. In: Dukor P et al. (eds) PAR Pseudo-allergic reactions. Involvement of drugs and chemicals. Karger, Basel, Vol 1, pp 56–107

Stendahl O, Molin L, Lindroth M (1983) Granulocyte-mediated release of histamine from mast cells. Effect of myeloperoxidase and its inhibition by antiinflammatory sulfone compounds. Int Arch Allergy Appl Immunol 70:277–284

Sterry W (1984) Enzyme der Mastzellen: Histochemische Nachweisbarkeit und mögliche funktionelle Bedeutung. Allergologie 7:16–19

Stevens RL, Austen KF (1981) Proteoglycans of the mast cell. In: Alan R (ed), Biochemistry of the acute allergic reactions. Liss Inc, New York, pp 69–88

Terano T, Salmon JA, Moncada S (1984) Biosynthesis and biological activity of leukotriene B_5. Prostaglandins 27:217–232

Tertian G, Yung YP, Guy-Grand D, Moore MAS (1981) Long-term in vitro culture of murine mast cells. I. Description of a growth factor-dependent culture technique. J Immunol 127:788–794

Thueson SO, Speck LS, Lett-Brown MA, Grant A (1979) Histamine-releasing activity (HRA). I. Production by mitogen- or antigen-stimulated human mononuclear cells. J Immunol 123:626–632

Ting S, Dunsky EH, Lavker RM, Zweiman B (1980) Patterns of mast cell alterations and in vivo mediator release in human allergic skin reactions. J Allergy Clin Immunol 66:417–423

Ting S, Zweiman B, Lavker RM (1983) Cromolyn does not modulate human allergic skin reactions in vivo. J Allergy Clin Immunol 71:12–17

Umemoto L, Poothullil J, Dolovich J, Hargreave FE (1976) Factors which influence late cutaneous allergic responses. J Allergy Clin Immunol 58:60–68

Vadas MA (1982) Genetic control of eosinophilia in mice: Genes expressed in bone marrow-derived cells control high responsiveness. J Immunol 128:691–695

Vargaftig BB, Chignard M, Mencia-Huerta JM, Arnoux B, Benveniste J (1981) Pharmacology of arachidonate metabolites and of platelet-activating factor (PAF-acether). In: Gordon (ed) Platelets in Biology and Pathology. Elsevier/North Holland, Biomedical Press, pp 373–406

Ward PA (1971) Chemotactic factors for neutrophils, eosinophils, mononuclear cells and lymphocytes. In: Austen KF, Becker EL (eds) Biochemistry of acute allergic reactions. Blackwell Scientific Oxford, pp. 229–241

Wasserman SI (1983) Mediators of immediate hypersensitivity. J Allergy Clin Immunol 72:101–116

Webb DR, Nowowiejski I, Healy C, Rogers TJ (1982) Immunosuppressive properties of leukotriene D_4 and E_4 in vitro. Biochem Biophys Res Com 104:1617–1622

Weller PF, Lee CW, Foster DW, Corey EJ, Austen KF, Lewis RA (1983) Generation and metabolism of 5-lipoxygenase pathway leukotrienes by human eosinophils: Predominant production of leukotriene C_4. Proc Natl Acad Sci 80:7626–7630

Wilhelms O-H, Roesch E (1981) Antigen-induced release of esterase (protease) activity from rat mast cells as a modulator of type I allergic reactions? Int Arch Allergy Appl Immunol 66 (Suppl 1):159–164

Winslow CM, Austen KF (1982) Enzymatic regulation of mast cell activation and secretion by adenylate cyclase and cyclic AMP-dependent protein kinases. Fed Proc 41:22–29

Yamamoto S, Greaves MW, Fairley VM (1973) Cyclic AMP-induced inhibition of IgE-mediated hypersensitivity in human skin. Immunology 24:77–83

Yecies LD, Kaplan AP (1980) Urticaria. In: Parker CW (ed) Clinical Immunology. Saunders, Philadelphia, pp 1283–1315

Chapter 3 (Acute and Chronic Urticaria)

Ackermann R (1983) Erythema chronicum migrans und durch Zecken übertragene Meningopolyneuritis (Garin-Bujadoux-Bannwarth): Borrelien-Infektionen? Dtsch Med Wschr 108:577–580

Africk JA, Halprin KM (1969) Infectious mononucleosis presenting as urticaria. JAMA 109:1524–1525

Ahlstedt S, Haag B, Wiklund SE (1980a) Antigenic high molecular weight material in penicillin preparations. Int Arch Allergy Appl Immunol 63:344–346

Ahlstedt S, Kristofferson A, Hall E (1980b) Antigens in penicillin allergy. V. On the relative allergenic potency of antigens carrying penicilloyl determinants derived from azidocillin, ampicillin and benzylpenicillin. Int Arch Allergy Appl Immunol 61:91–99

Altmeyer P, Welke S (1977) Waldenstrom's macroglobulinemia in association with a chronic urticaria exanthem. Akt Dermatol 3:71–76

Amblard P, Reymond JL, Pih J (1978) Urticaria, deafness and arthralgias: the Muckle and Wells syndrome; a new family study. Rev Fr Allergol Immunol Clin 18:147–150

Asboe-Hansen G (1950) A survey of the normal and pathological occurrence of mucinous substances and mast cells in the dermal connective tissue in man. Acta Dermatovenereol 30:338–347

Atkins FM (1983) The basis of immediate hypersensitivity reactions to foods. Nutrition Rev 41:229–234

Bäurle G, Haneke E (1980) Leitregeln für die Testung bei Penicillinallergie. Dtsch Med Wschr 105:625–627

Barriere H, Schnitzler L, Moulin G, Grolleau Y (1976) Chronic urticaria and macroglobulinemia. Report of 5 cases. Sem Hop Paris 52:221–227

Becker CG, Dubin T, Wiedeman HP (1976) Hypersensitivity to tobacco antigen. Proc Natl Acad Sci USA 73:1712–1716

Bierman CW, Pierson WE, Zeitz SJ, Hoffman LS, Van Arsdel PP Jr (1972) Reactions associated with penicillin therapy. JAMA 220:1098–1100

Blake PA, Merson MH, Weaver RE (1979) Disease caused by a marine Vibrio. New Engl J Med 300:1–5

Blum G, De Weck AL (1966) Über den Zusammenhang von Dermatomykosen mit der Penicillin-Überempfindlichkeit. Dermatologica 133:465–474

Bock SA (1982) The natural history of food sensitivity. J Allergy Clin Immunol 69:173–177

Boonk WJ, Van Ketel WG (1981) Skin testing in chronic urticaria. Dermatologica 163:151–159

Bork K, Wecker H, Theile U (1980) Heart involvement in urticaria. Hautarzt 31:150–153

Bourne G (1962) Toxemic rash of pregnancy. Proc R Soc Med 55:462–464

Bretag AH, Archer RS, Atkinson HM, Woods WH (1984) Circadian urticaria: Another camplobacter association. Lancet I:954

Brown EB, Hermance WE, Choi Y-C (1974) Serum immunoglobulin M in chronic urticaria. Ann Allergy 33:331–336

Buckley RH, Metcalfe D (1982) Food allergy. JAMA 248:2627–2631

Buisseret PD, Youlten LJF, Heinzelmann DI, Lessof MH (1978) Prostaglandin synthesis inhibitors in prophylaxis of food intolerance. Lancet I:906–908

Bywaters EGL (1971) Still's disease in the adult. Ann Rheum Dis 30:121–133

Callen JP, Dubin HV (1978) Urticaria and polymoysitis. Arch Dermatol 114:1545–1546

Campbell AMG, Clifton F (1950) Adult toxoplasmosis in one family. Brain 83:281–294

Canizares O (1951) Cutaneous lesions of rheumatic fever. Arch Dermatol 76:702–707

Castberg T, Sorenson CM (1949) Allergic examination of bakers and millers. Acta Allergol 1:283–296

Castelain PY, Besson J (1961) Role de l'allergie bacterienne dans l'etiologie de certaines urticaires. Bull Soc Fr Dermatol 68:72–74

Cauna N, Levine MI, Gralley A (1970) The fine morphology of the human skin in dermographism. J Allergy 45:266–285

Champion RH, Roberts SOB, Carpenter RG, Roger JH (1969) Urticaria and angio-oedema. A review of 554 patients. Br J Dermatol 81:588–597

Chapel TA, Krugel L, Chapel J, Segal A (1981) Scabies presenting as urticaria. JAMA 246:1440–1441

Cherry JD, Hurwitz ES, Welliver RC (1975) Mycoplasma pneumoniae infections and exanthemas. J Pediatr 87:369–373

Cherry JD, Lerner AM, Klein JO, Finland M (1963) Coxsackie A9 infections with exanthems with particular reference to urticaria. Pediatr 31:819–823

Chin TM, Fellner MJ (1980) Allergic hypersensitivity to lidocaine hydrochloride. Int J Dermatol 19:147–148

Clauvel JP, Brouet JC, Danon F, Leibowitch M, Seligmann

M (1982) Chronic urticaria with monoclonal IgM. A report of five cases. Clin Immunol Immunopathol 25:348–353

Cleare MJ, Hughes EG, Jacoby B, Pepys J (1976) Immediate (type 1) allergic responses to platinum compounds. Clin Allergy 6:183–195

Cohen SJ, Yunginger JW, Rosenberg N, Fink JN (1979) Acute allergic reaction after composite pollen ingestion. J Allergy Clin Immunol 64:270–274

Cowdrey SC, Reynolds JS (1969) Acute urticaria in infectious mononucleosis. Ann Allergy 27:182–187

Crovato F, Rebora A (1977) Alpha$_1$-antitrypsin deficiency. Arch Dermatol 113:236

Daniels LK (1973) Treatment of urticaria and severe headache by behavior therapy. Psychosomatics 14:347–351

Derbes VJ (1957) Osmylogenic urticaria. Arch Dermatol 76:103–104

Dienstag JL, Rhodes AR, Bhan AK, Dvorak AM, Mihm MC, Wands JR (1978) Urticaria associated with acute viral hepatitis type B. Studies of pathogenesis. Ann Int Med 89:34–30

Doeglas HMG (1975) Chronic urticaria. Clinical and pathogenetic studies on 141 patients. Dykstra Niemeyer, Groningen

Doeglas HMG, Bleumink E (1975) Protease inhibitors in plasma of patients with chronic urticaria. Arch Dermatol 111:979–985

Facey RV, Marsden PD (1960) Fascioliasis in man; an outbreak in Hampshire. Br Med J II:619–625

Farah FS, Shbaklu Z (1971) Autoimmune progesterone urticaria. J Allergy Clin Immunol 48:257–261

Fellner MJ, Baer RL (1967) Immunologic studies in patients with serum sickness-like reactions following penicillin therapy. J Invest Dermatol 48:384–390

Fikentscher R, Koester H, Spinar H (1971) Die routinemäßige Fokussuche bei Hauterkrankungen und ihre Trefferquote im HNO Bereich. Dermatol Mschr 157:564–569

Finke SR, Grieco MH, Connell JT, Smith EC, Sherman WB (1965) Results of comparative skin tests with penicilloyl-polylysine and penicillin in patients with penicillin allergy. Am J Med 38:71–82

Gloor M, Henkel K, Schulz U (1972) Zur pathogenetischen Bedeutung von Magenfunktionsstörungen bei allergisch bedingter chronischer Urtikaria. Dermatol Mschr 158:96–102

Golbert TM, Patterson R, Pruzansky JJ (1969) Systemic reactions to ingested antigens. J Allergy 44:96–107

Greaves MW, Plummer VM, McLaughlan P, Stanworth DR (1974) Serum and cell bound IgE in chronic urticaria. Clin Allergy 4:265–271

Green GR, Koelsche GA, Kierland RR (1965) Etiology and pathogenesis of chronic urticaria. Ann Allergy 23:30–32

Haddad ZH (1982) Clinical and immunological aspects of food hypersensitivity. Ann Allergy 49:29–34

Halpern SR (1965) Chronic hives in children. Ann Allergy 23:589–599

Haneke EG, Koerner E, Haneke E (1980) Klinische Bedeutung positiver Penicillintestreaktionen. Dtsch Med Wschr 105:635–639

Hannuksela M (1983) Food allergy and skin diseases. Ann Allergy 51:269–272

Hannuksela M, Lahti A (1977) Immediate reactions for fruits and vegetables. Contact Dermatitis 3:79–84

Harris RH, Mitchell JH (1949) Chronic urticaria due to Giardia Lamblia. Arch Dermatol 59:587–589

Harris A, Twarog FJ, Geha RS (1982) Chronic urticaria in children. A review of 90 patients. J Allergy Clin Immunol 69:109

Hart R (1977) Autoimmune progesterone dermatitis. Arch Dermatol 113:426–430

Hellgren L (1983) Urticaria, die Prävalenz in Geschlechts-, Alters- und Berufsgruppen in ganzen Bevölkerungsgruppen in Schweden. Akt Dermatol 9:189–190

Hellgren L, Hersle K (1964) Acute and chronic urticaria. Acta Allergol 19:406–420

Heng MCY, Kloss SG, Haberfelde GC (1984) Pathogenesis of papular urticaria. J Am Acad Dermatol 10:1030–1034

Holti G (1967) Management of pruritus and urticaria. Br Med J I:155–158

Horsfall FL Jr (1934) Formaldehyde hypersensitivity: an experimental study. J Immunol 27:569–581

Humphrey DM, Myers A (1975) Cytomegalovirus mononucleosis with urticaria. Postgrad Med J 51:404–406

Husz S, Berko G, Szabo R, Simon N (1974) Immunoelectrophoresis in the dermatologic practice. III. Dysproteinemias (chronic urticaria, drug allergy). Dermatol Mschr 160:93–100

Idsoe O, Guthe T, Willcox RR, deWeck AA (1968) Nature and extent of penicillin side reactions, with particular reference to fatalities from anaphylactic shock. Bull WHO 38:159–188

Illig L, Paul E (1978) Die Immunologie als Voraussetzung zum Verständnis von Pathogenese, Diagnostik und Therapie der Urticaria. Dtsch Dermatol 26:245–255

Isaacs NJ, Ertel MH (1971) Urticaria and pruritus: uncommon manifestations of hyperthyroidism. J Allergy Clin Immunol 48:73–81

James J, Warin RP (1971) An assessment of the role of candida albicans and food yeast in chronic urticaria. Br J Dermatol 84:227–237

Jegasothy BV (1980) Allergic reactions to insulin. Int J Dermatol 19:139–141

Juhlin L (1981) Recurrent urticaria: a clinical investigation of 330 patients. Br J Dermatol 104:309–318

Juhlin L, Johansson SGO, Bennich H, Högman C, Thyresson N (1969) Immunoglobulin E in dermatoses. Arch Dermatol 100:12–16

Kaufmann M (1950) Allergy to castor bean dust, with report of a case. Ann Allergy 10:690–694

Kauppingen K, Juntunen K, Lanki H (1984) Urticaria in children. Allergy 39:469–472

Kauppinen K, Kousa M, Reunala T (1980) Aromatic plants. A cause of severe attacks of angio-edema and urticaria. Contact Dermatitis 6:251–254

Key MM (1961) Some unusual allergic reactions in industry. Arch Dermatol 83:3–6

Koblenzer C (1983) Psychosomatic concepts in dermatology. Arch Dermatol 119:501–512

Kroon S (1980) Allergy to human seminal plasma. A presentation of six cases. Acta Derm Venereol 60:436–439

Lanigan SW, Adams SJ, Gilkes JJH, Robinson TWE (1984) Association between urticaria and hypothyroidism. Lancet I:1476

Lawley TJ, Hertz KC, Wade TR, Ackerman AB, Katz SI (1979) Pruritic urticarial papules and plaques of pregnancy. JAMA 241:1696–1699

Leech SH, Kumar P (1981) Cyclic urticaria. Ann Allergy 46:201–203

Levine BB (1966) Immunologic mechanisms of penicillin allergy. New Engl J Med 275:1115–1125

Levine MI, Geer JH, Kost PF (1966) Hypnotic suggestion and the histamine wheal. J Allergy 37:246–250

Leznoff A, Josse RG, Denburg J, Dolovich J (1983) Association of chronic urticaria and angioedema with thyroid autoimmunity. Arch Dermatol 119:636–640
Lieberman P (1971) Allergic reaction to insulin. JAMA 215:1106–1112
Lindemayr H, Gathmann P, Cermak T, Grunberger J (1981) Ist die chronische Urticaria eine psychosomatische Erkrankung? Z Hautkr 56:28–40
Majno G, Shea SM, Leventhal M (1969) Endothelial contraction induced by histamine type mediators. An electron microscopic study. J Cell Biol 42:647–672
Mamou H, Mamou JE, De Regnault DM (1974) Maladie periodique et syndrome de Muckle et Wells. Nouv Presse Med 3:1363–1364
Maru M, Mengistu M (1979) Acute urticaria due to Plasmodium falciparum infection: a report of two cases with a review of the English literature. East Afr Med J 56:288–290
Mathews KP (1974) A current view of urticaria. Med Clin North Am 58:195–205
Mathison DA, Arroyave CM, Bhat KN, Hurewitz DR, Marnell DJ (1977) Hypocomplementemia in chronic idiopathic urticaria. Ann Int Med 86:534–538
McGowen EM (1966) Menthol urticaria. Arch Dermatol 94:62–63
McKee WD (1966) The incidence and familial occurrence of allergy. J Allergy 38:226–235
Mekori YA, Giorno RC, Anderson P, Kohler PF (1983) Lymphocyte subpopulations in the skin of patients with chronic urticaria. J Allergy Clin Immunol 72:681–684
Midelfart K, Moseng D, Kavli G, Stenvold SE, Volden G (1983) A case of chronic urticaria and vitiligo, associated with thyroiditis, treated with PUVA. Dermatologica 167:39–41
Monroe EW, Schulz CI, Maize JC, Jordon RE (1981) Vasculitis in chronic urticaria. An immunopathological study. J Invest Dermatol 76:103–107
Moynihan NH (1955) Serum sickness and local reactions in tetanus prophylaxis. Lancet II:264
Much T, Wüthrich B, Toendury T (1978) Zur Klinik. Diagnose und Therapie der Nahrungsmittelallergie. Z Hautkr 53:141–149
Muckle TJ, Wells M (1962) Urticaria, deafness and amyloidosis. A new heredofamilial syndrome. Quart J Med 31:235–248
Natbony SF, Phillips ME, Elias JM, Godfrey HP, Kaplan AP (1983) Histologic studies of chronic idiopathic urticaria. J Allergy Clin Immunol 71:177–183
Nishioka K, Katayama I, Sano S (1983) Urticaria induced by d-psicose. Lancet II:1417–1418
Noguera J, Moreno A, deMoragas JM (1983) Pruritic urticarial papules and plaques of pregnancy (PUPPP). Acta Dermatovenereol 63:35–38
Numata T, Yamamoto S, Yamura T (1979) The role of mite allergen in chronic urticaria. Ann Allergy 43:356–358
Numata T, Yamamoto S, Yamura T (1980) The role of mite, house dust and candida allergens in chronic urticaria. J Dermatol (Tokyo) 7:197–202
O'Loughlin S, Schroeter AL, Jordon RE (1978) Chronic urticaria-like lesions in systemic lupus erythematosus. A review of 12 cases. Arch Dermatol 114:879–883
Ormerod AD, Holt PJA (1983) Acute urticaria due to alcohol. Br J Dermatol 108:723–724
Owen RL (1977) Sequential uptake of horseradish peroxidase by lymphoid follicle epithelium of Peyer's patches in the normal unobstructed mouse intestine. An ultrastructural study. Gastroenterol 72:440–444
Pace JL, Garretts M (1975) Urticaria and hyperthyroidism. Br J Dermatol 93:97–99
Parker CW (1975) Drug therapy: Drug allergy. New Engl J Med 292:511–514
Pasricha JS, Pasricha A, Prakash OM (1972) Role of gastrointestinal parasites in urticaria. Ann Allergy 30:348–351
Patterson R, Mellies CJ, Roberts M (1973) Immunologic reactions against insulin. II. IgE anti-insulin, insulin allergy and combined IgE and IgG immunologic insulin resistance. J Immunol 110:1135–1145
Paulsen HC (1961) Alimentary allergy. Allergy to fish. Acta Allergol 16:380–386
Pollowitz JA (1980) Acute urticaria with shigellosis. A case report. Ann Allergy 45:302–303
Rajka G, Skog E (1965) On the relation between drug allergy and atopy. Acta Allergol 20:387–394
Rappaport BZ, Hoffman MM (1941) Urticaria due to aliphatic aldehydes. JAMA 116:2656–2659
Rees L (1957) An aetiological study of chronic urticaria and angioneurotic oedema. J Psychosom Res 2:172–189
Reinhold M (1960) Relationship of stress to the development of symptoms in alopecia areata and chronic urticaria. Br Med J I:846–849
Resch CE, Evans RE (1958) Chronic urticaria and dental infections. Cleve Clin Q 25:147–150
Rives H, Pellerat J, Thivolet J (1972) Urticaria chronique et oedème de Quincke. Dermatologica 144:193–204
Rook A, Staughton R (1972) The cutaneous manifestations of toxocariasis. Dermatologica 144:129–143
Rorsman H (1962) Studies on basophil leucocytes with special reference to urticaria and anaphylaxis. Acta Dermatovenereol 42 (Suppl 48)
Routledge RC, De Kretser DMH, Wadsworth LD (1976) Severe anaphylaxis due to passive sensitization by donor blood. Br Med J 1:434
Rudzki E, Borkowski W, Czubalski K (1970) The suggestion effect of placebo on the intensity of chronic urticaria. Acta Allergol 25:70–73
Schade C, Kaben U, Westphal HJ (1975) Incidence of yeasts and therapeutic results in chronic urticaria. Dermatol Mschr 161:187–195
Schmidl M, Kern A (1964) Zur Pathogenese der Urticaria chronica. Dermatol Wschr 150:481–487
Schuller D, Elvey SM (1980) Acute urticaria associated with streptococcal infection. Pediatr 65:592–596
Serrano H (1975) Hypersensitivity to candida albicans and other yeasts in patients with chronic urticaria. Allergol Immunopathol 3:289–298
Sheldon JM, Mathews KP, Lovell RG (1954) The vexing urticaria problem. Present concepts of etiology and management. J Allergy 25:525–560
Shelley WB, Florence R (1961) Chronic urticaria due to mold hypersensitivity. A study in cross sensitization and autoerythrocyte sensitization. Arch Dermatol 83:549–558
Shoemaker RJ, Levine MI, Shipman WG, Mally MA (1962) A search for the affective determinants of chronic urticaria. Am J Psychiatry 119:358–359
Shore RN, Shelley WB, Kyle GC (1975) Chronic urticaria from isophane insulin therapy. Sensitivity associated with noninsulin components in commercial preparations. Arch Dermatol 111:94–97

Siegel SC, Bergeron JG (1954) Urticaria and angioedema in children and young adults. Ann Allergy 12:241–252
Singh M, Arora NK, Sroa HS (1980) Urticaria neonatorum. An earliest marker of atopy. Indian J Med Res 71:273–277
Small P, Barrett D, Biskin N, Champlin E (1982) Chronic urticaria and angioedema. Clin Allergy 12:131–136
Small P, Lerman MD (1981) Hyperthyroidism and polycythemia vera with chronic urticaria and angioedema. Ann Allergy 46:256–259
Speer F, Casas Carrasco L, Kimura CC (1978) The management of urticaria. Ann Allergy 40:387–392
Steck WD, Byrd RB (1969) Urticaria secondary to pulmonary melioidosis. Arch Dermatol 99:80–81
Stemmler M, Lischka G (1979) Urticaria: Sinnvolle Diagnostik. Akt Dermatol 5:131–134
Sutter MC, Beaulieu G, Birt AR (1962) Histamine liberation by codeine and polymyxin B in urticaria pigmentosa. Arch Dermatol 86:217–221
Sweet RD (1964) An acute febrile neutrophilic dermatosis. Br J Dermatol 76:349–356
Swinny B (1941) The atopic factor in urticaria. South Med J 34:855–858
Tay CH (1974) Pattern of allergic drug eruptions in hospital practice. Asian J Med 10:223–228
Thoburn R, Johnson JE III, Cliff LE (1966) Studies on the epidemiology of adverse drug reactions. IV. The relationship of cephalotin and penicillin allergy. JAMA 198:345–348
Tinkelman DG, Tinkelman CL (1979) An unusual etiology of urticaria. Pediatr 63:339
Török L (1928) Urticaria. In: Handbuch der Haut- und Geschlechtskrankheiten. Jadassohn J et al. (eds) Springer, Berlin, pp 145–215
Tuffanelli DL, Dubois EL (1964) Cutaneous manifestations of systemic lupus erythematosus. Arch Dermatol 90:377–386
Uhlin SR (1981) Pruritic urticarial papules and plaques of pregnancy. Involvement in mother and infant. Arch Dermatol 117:238–239
Vaida GA, Goldman MA, Bloch KJ (1983) Testing for hepatitis B virus in patients with chronic urticaria and angioedema. J Allergy Clin Immunol 72:193–198
Velcovsky HG, Beringhoff B, Federlin K (1978) Beitrag zur allergischen Sofortreaktion gegen Insulin. Immunol Infekt 6:146–152
Vivarelli I, Mancosu A (1967) Rilievi su due inderizzi terapeutici nella cura dell'orticaria. Minerva Dermatol 42:441–442
Waldbott GL, Merkle K (1952) Urticaria due to pollen. Ann Allergy 10:30–35
Walton S, DeSouza EJ (1983) Variation in mast cell numbers in psoriasis and lichen planus: Comparison with normal skin. Dermatologica 166:236–239
Warin RP, Champion RH (1974) Urticaria. Saunders, London
Watzig V, Lochno M, Watzig H (1979) Zur psychischen Disposition bei Patienten mit chronischer Urtikaria. Dermatol Mschr 165:580–582
Weary PE, Guerrant JL (1967) Chronic urticaria in association with dermatophytosis. Arch Dermatol 95:400–401
Weber G, Stetter H (1969) Zur Frage: hautbeschränkte Ornithoseformen. Hautarzt 20:60–63
Werman BS, Rietschel RL (1981) Chronic urticaria from tantalum staples. Arch Dermatol 117:438–439
Westphal HJ, Schade C, Kaben U (1976) Spezifische Desensibilisierung bei Patienten mit sprosspilzbedingter chronischer Urtikaria und intestinaler Sprosspilzbesiedlung. Dermatol Mschr 162:912–915
Wicher K, Reisman RE (1980) Anaphylactic reaction to penicillin (or penicillin-like substance) in a soft drink. J Allergy Clin Immunol 66:155–157
Wintroub BU, Shiffman NJ, Arndt KA (1979) Adverse cutaneous reaction to drugs. In: Fitzpatrick TB, Eisen AZ, Wolff K, Friedberg IM, Austen KF (eds) Dermatology in general medicine. McGraw-Hill, New York, pp 555–567
Wüthrich B, Häcki-Herrmann D (1980) Zur Ätiologie der Urticaria. Z Hautkr 55:102–111
Wüthrich B, Kopper E (1974) Ergebnisse der IgE-Serumspiegel-Bestimmung und ihre klinische Bedeutung. Schweiz Med Wschr 104:1437–1443
Yancey KB, Hall RP, Lawley TJ (1984) Pruritic urticarial papules and plaques of pregnancy. J Am Acad Dermatol 10:473–480
Zide N, Davis J, Ehrenkranz NJ (1974) Fulminating Vibrio parahaemolyticus septicemia: A syndrome of erythema multiforme, hemolytic anemia and hypotension. Arch Intern Med 133:479–481

Chapter 4 (Angioedema)

Beckmann M, Muehlenstedt D, Happle R (1979) Pregnancy and delivery combined with hereditary angioneurotic edema. Geburtshilfe Frauenheilkd 39:338–340
Bork K, Witzke G, Artmann K, Benes P, Böckers M, Kreuz (1984) Interaction between C1-INA, coagulation, fibrinolysis and kinin system in hereditary angioneurotic edema (HANE) and urticaria. Arch Dermatol Res 276:375–380
Brackertz D, Isler E, Kueppers F (1975) Half life of C1 INH in hereditary angioneurotic oedema (HAE). Clin Allergy 5:89–94
Brasher GW (1977) C1q levels in hereditary angioedema. J Allergy Clin Immunol 59:263–265
Brasher GW, Starr JC, Hall FF, Spiekerman AM (1975) Complement component analysis in angioedema. Arch Dermatol 111:1140–1142
Bretza J, Novey HS (1979) Hereditary angioedema and the Mallory-Weiss syndrome. Ann Allergy 42:83–85
Brickman CM, Tsokos GC, Balow JE, Lawley TL, Chused TM, Frank MM (1984) Immunoregulatory diseases associated with hereditary angioedema (HAE). J Allergy Clin Immunol 73:155 (abstract)
Caldwell JR, Ruddy S, Schur PH, Austen KF (1972) Acquired C1 inhibitor deficiency in lymphosarcoma. Clin Immunol Immunopathol 1:39–52
Champion RH, Roberts SOB, Carpenter RG, Roger JH (1969) Urticaria and angioedema. Br J Dermatol 81:588–597
Cicardi M, Bergamaschini L, Marasini B, Boccassini G, Tucci A, Agostini A (1982) Hereditary angioedema: an appraisal of 104 cases. Am J Med Sci 284:2–9
Cohen SH, Koethe SM, Kozin F, Rodey G, Arkins JA, Fink JN (1978) Acquired angioedema associated with rectal carcinoma and its response to danazol therapy. J Allergy Clin Immunol 62:217–221
Cullmann W, Kövary PM, Dick W, Czarnetzki B, Echternach-Happle K (1982a) A rapid method for functional determination of C1 esterase inhibitor in plasma. Clin Chim Acta 119:237–242
Cullmann W, Kövary PM, Müller N, Dick W (1982b) Complement, coagulation and fibrinolytic parameters in

hereditary angioedema/HAE. Clin Exp Immunol 49:618–622
Curd JG, Prograis LJ Jr, Cochrane CG (1980) Detection of active kallikrein in induced blister fluids of hereditary angioedema patients. J Exp Med 152:742–747
Dolovich J, Denberg J, Kwee YN, Belda T, Blajchman J, Hargreave FE (1983) Does non-immunologic mast cell mediator release/activation elicit a late cutaneous response? Ann Allergy 50:241–244
Donaldson VH (1968) Mechanism of activation of C1 esterase in hereditary angioneurotic edema plasma in vitro. The role of Hageman factor, a clot-promoting agent. J Exp Med 127:411–429
Donaldson VH, Evans HH (1963) A biochemical abnormality in hereditary angioneurotic edema. Am J Med 35:37–44
Donaldson VH, Merler E, Rosen FS (1978) Polypeptide kinin from hereditary angioneurotic edema plasma. Symposium on "Clinical aspects of the complement system". Thieme, Stuttgart, pp 130–133
Donaldson VH, Ratnoff OD, De Silva WD, Rosen FS (1969) Permeability-increasing activity in hereditary angioneurotic edema plasma II. Mechanism of formation and partial characterization. J Clin Invest 48:642–653
Fields T, Ghebrehiwet B, Kaplan AP (1983) Kinin formation in hereditary angioedema plasma: evidence against kinin derivation from C2 and in support of "spontaneous" formation of bradykinin. J Allergy Clin Immunol 72:54–60
Frank MM, Gelfand JA, Atkinson JP (1976) Hereditary angioedema: the clinical syndrome and its management. Ann Intern Med 84:580–593
Gadek JE, Hosea SW, Gelfand JA, Frank MM (1979) Response of variant hereditary angioedema phenotypes to danazol therapy. J Clin Invest 64:280–286
Gelfand JA, Boss GR, Conley CL, Reinhart R, Frank MM (1979) Acquired C1 esterase inhibitor deficiency and angioedema: A review. Medicine 58:321–328
Gleich GJ, Schroeter AL, Marcoux JP, Sachs MI, O'Connell EJ, Kohler PF (1984) Episodic angioedema associated with eosinophilia. N Eng J Med 310:1621–1626
Gordon EH, Beall GN, Klaustermeyer WB (1983) Angioedema and multiple myeloma. Ann Allergy 50:349–350 and 378–390
Granerus G, Hallberg L, Laurell AB, Wetterquist H (1967) Studies on histamine metabolism and the complement system in hereditary angioneurotic edema. Acta Med Scand 182:11–22
Harpel PC, Hugli TE, Cooper NR (1975) Studies on human plasma C1 inactivator enzyme interactions. II. Structural features of an abnormal C1 inactivator from a kindred with hereditary angioneurotic edema. J Clin Invest 55:605–611
Jackson CE, Sweet LC, Hayashi H, Paul TD (1978) Evidence for nonlinkage of genes for HLA and hereditary angioedema. J Allergy Clin Immunol 61:331–333
Johnson AM, Alper CA, Rosen RS (1971) C1 inhibitor: evidence for decreased hepatic synthesis in hereditary angioneurotic edema. Science 173:553–554
Jordon RE, McDuffie FC, Good RA, Day NK (1974) Diffuse normolipaemic plane xanthomatosis. An abnormal complement component profile. Clin Exp Immunol 18:407–415
Kaplan AP (1981) The pathogenic basic of urticaria and angioedema: Recent advances. Am J Med 70:755–757
Klemperer MR, Donaldson VR, Rosen FS (1968) Effect of C1 esterase on vascular permeability in man: studies in normal and complement deficient individuals and in patients with hereditary angioneurotic edema. J Clin Invest 47:604–611
Landerman NS, Webster ME, Becker EL, Ratcliffe HE (1962) Hereditary angioneurotic edema. II. Deficiency of inhibitor for serum globulin permeability factor and/or plasma kallikrein. J Allergy 33:330–341
Laurberg G (1978) Plasma kinin activation in tranexamic acid treated patients with hereditary angioneurotic edema. Arch Dermatol Res 262:153–156
Laurell AB, Martensson U (1971) C1 inactivator protein complexed with albumin in plasma from a patient with angioneurotic edema. Eur J Immunol 1:146–149
Lewkonia R, Pineo G (1982) Angioedema-like skin lesions associated with lymphoproliferative disease. Can Med Assoc J 127:867–871
Ohela K, Tiilikainen A, Kaakinen A, Rasanen J (1977) Hereditary angioneurotic edema (HANE): lack of close linkage between HLA haplotypes and C1 esterase inhibitor deficiency. Tissue Antigens 9:90–95
Ollier MP, Hartmann L, Brecy H (1978) The molecular expression of C1 esterase inhibitor in hereditary angioneurotic oedema. Study of 32 families (Fren). Nouv Presse Med 7:2933–2938
Opferkuch W, Bohn L, Wellek B, Berger J (1974) Die diagnostischen Möglichkeiten beim hereditären angioneurotischen Ödem. Imm Inf 2:154–159
Osler W (1888) Hereditary angioneurotic oedema. Am J Med Sci 95:362–367
Quincke H (1882) Über akutes umschriebenes Hautödem. Mschr Prakt Dermatol 1:129–131
Röhrich B, Endres P (1985) Hereditäres angioneurotisches Ödem (HANE). Med Welt, in press
Rosen FS, Alper CA, Pensky J, Klemperer MR, Donaldson V (1971) Genetically determined heterogeneity of the C1 esterase inhibitor in patients with hereditary angioneurotic edema. J Clin Invest 50:2143–2149
Rosen FS, Austen KF (1976) Androgen therapy in hereditary angioneurotic edema. N Engl J Med 295:1476–1477
Rosen FS, Charache P, Pensky J, Donaldson V (1965) Hereditary angioneurotic edema: two genetic variants. Science 148:957–958
Scherak O, Smolen JS, Menzel EJ, Kolarz G (1979) Essential cryoglobulinemia with acquired angioedema (Germ). Acta Med Austr 6:214–216
Sheffer AL, Austen KF, Rosen FS, Fearon DT (1985) Acquired deficiency of the inhibitor of the first component of complement: Report of five additional cases with commentary on the syndrome. J Allergy Clin Immunol 75:640–646
Shokeir MHK (1973) The genetics of hereditary angioedema: a hypothesis. Clin Genet 4:494–499
Soulier JP, Gozin D, Ollier-Hartmann MP, Hartmann L (1981) A study of coagulation-contact factors in hereditary angioneurotic acute oedema (Fren). Nouv Presse Med 10:1627–1631
Spitzer RE, Stitzel AE, Urmson JR (1980) Hereditary angioneurotic edema: Immunochemical activity without clinical expression. Int Arch Allergy Appl Immunol 61:286–292
Starr JC, Brasher GW (1974) Erythema marginatum preceding hereditary angioedema. J Allergy Clin Immunol 53:352–355

Tannenbaum H (1982) Angioedema provoked by olfactory stimuli. Can Med Assoc J 127:735–739

Tappeiner G, Hintner H, Glatzl J, Wolff K (1979) Hereditary angio-oedema: treatment with danazol. Br J Dermatol 100:207–212

Van Dellen RG, Myers RP (1980) Bladder involvement in hereditary angioedema. Mayo Clin Proc 55:277–278

Warin RP, Higgs ER (1982) Acute and recurrent abdominal pain due to hereditary angioedema. Br Med J 284:1912

Willms K, Rosen FS, Donaldson VH (1975) Observations on the ultrastructure of lesions induced in human and guinea pig skin by C1 esterase and polypeptide from hereditary angioneurotic edema (HANE) plasma. Clin Immunol Immunopathol 4:174–188

Yelvington M, Prograis LJ, Pizzo CJ, Curd JG (1983) Immunodiffusion assay for C1 inhibitor function in serum: Prospective analysis in angioedema – urticaria. Am J Clin Pathol 80:309–313

Chapter 5 (The Physical Urticarias)

Ado AD, Fdaletshina RM, Listovoi NA (1978) Cholinergic system changes in patients with different forms of bronchial asthma and chronic urticaria. Sun-Sov Med 41:74–76

Aoyama H (1971) IgE as a dermographism-inducing principle of urticaria factitia. Jap J Dermatol 81:266–271

Atkins PC, Zweiman B (1981) Mediator release in local heat urticaria. J Allergy Clin Immunol 68:286–289

Baart de la Faille H, Rottier PB, Baart de la Faille-Kuyper EH (1975) Solar urticaria. A case with possible increase of skin mast cells. Br J Dermatol 92:101–107

Back O, Larsen A (1978) Delayed cold urticaria. Acta Dermatovenereol 58:369–371

Bart RS, Ackerman AB (1966) Urticarial dermographism. Arch Dermatol 94:716–719

Baughman RD, Jillson OF (1963) Seven specific types of urticaria. Ann Allergy 21:248–255

Bentley-Phillips CB, Black AK, Greaves MW (1976) Induced tolerance in cold urticaria caused by cold evoked histamine release. Lancet I:63–66

Bonnetblanc JM, Andrieu-Pfahl F, Mereaud JP, Roux J (1979) Familial aquagenic urticaria. Dermatologica 158:468–470

Breathnach SM, Allen R, Ward AM, Greaves MW (1981) A clinical and investigational review of patients with symptomatic dermographism. Br J Dermatol 105:23–24

Brehm G (1957) Zur Pathogenese der Kälteurticaria. Dermatol Wschr 136:1020–1022

Burgoyne RD (1981) The loss of muscarinic acetylcholine receptors in synaptic membranes under phosphorylating conditions is dependent on calmodulin. FEBS Lett 127:144–148

Cauna N, Levine MI, Cralley A (1970) The fine morphology of the human skin in dermographism. J Allergy 45:266–285

Chalamidas SL, Charles R (1971) Aquagenic urticaria. Arch Dermatol 104:541–546

Champion RH, Roberts SOB, Carpenter RG, Roger JH (1969) Urticaria and angioedema. A review of 544 patients. Br J Dermatol 81:588–597

Chin TM, Fellner MJ (1980) Allergic hypersensitivity to lidocaine hydrochloride. Int J Dermatol 19:147–148

Commens CA, Greaves MW (1978) Tests to establish the diagnosis in cholinergic urticaria. Br J Dermatol 98:47–51

Commerford PJ, Meyers OL (1977) Arthropathy associated with familial cold urticaria. S Afr Med J 51:105–108

Costanzi JJ, Coltman CA Jr, Donaldson VH (1969) Activation of complement by a monoclonal cryoglobulin associated with cold urticaria. J Lab Clin Med 74:902–910

Cripps DJ (1981) Instrumentation and action spectra in light-associated diseases. J Invest Dermatol 77:20–31

Crow KD, Alexander E, Buch WHL (1961) Photosensitivity due to pitch. Br J Dermatol 73:220–232

Curnow JSH (1978) Stable low temperature source to test for cold urticaria. Med Biol Eng Comput 16:215–216

Czarnetzki BM, Frosch PJ, Sprekeler R (1981) Localized cold reflex urticaria. Br J Dermatol 104:83–87

Czarnetzki BM, Galinski C, Meister R (1984a) Cutaneous and pulmonary reactivity in cholinergic urticaria. Br J Dermatol 111:315–323

Czarnetzki BM, Meentken J, Kolde G, Bröcker EB (1985) Morphology of the cellular infiltrate in delayed pressure urticaria. J Am Acad Dermatol 12:253–259

Czarnetzki BM, Meentken J, Rosenbach T, Prokopp A (1984b) Clinical, pharmacological and immunological aspects of delayed pressure urticaria. Br J Dermatol 111:315–323

Daman L, Liebermann P, Ganier M, Hashimoto K (1978) Localized heat urticaria. J Allergy Clin Immunol 61:273–278

Davis KC, Mekori YA, Kohler PF, Schocket AL (1984) Late cutaneous reactions (LCR) in patients with delayed pressure urticaria (DPU). J Allergy Clin Immunol 73:183 (abstract)

Davis RS, Remigio LK, Schocket AL, Bock SA (1981) Evaluation of a patient with both aquagenic and cholinergic urticaria. J Allergy Clin Immunol 68:479–483

DeLaus FV, Winkelmann RK (1973) Cold urticaria: A clinical study – Part I. Dermatol Digest, pp 39–49

Delorme P (1969) Localized heat urticaria. J Allergy 53:284–291

Delorme P, Giroux JM (1966) Solar urticaria as the presenting manifestation of systemic lupus erythematosus. Can Med Ass J 95:339–342

de Moragas JM, Gimenez-Camarasa M, Norguera J (1973) Localized heat urticaria. Arch Dermatol 108:684–686

Doeglas HMG (1975a) Chronic urticaria. Dijkstra Niemeyer, Groningen

Doeglas HMG (1975b) Reaction to aspirin and food additives in patients with chronic urticaria, including the physical urticarias. Br J Dermatol 93:135–144

Doeglas HMG, Bleumink E (1974) Familial cold urticaria. Clinical findings. Arch Dermatol 110:382–388

Doeglas HMG, Bleumink E (1975) Protease inhibitors in plasma of patients with chronic urticaria. Arch Dermatol 111:979–985

Duke WW (1924) Urticaria caused specifically by the action of physical agents. JAMA 83:3–9

Duke WW (1926) Physical allergy as a cause of dermatoses. Arch Derm Syph 13:176–186

Eady RAJ, Keahey TM, Sibbald RG, Kobza Black A (1981) Cold urticaria with vasculitis: Report of a case with light and electron microscopic, immunofluorescence and pharmacological studies. Clin Exp Dermatol 6:355–366

Eftekhari N, Milford-Ward A, Allen R, Greaves MW (1980) Protease inhibitor profiles in urticaria and angio-edema. Br J Dermatol 101 (Suppl 17): 20–21

Engelhardt AW (1961) Zur Kenntnis der mechanischen Späturticaria. Derm Wschr 144:1084–1086

Estes SA, Young CU (1981) Delayed pressure urticaria. J Am Acad Dermatol 5: 25–31
Fisher AA, Schwartz S (1953) Low incidence of dermographism in subacute and chronic urticaria. Arch Dermatol 68: 553–555
Fitzpatrick TB (1963) Essential cold urticaria. Arch Dermatol 87: 495
Floegel K, Buchholz W (1977) Cryoglobulinemia and fundus of the eye. Folia Ophthalmol (Jena) 2: 16–19
Garretts M (1958) Cholinergic urticaria and miliaria. Br J Dermatol 70: 166–170
Gerhard HJ, Schöpf E (1974) Kobner phenomenon in socalled cold water or cold air urticaria. Hautarzt 25: 197–199
Granerus G, Svensson SE, Wetterquist H, White T (1969) The metabolism of histamine in a case of cold urticaria. Acta Allergol 24: 258–260
Grant JA, Findlay SR, Thueson DO, Fine DP, Krueger GG (1981) Local heat urticaria – angioedema – evidence for histamine release without complement activation. J Allergy Clin Immunol 67: 75–77
Grant JA, Schmalstieg F, Fine DP, Lord R (1982) Familial exercise-induced anaphylaxis (EIA). J Allergy Clin Immunol 69: 103 (abstract)
Grant RT, Pearson RSB, Corneau WJ (1936) Observation on urticaria provoked by emotion, by exercise, and by warming the body. Clin Sci 2: 253–272
Greaves MW, Eady RAJ, Kobza-Black A (1981) Water; a cause of acute contact reactions in skin. Br J Dermatol 105: 25 (abstract)
Greaves MW, Sneddon IB, Smith AK, Stanworth DR (1974) Heat urticaria. Br J Dermatol 90: 289–292
Greaves MW, Sondergaard J (1970) Urticaria pigmentosa and factitious urticaria. Arch Dermatol 101: 418–425
Harber LC, Holloway RM, Wheatley VR, Baer RL (1963) Immunologic and biophysical studies in solar urticaria. J Invest Dermatol 41: 439–443
Hasei K, Ichihashi M (1982) Solar urticaria. Determinations of action and inhibition spectra. Arch Dermatol 118: 346–350
Hauptmann G, Lang JH, North MC, Oberling F, Mayer G, Lachmann PJ (1975) Lymphosarcoma, cold urticaria, IgG_1, monoclonal cryoglobulins and complement abnormalities. Scand J Haematol 15: 22–26
Hawk JLM, Eady RAJ, Challoner AVJ, Kobza-Black A, Keahey TM, Greaves MW (1980) Elevated blood histamine levels and mast cell degranulation in solar urticaria. Br J Clin Pharmacol 9: 183–186
Haxthausen H (1941) Adiponecrosis e frigore. Br J Dermatol 53: 83–89
Herxheimer A (1956) The nervous pathway mediating cholinergic urticaria. Clin Sci 15: 195–204
Highet AS, Pye R, Felix RH (1981) Vibratory urticaria. Br J Dermatol 105: 40–41
Hopkins JG, Kesten BM, Hazel OG (1938) Urticaria provoked by heat or psychic stimuli. Arch Derm Syph 38: 679–691
Horio T (1975) Chlorpromazine photoallergy. Coexistence of immediate and delayed type. Arch Dermatol 111: 1469–1471
Horio T (1978) Photoallergic urticaria induced by visible light. Additional cases and further studies. Arch Dermatol 114: 1761–1764
Horio T, Minami K (1977) Solar urticaria. Arch Dermatol 113: 157–160
Horio T, Yoshioka A, Okamoto H (1984) Production and inhibition of solar urticaria by visible light sources. J Am Acad Dermatol 11: 1094–1099
Houser DD, Arbesman CE, Kohi ITO, Wicher K (1970) Cold urticaria (immunologic studies). Am J Med 49: 23–33
Ichihashi M, Hasei K, Hagashibe K (1985) Solar urticaria. Arch Dermatol 121: 503–507
Illig L (1967) Zur Pathogenese der cholinergischen Urticaria. I. Klinische Beobachtungen und histologische Untersuchungen. Arch klin exp Dermatol 229: 231–247
Illig L (1973) Physical urticaria. Its diagnosis and treatment. In: Mali JWH (ed) Current problems in dermatology. Karger, Basel, pp 79–116
Illig L, Heinicke A (1967a) Zur Pathogenese der cholinergischen Urticaria. II. Untersuchungen über die Beziehung der cholinergischen Urticaria zur Schweißsekretion mit Hilfe von verschiedenen Cholinomimetika. Arch klin exp Dermatol 229: 285–299
Illig L, Heinicke A (1967b) Zur Pathogenese der cholinergischen Urticaria. IV. Zur Frage einer echten Antigen-Antikörper-Reaktion. Arch klin exp Dermatol 229: 360–371
Illig L, Kunick J (1969) Klinik und Diagnostik der physikalischen Urticaria I. Hautarzt 20: 167–178
Illig L, Paul E, Brueck K, Schwennicke HP (1980) Experimental investigations on the trigger mechanism of the generalized type of heat and cold urticaria by means of a climate chamber. Acta Dermatovenereol 60: 373–380
Inou S, Teshima H, Ago Y, Nagata S (1980) Cold urticaria associated with immunoglobulin M serum factor. J Allergy Clin Immunol 66: 299–304
Irwin R, Lieberman P, Kaplan R, Kaliner M, Treadwell G, Yoo T (1984) Mediator release in local heat urticaria (LHU): Protection with combined H1 and H2 antagonists. J Allergy Clin Immunol 73: 181 (abstract)
Ive H, Lloyd J, Magnus IA (1965) Action spectra in idiopathic solar urticaria. A study of 17 cases with a monochromator. Br J Dermatol 77: 229–243
James J, Warin RP (1969) Factitous wealing at the site of previous cutaneous response. Br J Dermatol 81: 882–884
James MP, Eady RAJ, Kobza-Black A, Hawk JLM, Greaves MW (1980) Physical urticaria: A microscopical and pharmacological study of mast cell involvement. J Invest Dermatol 74: 451 (abstract)
Johansson EA, Reunala T, Koskimies S, Lagerstedt A, Kauppinen K, Timonen K (1984) Localized heat urticaria with a decrease in serum complement factor B (C3 proactivator). Br J Dermatol 110: 227–231
Juhlin L (1981) Cold urticaria with persistent weals. Br J Dermatol 104: 705–707
Juhlin L, Shelley WB (1961) Role of mast cell and basophil in cold urticaria with associated systemic reactions. JAMA 177: 371–377
Kalz F (1946) Dermographia: another side effect of penicillin therapy. Arch Dermatol Syph 54: 66
Kalz F, Bower CM, Prichard H (1950) Delayed and persistent dermographia. Arch Dermatol 61: 772–780
Kalz F, Prichard H (1952) Investigation of some side effects on syphilitic patients treated with penicillin. Arch Dermatol 65: 568–580
Kaplan AP (1984) Unusual cold-induced disorders: Cold-dependent dermographism and systemic cold urticaria. J Allergy Clin Immunol 73: 453–456
Kaplan AP, Beaven MA (1976) In vivo studies of the pathogenesis of cold urticaria, cholinergic urticaria and vibration-induced swelling. J Invest Dermatol 67: 327–332
Kaplan AP, Garofalo J (1981) Identification of a new

physically induced urticaria: Cold-induced cholinergic urticaria. J Allergy Clin Immunol 68:438–441

Kaplan AP, Garofalo J, Stigler R, Hauber T (1981a) Idiopathic cold urticaria: In vitro demonstration of histamine release upon challenge of skin biopsies. New Engl J Med 305:1074–1077

Kaplan AP, Gray L, Shaff RE, Horakova Z, Beaven MA (1975) In vivo studies of mediator release in cold urticaria and cholinergic urticaria. J Allergy Clin Immunol 55: 394–402

Kaplan AP, Horakova Z, Katz SI (1978) Assessment of tissue fluid histamine in patients with urticaria. J Allergy Clin Immunol 61:350–354

Kaplan AP, Natbony SF, Tauril AP, Fruchter L, Foster M (1981b) Exercise-induced anaphylaxis as a manifestation of cholinergic urticaria. J Allergy Clin Immunol 68: 319–324

Keahey TM, Greaves MW (1980) Cold urticaria. Dissociation of cold-evoked histamine release and urticaria following cold challenge. Arch Dermatol 116:174–177

Keahey TM, Indrisano J, Kaliner MA (1984) Delayed vibratory angioedema. J Allergy Clin Immunol 73:183 (abstract)

Keahey TM, Lavker RM, Kaidbey KH (1981) Solar urticaria: Induction of tolerance and demonstration of a photoreactive serum factor. J Invest Dermatol 76:322A (abstract)

Kidd JM III, Cohen SH, Sosman AJ, Fink JN (1983) Food-dependent exercise-induced anaphylaxis. J Allergy Clin Immunol 71:407–411

Kierland RR (1953) Physical allergies. Arch Dermatol 68:61–68

Kirby JD, Matthews CNA, James J, Duncan EHL, Warin RP (1971) The incidence and other aspects of factitious wealing (dermographism). Br J Dermatol 85:331–335

Kobza A, Ramsay CA, Magnus IA (1973) Oral β-carotene therapy in actinic reticuloid and solar urticaria. Br J Dermatol 88:157–166

Kobza-Black A, Keahey TM, Eady RAJ, Greaves MW (1981) Dissociation of histamine release and clinical improvement following treatment of acquired cold urticaria by prednisone. Br J Clin Pharmacol 12:327–331

Kochenar IE, Lamda AA, Giovinazzo VJ (1981) An instrument for action spectra studies in dermatology: Results on coal tar components. J Invest Dermatol 76:323 (abstract)

Koda H, Kanaide A, Asahi M, Urabe H (1978) Essential IgG cryoglobulinemia with purpura and cold urticaria. Arch Dermatol 114:784–786

Kounis NG, MacMahon RG (1975) Cholinergic urticaria with systemic manifestations. Ann Allergy 35:243–245

Lass N, Doron O, Gilat T (1980) Gastric acid secretion in cold urticaria. Dig Dis Sci 25:526–528

Lawrence CM, Jorizzo JL, Kobza-Black A, Coutts A, Greaves MW (1981) Cholinergic urticaria with associated angio-oedema. Br J Dermatol 195:543–550

Lehner E, Rajka E (1930) Der Nachweis der Allergie bei der Urticaria factitia. Arch Dermatol Syph 159: 172–179

Leigh LM, Ramsay CA (1975) Localized heat urticaria treated by inducing tolerance to heat. Br J Dermatol 92:191–194

Lemanske RF, Bush RK (1982) Cold urticaria in infectious mononucleosis. JAMA 247:1604

Lewis GM (1939) Urticaria (heat). Arch Dermatol 39: 365–366

Lewis J, Liebermann P, Treadwell G, Erffmeyer J (1981) Exercise-induced urticaria, angioedema and anaphylactic episodes. J Allergy Clin Immunol 68:432–437

Lewis T (1927) The blood vessels of the human skin and their responses. Shaw & Sons, LtD, London

Longley S, Scornick J, Panush R, Katz P (1982) Familial exercise-induced anaphylaxis. J Allergy Clin Immunol 69:103 (abstract)

Lorincz AL (1964) Solar urticaria. Illinois Med J 125: 626–631

Lorincz AL (1966) The physical urticarias. Jap J Dermatol 76:11–15

Magnus I, Porter A, McCree K, Moreland JD, Wright WD (1959) A monochrometer: An apparatus for the investigation of the skin to ultraviolet, visible and near infrared radiations. Br J Dermatol 71:261–266

Marcussen PV (1950) Dermographic prurigo: a syndrome with constitutional, psychic and mechanical etiology. Acta Dermatovenereol 30:95–113

Martens BPM, Berrens L (1975) Enzyme activation and inhibition induced by cold provocation in a patient with cold urticaria. Acta Dermatovenereol 55:121–125

Martin S, Eastern J, Knox JM (1981) Familial polymorphous cold eruption. Cutis 27:173–175

Mathews KP, Pan PM (1970) Postexercise hyperhistaminemia, dermographia and wheezing. Ann Int Med 72: 241–249

Matthews CNA, Kirby JD, James D, Warin RP (1973) Dermographism: Reduction in wheal size by chlorpheniramine and hydroxyzine. Br J Dermatol 88:279–286

Matthews CNA, Warin RP (1970) Cold urticaria and cold precipitable dermographism. Br J Dermatol 82:91

Maulitz RM, Pratt DS, Shockett AL (1979) Exercise-induced anaphylactic reactions to shellfish. J Allergy Clin Immunol 63:433–434

Metzger WJ, Kaplan AP, Beaven MA, Irons JS, Patterson R (1976) Hereditary vibratory angioedema. Confirmation of histamine release in a type of physical hypersensitivity. J Allergy Clin Immunol 57:605–608

Michaelsson G, Ros AM (1971) Familial localized heat urticaria of delayed type. Acta Dermatovenereol 51: 279–283

Misra RS, Singh R, Pandhi RK (1977) Urticaria calorica. Indian J Derm Venereol Leprol 43:138–142

Moore-Robinson M, Warin RP (1968) Some clinical aspects of cholinergic urticaria. Br J Dermatol 80:794–799

Morgan JK (1953) Observations on cholinergic urticaria. J Invest Dermatol 21:173–182

Murphy GM, Kobza-Black A, Greaves MW (1983) Persisting cholinergic erythema: a variant of cholinergic urticaria. Br J Dermatol 109:343–348

Newcomb RW, Nelson H (1973) Dermographia mediated by immunoglobulin E. Am J Med 54:174–180

Newman JC (1981) Neurotransmitters and urticaria: Primary acquired cold urticaria as a model-system for studying aspects of behavioural change in humans. Specul Sci Technol 4:231–248

Nilsson T, Bäck O (1984) On the role of C1-esterase inhibitor in cold urticaria. Acta Dermatovenereol 64:197–202

Nomland R (1944) Cholinergic urticaria and cholinergic itching. Arch Derm Syph 50:247–249

Panfilis G De (1969) Rilievi di ordine patogenetico a proposito di un caso di orticaria "colinergica" in gemelli. G Ital Dermatol e Minverva Dermatol 44:236–241

Parillo JE, Lawley TJ, Frank MM, Kaplan AP, Fauci AS (1979) Immunologic reactivity in the hypereosinophilic syndrome. J Allergy Clin Immunol 64:113–121

Pasricha JS, Nayyar KC (1975) Idiopathic acquired cold urticaria in North India. Ann Allergy 34:363–365

Patterson R, Mellies CJ, Blankenship ML, Pruzansky JJ (1972) Vibratory angioedema: a hereditary type of physical allergy. J Allergy Clin Immunol 50:174–182

Ramsay CA (1980) Solar urticaria. Int J Dermatol 19:233–236

Ratanen T, Suhonen R (1980) Solar urticaria. A case with increased skin mast cells and good therapeutic response to an antihistamine. Acta Derm Venereol (Stockh) 60: 363–365

Ravits M, Armstrong RB, Harber LC (1982) Solar urticaria. Clinical features and wavelength dependency. Arch Dermatol 118:228–231

Rawnsley HM, Shelley WB (1968) Cold urticaria with cryoglobulinemia in a patient with chronic lymphatic leukemia. Arch Dermatol 98:12–17

Rich WG (1949) Dermographia. Br Med J 2:600

Roed-Petersen J (1978) Localized cold urticaria. Contact. Dermatitis 4:59

Rose B (1941) Studies on blood histamine in cases of allergy. J Allergy 12:327–334

Ruiz-Maldonado R, Tamayo L, Ridaura C (1975) Diffuse dermographic mastocytosis without visible skin lesions. Int J Dermatol 14:126–129

Ryan TJ, Shim-Young N, Turk JL (1968) Delayed pressure urticaria. Br J Dermatol 80:485–490

Sahihi T, Esterly NB (1972) Atypical diffuse cutaneous mastocytosis. Amer J Dis Child 124:133–135

Sams WM Jr (1970) Solar urticaria, studies with the active serum factor. J Allergy 45:295–301

Sams WM Jr, Epstein JH, Winkelmann RK (1969) Solar urticaria. Investigation of pathogenetic mechanisms. Arch Dermatol 99:390–397

Sarkany I, Gaylarde PM (1971) Negative reactions to ice in cold urticaria. Br J Dermatol 85:46–48

Sheffer Al, Austen KF (1980) Exercise-induced anaphylaxis. J Allergy Clin Immunol 66:106–111

Sheffer AL, Murphy GF, McFadden ER, Shepard MA, Austen KF (1984) Exercise-induced anaphylaxis (EIA): A common serious form of physical allergy associated with mast cell (MC) degranulation. J Allergy Clin Immunol 73:112 (abstract)

Sheffer AL, Soter NA, McFadden ER, Austen KF (1983) Exercise-induced anaphylaxis: a distinct form of physical allergy. J Allergy Clin Immunol 71:311–316

Shelley WB, Caro WA (1962) Cold erythema. A new hypersensitivity syndrome. JAMA 180:639–642

Shelley WB, Florence R (1961) Chronic urticaria due to mold hypersensitivity. Arch Dermatol 83:549–558

Shelley WB, Rawnsley HM (1964) Aquagenic urticaria. Contact sensitivity reaction to water. JAMA 189:895–898

Shelley WB, Shelley ED, Ho AKS (1983) Cholinergic urticaria: acetylcholine-receptor-dependent immediate-type hypersensitivity reaction to copper. Lancet I:843–846

Sibbald RG, Black AK, Eady RA, James M, Greaves MW (1981) Aquagenic urticaria: evidence of cholinergic and histaminergic basis. Br J Dermatol 105:297–302

Sibbald RG, Eady RAJ, Kobza-Black A, Greaves MW (1979) Cold urticaria and complement C_2 deficiency. Br J Dermatol 101 (Suppl 17): 45

Sigler RW, Evans R III, Horakova Z, Ottensen E, Kaplan AP (1980) Role of cyproheptadine in treatment of cold urticaria. J Allergy Clin Immunol 65:309–312

Sigler RW, Lewinson AI, Evans R, Horakova Z, Kaplan AP (1979) Evaluation of a patient with cold and cholinergic urticaria. J Allergy Clin Immunol 63:35–38

Smith JA, Mansfield LE, Fokakis A, Nelson HS (1983) Dermographia caused by IgE mediated penicillin allergy. Ann Allergy 51:30–32

Solomon LM, Strauss H, Leznoff A (1966) Localized "secondary" cold urticaria. Arch Dermatol 94:156–160

Songsiridej V, Busse WW (1983) Exercise-induced anaphylaxis. Clin Allergy 13:317–321

Soter NA, Joshi NP, Twarog FJ, Zeiger KS, Rothman PM, Colton HR (1977) Delayed cold induced urticaria: A dominantly inherited disorder. J Allergy Clin Immunol 59:294–297

Soter NA, Wasserman SI, Austen KF (1976) Cold urticaria: Release into the circulation of histamine and eosinophil chemotactic factor of anaphylaxis during cold challenge. New Engl J Med 294:687–690

Soter NA, Wassermann SI, Austen KF, McFadden ER Jr (1980) Release of mast-cell mediators and alterations in lung function in patients with cholinergic urticaria. New Engl J Med 302:604–608

Soter NA, Wasserman SI, Pathak MA, Parrish JA, Austen KF (1979) Solar urticaria. Release of mast cell mediators into the circulation after experimental challenge. J Invest Dermatol 72:282 (abstract)

Starr JC, Brasher GW, Hammerschmidt DE (1980) Localized heat urticaria. Ann Allergy 44:164–165

Sussman GL, Harvey RP, Schocket AL (1982) Delayed pressure urticaria. J Allergy Clin Immunol 70:337–342

Tennenbaum JI, Lowney E (1973) Localized heat and cold urticaria: New phenomenon occurring in the same individual. J Allergy Clin Immunol 51:57–59

Thiers H, Moulin G (1969) Urticaire au froid et cryoglobulinemie révélatrice d'un myèlome. Bull Soc Franc Derm Syph 76:578–581

Thompson JS (1968) Urticaria and angioedema. Ann Int Med 69:361–380

Thueson DO, Speck LS, Lett-Brown MA, Grant JA (1979) Histamine-releasing activity (HRA) I. Production by mitogen- or antigen-stimulated human mononuclear cells. J Immunol 123:626–632

Torinuki W, Kumai N, Miura T (1983) Solar urticaria inhibited by visible light. Dermatologica 166:151–155

Tronovitch TA (1967) Urticaria from contact with water. Calif Med 106:400–401

Tuffanelli DL, Dubois EL (1969) Cutaneous manifestations of systemic lupus erythematosus. Arch Dermatol 99: 390–397

Tyson CJ, Czarny D (1981) Cold-induced urticaria in infectious mononucleosis. Med J Aust 1:33–35

Udassin R, Harari Z, Schoenfeld Y, Keren G (1981) Cholinergic urticaria: a seasonal disease. Arch Int Med 141:1029–1030

Urbach E, Fasal P (1929) Mechanische Späturticaria. Ein weiterer Beitrag zur physikalischen Allergie der Haut. Klin Wschr 8:2368–2371

Van Hecke E (1979) Solar urticaria. Arch Dermatol 115:759

Vlagopoulos T, Townley R, Villacorte G (1975) Familial cold urticaria. Ann Allergy 34:366–369

Walzer A (1928) Urticaria III. Experimental urticaria factitia. Arch Dermatol 18:868–886

Wager O, Kimmo K, Räsänen JA (1968) Mixed IgA-IgG cryoglobulinemia. Am J Med 44:179–187

Wanderer A, Maselli R, Ellis EF, Ishizaka K (1971) Immunologic characterization of serum factors responsible for cold urticaria. J Allergy Clin Immunol 48:13–22

Wanderer AA, Nuss DD, Torney AD, Giclas PC (1983) Urticaria leukocytoclastic vasculitis with cold urticaria. Arch Dermatol 119:145–151

Warin RP (1976) Clinical aspects of mast cell disorders in man and consideration of factitious urticaria. Clin Exp Dermatol 1: 323–326

Warin RP (1977) Auslösende Faktoren bei chronischer Urtikaria. Hautarzt 28: 511–515

Warin RP (1981) Factitious urticaria: Red dermographism. Br J Dermatol 104: 285–288

Warin RP, Champion RH (1974) Urticaria. Saunders, London

Wasserman SI, Soter NA, Center DM, Austen KF (1977) Cold urticaria. J Clin Invest 60: 189–196

Willis I, Epstein JH (1974) Solar vs heat-induced urticaria. Arch Dermatol 110: 389–392

Winkelmann RK, Wilhelmy CM, Horner FA (1965) Experimental studies in dermographism. Arch Dermatol 92: 436–440

Wise RD, Malkinson FD, Luskin A, Gewurs AT, Zeitz HJ (1978) Localized heat urticaria. Arch Dermatol 114: 1079–1080

Wüthrich B (1979) Clinical and immunological studies on acquired heat contact urticaria. Dermatologica (Basel) 158: 371–376

Chapter 6 (Contact Urticaria)

Andersen KE, Lowenstein H (1978) An investigation of the possible immunological relationship between allergen extracts from birch pollen, hazelnut, potatoe and apple. Contact Dermatitis 4: 73–79

Andersen KE, Maibach HI (1984) Multiple application delayed onset urticaria: possible relation to certain unusual formalin and textile reactions. Contact Dermatitis 10: 227–234

Bernstein DI, Gallagher JS, Bernstein IL (1983) Mealworm asthma: clinical and immunological studies. J Allergy Clin Immunol 72: 475–480

Bjorkner B (1980) Contact urticaria and asthma from denatonium benzoate (Bitrex[R]). Contact Dermatitis 6/7: 466–471

Brubaker MM (1972) Urticarial reaction to ammonium persulfate. Arch Dermatol 106: 413–414

Burnett JW, Calton GJ (1981) Use of IgE antibody determinations in cutaneous coelenterate envenomations. Cutis 27: 50–52

Calnan D, Shuster S (1963) Reaction to ammonium persulfate. Arch Dermatol 80: 812–815

Dorrestein DM, Van Bronswijk JEMH (1979) Trixacarus caviae Fain, Fowell and Hyatt (Acari: Sarcoptidae) as a cause of mange in guineapigs and papular urticaria in man. Vet Parasitol 5: 389–398

Emmelin M, Feldberg W (1947) The mechanism of the sting of the common nettle (urtica urens). J Physiol 106: 440–455

Emmett EA (1983) Occupational skin diseases. J Allergy Clin Immunol 72: 649–656

Fisher AA (ed) (1973) Noneczematous contact dermatitis. In: Contact dermatitis. 2nd ed, Lea & Febiger, Philadelphia, pp 283–291

Fisher AA (1978) Immediate and delayed allergic contact reactions to polyethylene glycol. Contact Dermatitis 4: 135–138

Fisher AA, Dooms-Goossens A (1976) Persulfate hair bleach reactions. Cutaneous and respiratory manifestations. Arch Dermatol 112: 1407–1409

Habermann E (1972) Bee and wasp venom. Science 177: 314–316

Hannuksela M (1980) Atopic contact dermatitis. Contact Dermatitis 6: 30–32

Hannuksela M, Lahti A (1977) Immediate reactions to fruits and vegetables. Contact Dermatitis 3: 79–84

Hatch KL, Maibach HI (1985) Textile fiber dermatitis. Contact Dermatitis 12: 1–11

Helander I (1977) Contact urticaria from leather containing formaldehyde. Arch Dermatol 113: 1443

Henry JC, Tschen EH, Becker LE (1979) Contact urticaria to parabens. Arch Dermatol 115: 1231–1232

Herrmann F, Sulzberger MB, Baer RL (1944) Penetration of allergens into the human skin. NY State Med J 44: 2452–2459

Jacques R, Schacter M (1954) The presence of histamine, 5-hydroxytryptamine and a potent, slow contracting substance in wasp venom. Br J Pharmacol 9: 54–58

Kallos P, Kallos L (1980) Histamine and some other mediators of pseudoallergic reactions. In: Dukor K, Kallos P, Schlumberger HD, West GB (eds) PAR pseudoallergic reactions. Involvement of drugs and chemicals. Vol I, Karger, Basel, pp 28–55

Kalveram KJ, Forck G, Beck M, Fuchs E (1984) In-vitro-Untersuchungen zum kreuzreaktiven Verhalten von Birken-, Erlen- und Haselnußpollenallergenen einerseits und Apfelfruchtallergenen andererseits. Allergologie 7: 146–147

Kligman AM (1965) Topical pharmacology and toxicology of dimethyl sulfoxide. Part I. JAMA 193: 796–802

Lahti A (1980) Non-immunologic contact urticaria. Acta Dermatovenereol 60 (Suppl 91): 1–49

Lahti A, Hannuksela M (1978) Hypersensitivity to apple and carrot can be reliably detected with fresh material. Allery 33: 143–146

Langeland T, Nyrud M (1982) Contact urticaria to wheat bran bath: A case report. Acta Dermatovenereol 62: 82–83

Maibach HI (1976) Immediate hypersensitivity in hand dermatitis. Role of food contact dermatitis. Arch Dermatol 112: 1289–1291

Maibach HI, Johnson HL (1975) Contact urticaria syndrome. Contact urticaria to diethyltoluamide. Arch Dermatol 111: 726–730

Nagano T, Kanoa K, Sugai T (1984) Allergic contact urticaria caused by raw prawns and shrimps: three cases. J Allergy Clin Immunol 74: 489–493

Osmundsen PE (1980) Contact urticaria from nickel and plastic additives (butylhydroxytoluene, oleylamide). Contact Dermatitis 6: 425–454

Paton WDM (1951) Compound 48/80: A potent histamine liberator. Br J Pharmacol 6: 499–508

Ramsay DL, Cohen HJ, Baer RL (1972) Allergic reaction to benzophenone. Simultaneous occurrence of urticaria and contact sensitivities. Arch Dermatol 105: 906–908

Ray MC, Tharp MD, Sullivan TJ, Tigelaar RE (1983) Contact hypersensitivity reactions to dinitrofluorobenzene mediated by monoclonal IgE anti-DNP antibodies. J Immunol 131: 1096–1102

Rietschel RL (1978) Contact urticaria from synthetic cassia oil and sorbic acid limited to the face. Contact Dermatitis 4: 347–349

Rilliet A, Hunziker N, Brun R (1980) Alcohol contact urticaria syndrome (immediate type hypersensitivity). Dermatologica 161: 361–364

Ryan ME, Davis BM, Marks JG (1980) Contact urticaria and allergic contact dermatitis to benzocaine gel. J Am Acad Dermatol 2: 221–223

Schechter JA, Wilkinson RD, Del Carpio R (1984)

Anaphylaxis following the use of bacitracin ointment. Arch Dermatol 120:909–911
Schneider R (1953) Erfahrungen mit Trafuril-Liniment. Wien Med Wschr 103:30–35
Stanworth DR (1980) Oligopeptide-induced release of histamine. In: Dukor P, Kallos P, Schlumberger HD, West GB (eds) PAR. Pseudoallergic reactions. Involvement of drugs and chemicals. Karger, Basel, Vol. 1, pp 56–107
Strehler E (1949) Über die Wirkungsweise eines neuen Hauthyperämiemittels Trafuril (Nikotinsäure-tetrahydrofurfurylester). Schweiz Med Wschr 79:144–149
Thurston EL, Lersten NR (1969) The morphology and toxicology of plant stinging hairs. Bot Rev 35:393–410
Togias AG, Burnett JW, Kagey-Sobotka A, Lichtenstein LM (1985) Anaphylaxis after contact with a jellyfish. J Allergy Clin Immunol 75:672–675
Tuft L, Blumenstein GI (1942) Studies in food allergy. II. Sensitization to fresh fruits: Clinical and experimental observations. J Allergy 13:574–581
Vaillancourt G de (1954) The cutaneous application of a nicotinic acid cream as a diagnostic aid in various rheumatic diseases. Can Med Ass J 71:283–285
Von Krogh G, Maibach HI (1981) The contact urticaria syndrome: An updated review. J Am Acad Dermatol 5:328–342

Chapter 7 (Anaphylactoid Reactions)

Ansell G (1970) Adverse reactions to contrast agents. Scope of problem. Invest Radiol 5:374–384
Arroyave CM, Stevenson DD, Vaughan JH, Tan EM (1977) Plasma complement changes during bronchospasm provoked in asthmatic patients. Clin Allergy 7:173–182
Assem ESK, Bray K, Dawson P (1983) The release of histamine from human basophils by radiological contrast agents. Br J Radiol 56:647–652
Attallah AA, Lee JB (1980) Indomethacin, salicylates and prostaglandin binding. Prostaglandins 19:311–318
Bochner BS, Thomas LL, Godnik L, Samter M (1984) Effect of the calcium ionophore A 23187 and aspirin on histamine release in vitro from leukocytes of aspirin-intolerant donors. Int Arch Allergy Appl Immunol 74:104–107
Chafee FH, Settipane GA (1974) Aspirin intolerance: I. Frequency in an allergic population. J Allergy Clin Immunol 53:193–199
Condemi JJ (1981) Aspirin and food dye reactions. Bull NY Acad Med 57:600–607
Cooke RA (1919) Allergy in drug idiosyncrasy. JAMA 73:759–760
Czarnetzki BM (1983) Release of eosinophil chemotactic leukotriene from neutrophils of patients with pseudoallergic reactions. Int Arch Allergy Appl Immunol 70:78–82
Czerniawska-Mysik G, Szczeklik A (1981) Idiosyncrasy to pyrazolone drugs. Allergy 36:381–384
Delaney JC (1973) Asthma, nasal polyposis, and aspirin idiosyncrasy. Ann Intern Med 79:761
Delaney JC, Kay AB (1976) Complement components and IgE in patients with asthma and aspirin idiosyncrasy. Thorax 31:425–427
De Weck AL (1971) Immunological effects of aspirin anhydride, a contaminant of commercial acetylsalicylic acid preparations. Int Arch Allergy 41:393–418
Doeglas HMG (1975) Reactions to aspirin and food additives in patients with chronic urticaria, including physical urticarias. Br J Dermatol 93:135–144
Doenicke A (1980) Pseudo-allergic reactions due to histamine release during intravenous anesthesia. In: Dukor P, Kallos P, Schlumberger HD, West GB (eds) PAR. Pseudoallergic reactions. Involvement of drugs and chemicals. Karger, Basel, Vol 1, pp 224–250
Dukor P, Kallos P, Schlumberger HD, West GB (1980) PAR Pseudo-allergic reactions. Karger, Basel, Vol 1–3
Farr RS (1970) Presidential message: The need to re-evaluate acetylsalicylic acid (aspirin). J Allergy Clin Immunol 45:321–324
Findlay SR, Dvorak A, Kagey-Sobotka A, Lichtenstein LM (1981) Hyperosmolar triggering of histamine release from human basophils. J Clin Invest 67:1604–1613
Findlay SR, Kagey-Sobotka A, Lichtenstein LM (1984) In vitro basophil histamine release induced by mannitol in a patient with a mannitol-induced anaphylactoid reaction. J Allergy Clin Immunol 73:578–583
Fisherman EW, Cohen GN (1973a) Test for aspirin intolerance (hypersensitivity) and adrenergic stimulators. Ann Allergy 31:182–194
Fisherman EW, Cohen GN (1973b) Chemical intolerance to butylated-hydroxyanisole (BHA) and butylated-hydroxytoluene (BHT) and vascular response as an indicator and monitor of drug intolerance. Ann Allergy 31:126–133
Fisherman EW, Cohen GN (1973c) Aspirin and other cross-reacting small chemicals in known aspirin intolerant patients. Ann Allergy 31:476–484
Fisherman EW, Cohen GN (1976) Recurring and chronic urticaria: Identification of etiologies. Ann Allergy 36:400–409
Fisherman EW, Cohen GN (1977) Chronic and recurrent urticaria: New concepts of drug-group sensitivity. Ann Allergy 39:404–414
Gerber JG, Payne NA, Oelz O, Nies AS, Oates JA (1979) Tartrazine and the prostaglandin system. J Allergy Clin Immunol 63:289–294
Gibson A, Clancy R (1980) Management of chronic idiopathic urticaria by the identification and exclusion of dietary factors. Clin Allergy 10:699–704
Giraldo B, Blumenthal MN, Spink WW (1969) Aspirin intolerance and asthma. A clinical and experimental study. Ann Intern Med 71:479–496
Greenberger PA, Patterson R, Radin RC (1984) Two pretreatment regimens for high-risk patients receiving radiographic contrast media. J Allergy Clin Immunol 74:540–543
Hänsch GM, Voigtländer V, Rother U (1980) Effect of aspirin on the complement system in vitro. Int Arch Allergy Appl Immunol 61:150–158
Hansen-Pruss OC (1949) Studies on drug sensitivity. Ann Allergy 7:219–229
Hirschberg L (1902) Mitteilung über einen Fall von Nebenwirkung des Aspirins. Dtsch Med Wschr 28:416
Illig L (1980) Urticaria und Intoleranz-Syndrom vom "Aspirin-Typ". Zentralbl Haut Geschlkr. 144:43–53
Juhlin L (1980) Incidence of intolerance to food additives. Int J Dermatol 19:548–551
Juhlin L (1981) Recurrent urticaria: clinical investigation of 330 patients. Br J Dermatol 104:369–381
Juhlin L, Michaelsson G, Zetterström O (1972) Urticaria and asthma induced by food and drug additives in patients with aspirin hypersensitivity. J Allergy Clin Immunol 50:92–98
Kallos P, Schlumberger HD (1980) The pathomechanism of acetylsalicylic acid intolerance. A hypothesis. Med Hypotheses 6:487–490

Kreindler JJ, Slutsky J, Haddad ZH (1980) The effect of food colors and sodium benzoate on rat peritoneal mast cells. Ann Allergy 44:76–81

Krilis S, Gregson RP, Basten A, Baldo BA (1981) Investigation of the possible involvement of IgE anti-salicyloyl antibodies in patients with urticaria. Int Arch Allergy Appl Immunol 64:293–301

Lahti A (1980) Non-immunological contact urticaria. Acta Dermatovenereol 60 (Suppl 91), pp 1–49

Lasser EC, Lang JH, Lyon SG, Hamblin BS (1979) Complement and contrast material reactors. J Med Eng Technol 3:105–112

Lindemayr H, Schmidt J (1979) Intolerance to acetylsalicylic acid and food additives in patients suffering from recurrent urticaria. Wien Klin Wschr 91:817–822

Lockey SD (1959) Allergic reactions due to FD and C yellow No 5, tartrazine, and aniline dye used as colouring and identifying agent in various steroids. Ann Allergy 17: 719–721

Lockey SD (1971) Reactions to hidden agents in foods, beverages and drugs. Ann Allergy 29:461–466

Lockey RF, Rucknagel DL, Vanselow NA (1973) Familial occurrence of asthma, nasal polyps and aspirin intolerance. Ann Intern Med 78:57–63

Lumry WR, Curd JG, Brocklehurst WE, Simon RA, Stevenson DD (1982) Benoxaprofen, an inhibitor of arachidonic and lipoxygenase, does not prevent aspirin sensitive asthma. J Allergy Clin Immunol 69:93 (abstract)

Mathews KP, Lovell RG, Sheldon JM (1950) The problem of aspirin allergy with a report on skin testing with salicylate-containing human sera. J Lab Clin Med 36:416–421

Maucher OM, Fuchs A (1984) Pyrazolonallergie. Allergologie 7:142

McDonald JR, Mathison DA, Stevenson D (1972) Aspirin intolerance in asthma: detection by oral challenge. J Allergy Clin Immunol 50:198–207

Michaelsson G, Juhlin L (1973) Urticaria induced by preservative and dye additives in food and drugs. Brit J Dermatol 88:525–532

Miller FF (1971) Aspirin-induced bronchial asthma in sisters. Ann Allergy 29:263–265

Miller WA, Doppman JL, Kaplan AP (1975) Renal arteriography following systemic reaction to contrast material. J Allergy 56:291–295

Moneret-Vautrin DA, De Korwin JD, Tisserant J, Grignon M, Claudot N (1984) Ultrastructural study of the mast cells of the human duodenal mucosa. Clin Allergy 14:471–481

Moore-Robinson M, Warin RP (1967) Effect of salicylates in urticaria. Brit Med J 4:262–264

Patrono G, Ciabattoni G, Venuti A, Pugliese F, Schiavino D, Patriarca G (1978) Aspirin intolerance: Unaltered susceptibility of platelet cyclo-oxygenase to inhibition by aspirin in vitro. J Allergy Clin Immunol 62:271–275

Paul E, Illig L (1983) Zur Intoleranz-Diagnostik bei chronischer Urtikaria – Neue Erkenntnisse aufgrund eines veränderten Provokationsprogramms. Hautarzt 34 (Suppl VI), pp 367–368

Pleskow WW, Chenoweth DE, Simon RA, Stevenson DD, Curd JG (1983) The absence of detectable complement activation in aspirin-sensitive asthmatic patients during aspirin challenge. J Allergy Clin Immunol 72:462–468

Pleskow WW, Stevenson DD, Mathison DA, Simon RA, Schatz M, Zeiger RS (1982) Aspirin desensitization in aspirin-sensitive asthmatic patients: clinical manifestations and characterization of the refractory period. J Allergy Clin Immunol 69:11–19

Quick AJ (1966) Effect of aspirin on the bleeding time. Fed Proc 25:498

Rice MC, Lieberman P, Siegle RL, Mason J (1983) In vitro histamine release induced by radiocontrast media and various chemical analogs in reactor and control subjects. J Allergy Clin Immunol 72:180–186

Richter AW, Granath K, Östling G (1976) Anaphylactoid reactions in connection with infusion of invert sugar solutions are due to macromolecular contaminants. Int Arch Allergy Appl Immunol 50:606–612

Ring J (1980) Pseudo-allergic (anaphylactoid) reactions to colloid volume substitutes. In: Dukor P, Kallos P, Schlumberger HD, West GB (eds) PAR. Pseudo-allergic reactions. Karger Basel, Vol. 1, pp 251–272

Ring J (1981) Ätiopathogenese pseudoallergischer (anaphylactoider) Reaktionen. Allergologie 4:174–183

Ring J (1985) Pseudo-allergische Arzneimittelreaktionen: Überlegungen zur Pathophysiologie, Klinik und Diagnostik am Beispiel von Röntgenkontrastmitteln und Lokalanästhetika. Allergologie, in press

Ring J, Simon RA, Arroyave CM (1978) Increased in vitro histamine release by radiographic contrast media in patients with a history of incompatibility. Clin Exp Immunol 34:302–309

Ring J, Sovak M (1981) Release of serotonin from human platelets in vitro by radiographic contrast media. Invest Radiol 16:245–248

Rockoff SD, Brasch R, Kuhn C, Chraplyvy M (1970) Contrast media as histamine liberators. I. Mast-cell histamine release in vitro by sodium salts of contrast media. Invest Radiol 5:503–509

Ros AM, Juhlin L, Michaelsson G (1976) A follow up study of patients with recurrent urticaria and hypersensitivity to aspirin, benzoates and azo dyes. Brit J Derm 95:19–24

Samter M, Beers RF (1967) Concerning the nature of intolerance to aspirin. J Allergy 40:281–283

Samter M, Beers RF (1968) Intolerance to aspirin. Clinical studies and consideration of its pathogenetis. Ann Intern Med 68:975–983

Schatz M (1984) Skin testing and incremental challenge in the evaluation of adverse reactions to local anesthetics. J Allergy Clin Immunol 74:606–616

Schlumberger HD (1980) Drug-induced pseudo-allergic syndrome as exemplified by acetylsalicylic acid intolerance. In: Dukor P, Kallos P, Schlumberger HD, West GB (eds) PAR. Pseudo-allergic reactions. Involvement of drugs and chemicals. Karger Basel, Vol. 1, pp 125–203

Schlumberger HD (1983) Pseudo-allergic reactions to drugs and chemicals. Ann Allergy 51:317–324

Settipane GA (1981) Adverse reactions to aspirin and related drugs. Arch Int Med 141:328–332

Settipane GA, Chafee FH, Postman IM, Levine MI, Saker JH, Barrick RH, Nicholas SS, Schwartz HJ, Honsinger RW, Klein DE (1976) Significance of tartrazine sensitivity in chronic urticaria of unknown etiology. J Allergy Clin Immunol 57:541–546

Settipane GA, Pudupakkam RK (1975) Aspirin intolerance. III. Subtypes, familial occurrence, and cross-reactivity with tartrazine. J Allergy Clin Immunol 56:215–221

Settipane RA, Constantine HP, Settipane GA (1980) Aspirin intolerance and recurrent urticaria in normal adults and children. Allergy 35:149–154

Siegel MI, McConnell RT, Cuatrecasas P (1979) Aspirin-like

drugs interfere with arachidonate metabolism by inhibition of the 12-hydroperoxy-5,8,10,14-eicosatetraenoic acid peroxidase activity of the lipoxygenase pathway. Proc Natl Acad Sci USA 76: 3774–3778

Siegle RL, Lieberman P (1976) Measurement of histamine, complement components and immune complexes during patient reactions to iodinated contrast media. Invest Radiol 11: 98–101

Simon RA (1984) Adverse reactions to drug additives. J Allergy Clin Immunol 74: 623–630

Smith L, Slavin RG (1976) Drugs containing tartrazine dye. J Allergy Clin Immunol 58: 456–470

Storm van Leeuwen W (1928) Pathognomonische Bedeutung der Überempfindlichkeit gegen Aspirin bei Asthmatikern. Münch Med Wschr 75: 1588–1590

Szczeklik A, Gryglewski RJ, Czerniawska-Mysik G (1967) Relationship of inhibition of prostaglandin biosynthesis to asthma attacks in aspirin-sensitive patients. Br Med J 1: 67–69

Szczeklik A, Gryglewski RJ, Czerniawska-Mysik G (1977) Clinical patterns of hypersensitivity to nonsteroidal anti-inflammatory drugs and their pathogenesis. J Allergy Clin Immunol 60: 276–284

Thune P, Granholt A (1975) Provocation tests with antiphlogistica and food additives in recurrent urticaria. Dermatologica 151: 360–367

Till G (1981) Pathogenese pseudoallergischer Reaktionen. Hautarzt 32 (Suppl V): 116–118

Valverde E, Vich JM, Garcia-Calderon JV, Garcia-Calderon PA (1980) In vitro stimulation of lymphocytes in patients with chronic urticaria induced by additives and food. Clin Allergy 10: 691–698

Vervloet D, Arnaud A, Vellieux P, Kaglanski S, Charpin J (1979) Anaphylactic reactions to muscle relaxants under general anesthesia. J Allergy Clin Immunol 63: 348–353

Vervloet D, Senft M, Dugue P, Arnaud A, Charpin J (1983) Anaphylactic reactions to modified fluid gelatins. J Allergy Clin Immunol 71: 535–540

Voigtländer W, Hänsch GM, Rother U (1980) Effect of aspirin on complement in vivo. Int Arch Allergy Appl Immunol 61: 145–149

Von Maur K, Adkinson NF, Metre TE van, Marsh DG, Norman PS (1974) Aspirin intolerance in a family. J Allergy Clin Immunol 54: 380–395

Waldenström JG (1980) Urticaria pigmentosa and acetylsalicylic acid intolerance. In: Dukor P, Kallos P, Schlumberger HD, West GB (eds) PAR. Pseudo-allergic reactions. Involvement of drugs and chemicals. Karger Basel, Vol 1, pp 204–218

Wasserman SI, Sheffer AL, Soter NA, Austen KF, McFadden ER (1978) Assessment of mast cell mediators and pulmonary function in aspirin (ASA)-induced bronchospasm. J Allergy Clin Immunol 61: 139

Weber RW, Hoffman M, Raine DA, Nelson HS (1979) Incidence of bronchoconstriction due to aspirin, azo dyes, non-azo dyes, and preservatives in a population of perennial asthmatics. J Allergy Clin Immunol 64: 32–37

Weliky N, Heiner DC (1980) Hypersensitivity to chemicals. Correlation of tartrazine hypersensitivity with characteristic serum IgD and IgE immune response patterns. Clin Allergy 10: 375–394

Weltman JK, Szaro RP, Settipane GA (1978) An analysis of the role of IgE in intolerance to aspirin and tartrazine. Allergy 34: 273–281

Wojnar RJ, Hearn T, Starkweather S (1980) Augmentation of allergic histamine release from human leukocytes by nonsteroidal anti-inflammatory analgesic agents. J Allergy Clin Immunol 66: 37–45

Wüthrich B, Fabro L (1981) Acetylsalicylsäure- und Lebensmitteladditiva-Intoleranz bei Urtikaria, Asthma bronchiale und chronischer Rhinopathie. Schweiz Med Wschr 111: 1445–1450

Chapter 8 (The Urticarial Vasculitis Syndrome)

Agnello V, Gabriel A, Tai M (1976) Detection of immune complexes. J Invest Dermatol 76: 339–345

Agnello W, Ruddy S, Winchester RJ, Christian CL, Kunkel HG (1975) Hereditary C2 deficiency in systemic lupus erythematosus and acquired complement abnormalities in an unusual SLE-related syndrome. Birth Defects 2: 312–317

Ballow M, Ward GW Jr, Gershwin ME, Day NK (1975) C1-bypass complement activation pathway in patients with chronic urticaria and angioedema. Lancet II: 248–250

Brasher GW, Starr JC, Hull FF, Spiekerman AM (1975) Complement component analysis in angioedema. Arch Dermatol 111: 1140–1142

Braverman IM, Yen A (1975) Demonstration of immune complexes in spontaneous and histamine-induced lesions and in normal skin of patients with leukocytoclastic angiitis. J Invest Dermatol 64: 105–112

Callen JP, Kalbfleisch S (1982) Urticarial vasculitis: a report of nine cases and review of the literature. Br J Dermatol 107: 87–94

Crawford JP, Movat HZ, Ranadive NS, Hay JB (1982) Pathways to inflammation induced by immune complexes: development of the Arthus reaction. Fed Proc 41: 2583–2587

Cream JJ, Bryceson ADM, Ryder G (1971) Disappearance of immunoglobulin and complement from the Arthus reaction and its relevance to studies of vasculitis in man. Br J Dermatol 84: 106–109

De Shazo CV, Henson PM, Cochrane CG (1972) Acute immunologic arthritis in rabbits. J Clin Invest 51: 50–57

Devey ME, Bleasdale K, Collins M, Steward MW (1982) Experimental antigen-antibody complex disease in mice. The role of antibody levels, antibody affinity, and circulating antigen-antibody complexes. Int Archs Allergy Appl Immunol 68: 47–53

Dienstag JL, Rhodes AR, Bhan AH, Dvorak AM, Mihm MC, Wands JR (1978) Urticaria associated with acute viral hepatitis type B. Studies of pathogenesis. Ann Int Med 89: 34–40

Ekenstam E af, Callen JP (1984) Cutaneous leukocytoclastic vasculitis. Arch Dermatol 120: 484–489

Falk DK (1984) Pulmonary disease in idiopathic urticarial vasculitis. J Am Acad Dermatol 11: 346–352

Fauci AS (1983) Vasculitis. J Allergy Clin Immunol 72: 311–323

Feig PU, Soter NA, Yager HM, Caplan L, Rosen S (1976) Vasculitis with urticaria, hypocomplementemia and multiple system involvement. JAMA 236: 2065–2068

Fellner MJ (1976) Penicillin allergy 1976: a review of reactions, detection and current management. Int J Dermatol 15: 497–504

Gammon WR, Wheeler CE Jr (1979) Urticarial vasculitis. Report of a case and review of the literature. Arch Dermatol 115: 76–80

Guillet G, Jeune R (1983) Urticarial vasculitis with shock, leukopenia and thrombocytopenia possibly due to anaphylatoxin release. Br J Dermatol 108: 605–608

Hintner H, Tappeiner G (1979) Nekrotisierende Vaskulitis-Manifestation als Urtikaria. Hautarzt 30:484–488

Horvath A, Kramer M, Ablonczy E (1981) Clinical evaluation and pathomechanisms of urticaria-like skin eruptions in systemic lupus erythematosus. Acta Dermatovenereol (Stockh) 62:253–256

Jones RR, Bhogal B, Dash A, Schifferli J (1983) Urticaria and vasculitis: a continuum of histological and immunopathological changes. Br J Dermatol 108:695–703

Jones RR, Eady RAJ (1984) Endothelial cell pathology as a marker for urticarial vasculitis: a light microscopic study. Br J Dermatol 110:139–149

Marder RJ, Burch FX, Schmid FR, Zeiss LR, Gewurz H (1978) Low molecular weight Clq-precipitins in hypocomplementemic vasculitis-urticaria syndrome: partial purification and characterization as immunoglobulin. J Immunol 121:613–618

McCoombs RP (1965) Systemic "allergic" vasculitis. JAMA 194:1059–1065

McDuffie FC, Sams WM, Maldonado JE, Andreini PH, Conn DL, Samayoa EA (1973) Hypocomplementemia with cutaneous vasculitis and arthritis. Possible immune complex syndrome. Mayo Clin Proc 48:340–348

McLean RH, Weinstein A, Chapitis J, Lowenstein M, Rothfield NF (1980) Familial partial deficiency of the third component of complement (3) and the hypocomplementaemic cutaneous vasculitis syndrome. Am J Med 68:549–558

Monroe EW (1981) Urticarial vasculitis: an updated review. J Am Acad Dermatol 5:88–95

Monroe EW, Schulz CI, Maize JC, Jordon RE (1981) Vasculitis in chronic urticaria: an immunopathologic study. J Invest Dermatol 76:103–107

Natbony SF, Phillips ME, Elias JM, Godfrey HP, Kaplan AP (1983) Histologic studies of chronic idiopathic urticaria. J Allergy Clin Immunol 71:177–183

Neumann HAM, Berretty PJM, Reinders Folmer SCC, Cormane RH (1981) Hepatitis B surface antigen deposition in the blood vessel walls of urticarial lesions in acute hepatitis B. Br J Dermatol 104:383–388

O'Loughlin S, Shroeter AL, Jordon RE (1978) Chronic urticaria-like lesions in systemic lupus erythematosus. A review of 12 cases. Arch Dermatol 114:879–883

Phanuphak P, Kohler PF, Stanford RE, Schocket AL, Carr RI, Claman HN (1980) Vasculitis in chronic urticaria. J Allergy Clin Immunol 65:436–444

Provost TT, Zone JJ, Synkowski O, Maddison PJ, Reichlin M (1980) Unusual cutaneous manifestations of systemic lupus erythematosus: I. urticaria-like lesions. Correlation with clinical and serological abnormalities. J Invest Dermatol 75:495–499

Pussell BA, Lockwood CM, Scott DM, Pinching AJ, Peters DK (1978) Value of immune complex assay in diagnosis and management. Lancet II:359–363

Sanchez NP, Winkelmann RK, Schroeter AL, Dicken CH (1982) The clinical and histopathologic spectrums of urticarial vasculitis: study of forty cases. J Am Acad Dermatol 7:599–605

Sissons JGP, Williams DG, Peters DK, Boulton-Jones JM, Goldsmith HJ (1974) Skin lesions, angioedema and histocomplementemia. Lancet II:1350–1352

Small P, Barrett D, Champlin E (1982) Chronic urticaria and vasculitis. Ann Allergy 48:172–174

Soter NA (1977) Chronic urticaria as a manifestation of necrotizing vasculitis. New Engl J Med 296:1440–1442

Soter NA, Austen KF, Gigli I (1974) Urticaria and arthralgias as a manifestation of necrotizing angiitis (vasculitis). J Invest Dermatol 63:485–490

Synkowski DR, Levine MI, Pabin BS, Unis EJ (1979) Urticaria: an immunofluorescence and histopathologic study. Arch Dermatol 115:1192–1194

Tuffanelli DL, Dubois EL (1964) Cutaneous manifestations of necrotizing vasculitis. Arch Dermatol 90:377–386

Wanderer AA, Nuss DD, Torney AD, Gidas PC (1983) Urticaria leukocytoclastic vasculitis with cold urticaria. Arch Dermatol 119:145–151

Wands JR, Perrotto JL, Isselbacher KJ (1976) Granulating immune complexes and complement sequence activation in infectious mononucleosis. Am J Med 60:269–272

Wechsler HL (1983) Lupus erythematosus: a clinician's coign of vantage. Arch Dermatol 119:877–882

Wolff HH, Maciejewski W, Scherer R, Braun-Falco O (1978) Immunoelectronmicroscopic examination of early lesions in histamine induced immune complex vasculitis in man. Br J Dermatol 99:13–24

Wüthrich B (1979) Immunglobuline (IgG, IgA, IgM und IgE) und Komplementfaktoren (C3, C4 und C1-Inhibitor) bei Urticaria chronica. Dermatol Mschr 165:191–197

Zeiss CR, Burch FX, Marder RJ, Furey NL, Schmid FR, Gewurz H (1980) Hypocomplementemic vasculitic urticarial syndrome: report of four new cases and definition of disease. Am J Med 68:867–875

Chapter 9 (Mastocytosis)

Ammann R, Spycher Ch (1972) Malabsorptionssyndrom bei generalisierter Mastocytose (Urticaria pigmentosa). Schweiz Med Wschr 102:213–220

Bakos L, Storck R, Silveiro Netto E (1972) Congenital macular urticaria pigmentosa, complicated by massive nodular mastocytosis with systemic involvement. Br J Dermatol 87:635–641

Caplan RM (1963) The natural course of urticaria pigmentosa. Analysis and follow-up of 112 cases. Arch Dermatol 87:146–157

Cook JE (1969) Canine mast cell diseases. In: Lingemann CH, Garner FM (eds) Comparative morphology of hematopoietic neoplasms. Natl Cancer Inst Monogr 32:267–283

Czarnetzki BM, Figdor CG, Kolde G, Vroom T, Aalberse R, de Vries JE (1984) Development of human connective tissue mast cells from purified blood monocytes. Immunology 51:549–554

Czarnetzki BM, Rosenbach T, Kolde G, Frosch PJ (1985) Phototherapy of urticaria pigmentosa: Clinical response and changes of cutaneous reactivity, histamine and chemotactic leukotrienes. Arch Dermatol Res 277:105–113

Czarnetzki BM, Sterry W, Bazin M, Kalveram KJ (1982) Evidence that tissue mast cell derive from mononuclear phagocytes. Int Archs Allergy Appl Immunol 67:44–48

Demis DJ (1963) The mastocytosis syndrome: Clinical and biological studies. Ann Intern Med 59:194–206

Demis DJ, Walton MD, Higdon RS (1961) Histaminuria in urticaria pigmentosa. Arch Dermatol 83:127–138

Desmons F (1980) Kutane Manifestation der Mastozytosen beim Kind anhand von 18 Beobachtungen. Hautarzt 31:56–62

Drennan JM, Beare JM (1954) Solitary mast cell nevus. J Path Bact 68:345–358

Freeman RG (1967) Diffuse urticaria pigmentosa. An ultrastructural study before and after whealing. Am J Clin Pathol 48:187–199

Granerus G, Olafsson JH, Roupe G (1983) Studies on histamine metabolism in mastocytosis. J Invest Dermatol 80:410–416

Hughes J, Warin RP (1963) Diffuse cutaneous mastocytosis. Br J Dermatol 75:296–297

James MP, Eady RAJ (1981) Familial urticaria pigmentosa with giant mast cell granules. Arch Dermatol 117:713–718

Johnson WC, Helwig RB (1961) Solitary mastocytosis (urticaria pigmentosa). Arch Dermatol 84:806–815

Kitamura Y, Shimada M, Hatanaka K, Miyano Y (1977) Development of mast cells from grafted bone marrow cells in irradiated mice. Nature 268:442–443

Klaus SN, Winkelmann RK (1962) Course of urticaria pigmentosa in children. Arch Dermatol 86:68–71

Kolde G, Frosch PJ, Czarnetzki BM (1984) Response of cutaneous mast cells to PUVA in patients with urticaria pigmentosa. Histomorphometric, ultrastructural and biochemical investigations. J Invest Dermatol 83:175–178

Lennert K (1962) Zur pathologischen Anatomie von Urticaria pigmentosa und Mastzellenretikulose. Klin Wschr 40:61–67

Ludatscher RM, Haim S, Gellei B, Cohen A (1977) Comparative ultrastructural study of mast cells in mastocytoma and mastocytosis. Dermatologica 155:80–89

Mihm MC, Clark WH, Reed RJ, Caruso MG (1973) Mast cell infiltrates of the skin and the mastocytosis syndrome. Hum Pathol 4:231–239

Nettleship E (1869) Rare forms of urticaria. Br Med J 2: 323–324

Ouwendijk RJT, Zijlstra FJ, Wilson JHP, Bonta IL, Vincent JE, Stolz E (1983) Raised plasma levels of thromboxane B_2 in systemic mastocytosis. Eur J Clin Invest 13:227–229

Roberts LJ, Sweetman BJ, Lewis RA, Austen KF, Oates JA (1980) Increased production of prostaglandin D_2 in patients with systemic mastocytosis. New Engl J Med 303:1400–1404

Robinson HM Jr, Kile RL, Hitch JM, Raleigh NC, Robinson RCV (1962) Bullous urticaria pigmentosa. Arch Dermatol 85:346–354

Rodermund OE, Biersack HJ, Rohner HG (1978) Szintigraphische Veränderungen an Leber und Milz bei Urticaria pigmentosa. Hautarzt 29:478–480

Sagher F, Even-Paz Z (1967) Mastocytosis and the mast cell. Karger, Basel-New York

Sahihi T, Esterly NB (1972) Atypical diffuse cutaneous mastocytosis. Am J Dis Child 124:133–135

Thueson SO, Speck LS, Lett-Brown MA, Grant A (1979) Histamine-releasing activity (HRA). I. Production by mitogen- or antigen-stimulated human mononuclear cells. J Immunol 123:628–632

Unna PG (1887) Beiträge zur Anatomie und Pathogenese der Urtikaria simplex und pigmentosa. Dermatol Studien H3, Voss, Hamburg Leipzig

Vella-Briffa D, Eady RAJ, James MP, Gatti S, Bleehen SS (1983) Photochemotherapy (PUVA) in the treatment of urticaria pigmentosa. Br J Dermatol 109:67–75

Webb TA, Lai CH, Lung TY (1982) Systemic mast cell disease: A clinical and hematopathologic study of 26 cases. Cancer 49:927–938

Willemze R, Reuter DJ, Scheffer E, Van Vloten WA (1980) Diffuse cutaneous mastocytosis with multiple cutaneous mastocytomas. Br J Dermatol 102:601–607

Chapter 10 (Diagnosis)

Adkinson NF (1980) The radioallergosorbent test: Uses and abuses. J Allergy Clin Immunol 65:1–4

American Academy of Allergy (1981) Position statement – controversial techniques. J Allergy Clin Immunol 67:333–338

Bar-Sela S, Shalit M, Kalbfleisch JH, Fink JN (1983) The relative value of skin tests and radioallergosorbent test in the diagnosis of bee sting hypersensitivity. J Allergy Clin Immunol 72:690–694

Cook TJ, MacQueen DM, Wittig HJ, Thornby JI, Lautos RL, Virtue CM (1973) Degree and duration of skin test suppression and side effects with antihistamines. J Allergy Clin Immunol 51:71–77

David TJ (1984) Anaphylactic shock during elimination diets for severe atopic eczema. Arch Dis Childhood 59:983–986

Diamant B, Patkar S (1982) Histamine release from washed whole blood. Int Arch Allergy Appl Immunol 67:13–17

Doeglas HMG, Nater JP (1968) Histamine in foods causing false positive scratch tests. J Allergy 42:164–168

Doyle AC (1901) The complete adventures and memoirs of Sherlock Holmes. Strand Magazine (Facsimile) Avenel Books Crown Publishers Inc 1976, New York

Galant S, Zippin C, Bullock J, Crisp J (1972) Allergy skin test: I Antihistamine inhibition. Ann Allergy 30:53–63

Galant SP, Bullock J, Wong D, Maibach HI (1973) The inhibitory effect of anti-allergy drugs on allergen and histamine induced wheal and flare response. J Allergy Clin Immunol 51:11–21

Gronemeyer W, Debelic M (1967) Der sogenannte "Reibtest", seine Anwendung und klinische Bedeutung. Dermatologica 134:208–218

Hirsch SR, Zastrow JE (1972) Basophil degranulation: A new method of observation and its correlation to skin testing. J Allergy Clin Immunol 50:338–347

Illig L (1977) Moderne Aspekte der Urticariapathogenese unter besonderer Berücksichtigung des Intoleranz-Phänomens. Hautarzt 28:102–112

Kraig M, Jacobson KW, Branch LB, Nelson HS (1980) Laboratory tests in chronic urticaria. JAMA 243: 1644–1646

Lee RE, Smolensky MH, Leach CS, McGovern JP (1977) Circadian rhythms in the cutaneous reactivity to histamine and selected antigens, including phase relationship to urinary cortisol excretion. Ann Allergy 38:231–236

Lichtenstein LM, Osler AG (1964) Studies on the mechanism of hypersensitivity phenomena. IX. Histamine release from human leukocytes by ragweed pollen allergens. J Exp Med 120:507–530

Ménardo JL, Bousquet J, Rodière M, Astruc J, Michel F-B (1985) Skin test reactivity in infancy. J Allergy Clin Immunol 75:646–651

Merget R, Schultze-Werninghaus G (1983) Allergiehauttest trotz antiallergischer Therapie. Dtsch Med Wschr 108:1250–1253

Metcalfe DD (1984) Food hypersensitivity. J Allergy Clin Immunol 73:749–762

Nelson HS (1981) Effect of preservatives and conditions of storage on the potency of allergy extracts. J Allergy Clin Immunol 67:64–69

Nelson HS (1983) Diagnostic procedures in allergy. I. Allergy skin testing. Ann Allergy 51:411–418

Nyfors A, Heegaard H (1968) The influence of corticosteroids on the allergic skin wheal reaction. Acta Allergologica 23:130–135

Shelley WB, Juhlin L (1961) A new test for detecting anaphylactic sensitivity: The basophil reaction. Nature 191:1056–1058

Shereff RH, Harwell W, Lieberman P, Rosenberg EW, Robinson H (1973) Effect of beta adrenergic stimulation and blockade on immediate hypersensitivity skin test reactions. J Allergy Clin Immunol 52:328–333

Siraganian RP (1977) Automated histamine analysis for in vitro allergy testing. J Allergy Clin Immunol 59:214–222

Slott RI, Zweiman B (1974) A controlled study of the effect of corticosteroids on immediate skin test reactivity. J Allergy Clin Immunol 54:229–234

Speer F, Casas Carrasco L, Kimura CC (1978) The management of urticaria. Ann Allergy 40:387–392

Stemmler M, Lischka G (1979) Urticaria – reasonable diagnostic proceeding. Akt Dermatol 5:131–134

Voorhorst R, van Krieken H (1973a) Atopic skin test reevaluated. I. Perfection of skin testing technique. Ann Allergy 31:137–142

Voorhorst R, van Krieken H (1973b) Atopic skin test reevaluated. II. Variability in results of skin testing done in octuplicate. Ann Allergy 31:195–204

Wide L, Bennich H, Johansson SGO (1967) Diagnosis of allergy by an in vitro test for allergen antibodies. Lancet II:1105–1107

Wortmann F (1984) Allergie-Diagnostik in der Praxis und ihre pathophysiologischen Grundlagen. Z Allg Med 60:45–50

Wüthrich B, Kopper E (1978) Bedeutung des radio-allergosorbens-tests (RAST) in der spezifischen Diagnostik des atopischen asthma bronchiale. Dtsch Med Wschr 103:603–609

Chapter 11 (Therapy)

Agostini A, Bergamaschini L, Martignoni G, Cicardi M, Marasini B (1980) Treatment of acute attacks of hereditary angioedema with C1 inhibitor concentrate. Ann Allergy 44:299–301

Agostini A, Marasini B, Cicardi M, Martignoni G, Uziel L, Pietrogrande M (1978) Hepatic function and fibrinolysis in patients with hereditary angioedema undergoing long-term treatment with tranexamic acid. Allergy 33:216–221

Altounyan REC (1980) Review of clinical activity and mode of action of sodium cromoglycate. Clin Allergy 10 (suppl): 481–489

Ash AS, Schild HO (1966) Receptors mediating some actions of histamine. Br J Pharmac Chemother 27:427–439

Atkins PC, Zweiman B (1981) Mediator release in local heat urticaria. J Allergy Clin Immunol 68:286–289

Baart de la Faille H, Rottier PB, Baart de la Faille-Kuyper EH (1975) Solar urticaria. A case with possible increase of skin mast cells. Br J Dermatol 92:101–107

Bacal E, Patterson R, Zeiss CR (1978) Evaluation of severe (anaphylactic) reactions. Clin Allergy 8:295–304

Bentley-Phillips CB, Kobza-Black A, Greaves MW (1976) Reduced intolerance in cold urticaria caused by cold-evoked histamine release. Lancet II:63–66

Bernhard JD, Jaenicke K, Khosnow Momtza T, Parrish JA (1984) Ultraviolet-A phototherapy in the prophylaxis of solar urticaria. J Am Acad Dermatol 10:29–33

Berova N, Petkow I, Andreev VC (1974) Treatment of chronic urticaria with a proteinase (kallikrein) inhibitor. Br J Dermatol 90:431–434

Black JW, Duncan WAM, Durant CJ, Ganellin CR, Parsons EM (1972) Definition and antagonism of histamine H_2-receptors. Nature 236:385–390

Blohmé G (1972) Treatment of hereditary angioneurotic oedema with tranexamic acid. A random double-blind cross-over study. Acta Med Scand 192:293–298

Boot JR, Sweatman WJF, Cox BA, Stone K, Dawson W (1982) The anti-allergic activity of benoxaprofen [2-(4-chlorophenyl)-α-methyl-5-benzoxazole acetic acid] – a lipoxygenase inhibitor. Int Arch Allergy Appl Immunol 67:340–343

Bork K, Kreuz W, Witzke G (1984) Hereditäres angioneurotisches Ödem. Dtsch Med Wschr 109:1331–1335

Boxer LA, Allen JM, Baehner RL (1980) Diminished polymorphonuclear leukocyte adherence. J Clin Invest 66:268–274

Brackertz D (1974) Hereditäres angioneurotisches Ödem: therapeutische Aspekte. Schweiz Med Wschr 104:403–405

Breathnach SM, Allen R, Ward AM, Greaves MW (1983) Symptomatic dermographism: Natural history, clinical features, laboratory investigations and response to therapy. Clin Exp Dermatol 8:463–476

Businco L, Cantani A, Businco E, Pepys J (1984) Systemic mastocytosis in a 5-year-old child: successful treatment with disodium cromoglycate. Clin Allergy 14:147–152

Callen JP, Kalbfleisch S (1982) Urticarial vasculitis: a report of nine cases and review of the literature. Br J Dermatol 107:87–94

Cap JP, Schwanitz HJ, Czarnetzki BM (1985) Die Wirkung von Ketotifen bei der Urticaria factitia und der Urticaria cholinergica im gekreuzten Doppelblindversuch. Hautarzt, 36:509–511

Casale TB, Shelhamer JH, Parrillo JE, Kaliner MA (1984) Dopamine inhibition of histamine-mediated cutaneous responses. J Allergy Clin Immunol 73:837–841

Cerio R, Lessof MH (1984) Treatment of chronic idiopathic urticaria with terfenadine. Clin Allergy 14:139–141

Champion RH, Lachmann PJ (1969) Hereditary angiooedema treated with ε-aminocaproic acid. Br J Dermatol 81:763–765

Chang HK, Morrison SL (1979) Bone marrow suppression associated with cimetidine. Ann Int Med 91:580

Christophers E, Hönigsmann H, Wolff K, Langner A (1978) PUVA-treatment of urticaria pigmentosa. Brit J Dermatol 98:701–702

Cicardi M, Bergamaschini L, Tucci A, Agostini A, Tornaghi G, Coggi G, Colombi R, Viale G (1983) Morphologic evaluation of the liver in hereditary angioedema patients on long-term treatment with androgen derivatives. J Allergy Clin Immunol 72:294–298

Claman HN (1975) How corticosteroids work. J Allergy Clin Immunol 55:145–151

Cohen G, Peterson A (1972) Treatment of hereditary angioedema with frozen plasma. Ann Allergy 30:690–692

Cohen SH, Koethe SM, Kozin F, Rodey G, Arkins JA, Fink JN (1978) Acquired angioedema associated with rectal carcinoma and its response to danazol therapy. J Allergy Clin Immunol 62:217–221

Commens CA, Greaves MW (1978) Cimetidine in chronic idiopathic urticaria: a randomized double-blind study. Br J Dermatol 99:675–679

Cook J, Shuster S (1983a) The effect of H1 and H2 recepter

antagonists on the dermographic response. Acta Derm Venereol (Stockh) 63:260–262
Cook LJ, Shuster S (1983b) Lack of effect of cimetidine in chronic-idiopathic urticaria. Acta Derm Venereol (Stockh) 63:265–267
Curtis AC, Brechner Owens B (1945) Beta dimethylaminoethyl benzhydryl ether hydrochloride (Benadryl) in treatment of urticaria. Arch Derm Syphilol 52:239–242
Czarnetzki BM (1983) A double-blind cross-over study of the effect of ketotifen in urticaria pigmentosa. Dermatologica 166:44–47
Czarnetzki BM, Behrendt H (1981) Urticaria pigmentosa: clinical picture and response to oral disodium cromoglycate. Brit J Dermatol 105:563–567
Czarnetzki BM, Rosenbach T, Kolde G, Frosch PJ (1985) Phototherapy of urticaria pigmentosa: Clinical response and changes of cutaneous reactivity, histamine and chemotactic leukotrienes. Arch Dermatol Res 277:105–113
Daëron M, Sterk AR, Hirata F, Ishizaka T (1982) Biochemical analysis of glucocorticoid-induced inhibition of IgE-mediated histamine release from mouse mast cells. J Immunol 129:1212–1218
Daman L, Lieberman P, Ganier M, Hashimoto K (1978) Localized heat urticaria. J Allergy Clin Immunol 61:273–278
Davis KC, Mekori YA, Kohler PF, Schocket AL (1984) Late cutaneous reactions (LCR) in patients with delayed pressure urticaria (DPU). J Allergy Clin Immunol 73:183 (abstract)
Davis PJ, Davis FB, Charache P (1974) Long-term therapy of hereditary angioedema (HAE). Preventive management with fluoxymesterone and oxymetholone in severely affected males and females. U Hopk Med J 135:391–398
Demaubeuge J, Tennstedt D, Broux R (1982) Does mast cell protection plus mediator antagonism surpass the effect of a classic antihistaminic in the treatment of chronic urticaria? A double-blind comparison of oxatomide and mequitazine. Dermatologica 164:386–394
de Moragas JM, Giménez-Camarasa M, Norguera J (1973) Localized heat urticaria. Arch Dermatol 108:684–686
Doeglas HMG (1975) Chronic Urticaria. Proefschrift, Rijksuniversiteit Groningen, Dijkstra Niemeyer, Groningen
Domschke S, Domschke W (1980) New Histamine H2-receptor antagonists. Hepato-Gastroenterology 27:163–168
Duke WW (1924) Urticaria caused specifically by the action of physical agents. JAMA 83:3–9
Evans S, Vickers CFH (1981) Bullous urticaria pigmentosa (cutaneous mastocytosis) and sodium cromoglycate. Acta Derm Venereol 61:572–575
Fairley JA, Pentland AP, Voorhees JJ (1984) Urticaria pigmentosa responsive to nifedipine. J Am Acad Dermatol 11:740–743
Farnam J, Grant JA, Guernsey BG, Jorizzo JL, Petrusa ER (1984) Successful treatment of chronic idiopathic urticaria and angioedema with cimetidine alone. J Allergy Clin Immunol 73:842–845
Fenske NA, Lober CW, Pautler SE (1985) Congenital bullous urticaria pigmentosa. Arch Dermatol 121:115–118
Fields DAS, Pillar J, Diamantis W, Perhach JL, Sofia RD, Chand N (1984) Inhibition by azelastine of nonallergic histamine release from rat peritoneal mast cells. J Allergy Clin Immunol 73:400–403
Finn R, Cohen HN (1978) Food Allergy: Fact or fiction? Lancet I:426–428
Frank MM, Gelfand JA, Atkinson JP (1976) Hereditary angioedema: the clinical syndrome and its management. Ann Intern Med 84:580–593
Frank MM, Sergent JS, Kane MA, Alling DW (1972) Epsilon aminocaproic acid therapy of hereditary angioneurotic edema. New Engl J Med 286:808–812
Gadek JE, Hosea SW, Gelfand JA, Frank MM (1979) Response of variant hereditary angioedema phenotypes to danazol therapy. J Clin Invest 64:280–286
Gadek JE, Hosea SW, Gelfand JA, Santaella M, Wickerhauser M, Triantaphyllopoulos DC, Frank MM (1980) Replacement therapy in hereditary angioedema. Successful treatment of acute episodes of angioedema with partly purified C1 inhibitor. N Engl J Med 302:542–546
Gee JBL, Stevens CA, Hinman LM (1980) Elastase and lysozyme secretion by peritoneal macrophages: Effects of dexamethasone and rifampin. Bull Europ Physiopath Resp 16 (Suppl): 415–421
Gelfand JA, Sherins RJ, Alling DW, Frank MM (1976) Treatment of hereditary angioedema with danazol. N Engl J Med 295:1444–1448
Gibson A, Clancy R (1980) Management of chronic idiopathic urticaria by the identification and exclusion of dietary factors. Clin Allergy 10:699–704
Gibson JR, Harvey SG, Barth JH, Moss MY, Burke CA (1984) An assessment of the novel antihistamine BW 825 C in the treatment of chronic idiopathic urticaria. Dermatologica 169:179–183
Glowania HJ, Schulz KH (1981) Zur Hyposensibilisierungsbehandlung mit Bienen- und Wespengift. Allergologie 4:60–66
Goodman LS, Gilman A (1980) The pharmacological basis of therapeutics. Macmillan Publishing Co, New York
Grant JA, Findlay SR, Thueson DO, Fine DP, Krueger GG (1981) Local heat urticaria/ angioedema: Evidence for histamine release without complement activation. J Allergy Clin Immunol 67:75–77
Greaves MW, Sneddon IB, Smith AK, Stanworth DR (1974) Heat urticaria. Br J Dermatol 90:289–292
Greenberger PA, Patterson R, Radin RC (1984) Two pretreatment regimens for high-risk patients receiving radiographic contrast media. J Allergy Clin Immunol 74:540–543
Gurd JG, Zuraw BL (1984) Efficacy of hydroxychloroquine treatment on urticarial vasculitis. J Allergy Clin Immunol 73:181 (abstract)
Gwynn CM (1974) Therapy in hereditary angioneurotic oedema. Arch Dis Childhood 49:636–640
Halpern BN (1942) Les antihistaminiques de synthèse: essais de chimiothérapie des états allergiques. Arch Int Pharmacodyn Thér 68:339–408
Harries MG, O'Brien IM, Burge PS, Pepys J (1978) Effects of orally administered sodium cromoglycate in asthma and urticaria due to foods. Clin Allergy 8:423–427
Harvey RP, Schocket AL (1980) The effect of H1 and H2 blockade on cutaneous histamine response in man. J Allergy Clin Immunol 65:136–139
Harvey RP, Wegs J, Schocket AL (1981) A controlled trial of therapy in chronic urticaria. J Allergy Clin Immunol 68:262–266
Hasei K, Ichihashi M (1982) Solar urticaria. Determinations of action and inhibition spectra. Arch Dermatol 118:346–350

Haustein UF, Kirchhoff B (1984) Die Behandlung der erworbenen Kälteurtikaria mit Ketotifen. Dermatol Mschr 170:536–537

Highet AS (1980) Urticarial vasculitis resembling systemic lupus erythematosus: efficacy of prednisone and dapsone combined. Br J Dermatol 102:358–360

Hindson C, Daymond T, Diffey B, Lawlor F (1982) Side effects of benoxaprofen. Brit Med J 284:138–139

Hintner H, Tappeiner G (1979) Nekrotisierende Vaskulitis-Manifestation als Urtikaria. Hautarzt 30:484–488

Hintner H, Tappeiner G, Gschnait F, Schwarz S, Wolff K (1979) Danazoltherapie des hereditären Angioödems. Dtsch Med Wschr 36:1269–1273

Hirata F (1981) The regulation of lipomodulin, a phospholipase inhibitory protein in rabbit neutrophils by phosphorylation. J Biol Chem 246:7730–7733

Hirata F, Axelrod J, Crews FT (1979) Concanavalin A stimulates phospholipid methylation and phosphatidylserine decarboxylation in rat mast cells. Proc Natl Acad Sci USA 76:4813–4816

Hirata F, Notsu Y, Iwata M, Parente L, DiRosa M, Flower RJ (1982) Identification of several species of phospholipase inhibitory proteins by radioimmunoassay for lipomodulin. Biochem Biophys Res Commun 109:223–230

Hirata F, Toyoshima S, Axelrod J, Waxdal MJ (1980) Phospholipid methylation: A biochemical signal modulating lymphocyte mitogenesis. Proc Natl Acad Sci USA 77:862–865

Horio T (1978) Photoallergic urticaria induced by visible light. Additional cases and further studies. Arch Dermatol 114:1761–1764

Horio T, Minami K (1977) Solar urticaria: Photoallergen in a patient's serum. Arch Dermatol 113:157–160

Horton BT, Brown GE, Roth GM (1936) Hypersensitiveness to cold. JAMA 107:1263–1269

Hosea SW, Frank MM (1980) Danazol in the treatment of hereditary angioedema. Drugs 19:370–372

Hutchcroft BJ, Moore EG, Orange RP (1979) The effect of H1 and H2 receptor antagonism on the response of monkey skin to intradermal histamine, reverse-type anaphylaxis, and passive cutaneous anaphylaxis. J Allergy Clin Immunol 63:376–382

Ignarro LJ (1977) Glucocorticosteroid inhibition of nonphagocytic discharge of lysosomal enzymes from human neutrophils. Arthritis Rheum 19:73–83

Illig L, Paul E (1978) Die Stellung der Antihistaminika in der Urtikariatherapie. Hautarzt 29:407–415

Irwin R, Lieberman P, Kaplan R, Kaliner M, Treadwell G, Yoo T (1984) Mediator release in local heat urticaria (LHU): Protection with combined H1 and H2 antagonists. J Allergy Clin Immunol 73:181 (abstract)

Ishizaka K (1984) Regulation of IgE synthesis. Ann Rev Immunol 2:159–182

Jaffe CJ, Atkinson JP, Gelfand JA, Frank MM (1975) Hereditary angioedema: The use of fresh frozen plasma for prophylaxis in patients undergoing oral surgery. J Allergy Clin Immunol 55:386–393

Johansson EA, Reunala T, Koskimies S, Lagerstedt A, Kauppinen K, Timonen K (1984) Localized heat urticaria associated with a decrease in serum complement factor B (C_3 proactivator). Brit J Dermatol 110:227–231

Johnson GJ, Silvis SE, Roitman B, Blumenthal M, Gilbert HS (1980) Long-term treatment of systemic mastocytosis with histamine H_2 receptor antagonists. Am J Gastroenterol 74:485–489

Jones RR, Bhogal B, Dash A, Schifferli J (1983) Urticaria and vasculitis: a continuum of histological and immunopathological changes. Brit J Dermatol 108:695–703

Juhlin L, Michaelsson G (1969) Use of a kallikrein inhibitor in the treatment of urticaria and hereditary angioedema. Acta Derm Venereol 49:37–44

Kaiser HB, Weisberg SC, Morris RJ (1980) Cimetidine in chronic urticaria. Lancet II:206

Kalimo K, Jansen CT (1980) Treatment of chronic urticaria with an inhibitor of complement activation (Cinnarizine). Ann Allergy 44:34–37

Kaliner M, Shelhamer JH, Ottesen EA (1982) Effects of infused histamine: Correlation of plasma histamine levels and symptoms. J Allergy Clin Immunol 69:283–289

Katz HI (1975) Anaphylactic syndromes. In: Moschella SL, Pillsburg DM, Harley HJ (eds) Dermatology. WB Saunders Co, Philadelphia, pp 219–238

Kaur S, Greaves M, Eftekhari N (1981) Factitious urticaria (dermographism) – treatment by cimetidine and chlorpheniramine in a randomized double-blind study. Br J Dermatol 104:185–190

Keahey TM, Lavker RM, Kaidbey KH, Atkins PC, Zweiman B (1984) Studies on the mechanism of clinical tolerance in solar urticaria. Br J Dermatol 110:327–338

Kennes B, De Maubeuge J, Delespesse G (1977) Treatment of chronic urticaria with a $beta_2$-adrenergic stimulant. Clin Allergy 7:35–39

Kobza A, Ramsay CA, Magnus IA (1973) Oral β carotene therapy in actinic reticuloid and solar urticaria. Br J Dermatol 88:157–166

Kobza-Black A, Keahey TM, Eady RAJ, Greaves MW (1981) Dissociation of histamine release and clinical improvement following treatment of acquired cold urticaria by prednisone. Br J Clin Pharmac 12:327–331

Kolde G, Frosch PJ, Czarnetzki BM (1984) Response of cutaneous mast cells to PUVA in patients with urticaria pigmentosa. Histomorphometric, ultrastructural and biochemical investigations. J Invest Dermatol 83:175–178

Kövary PM, Opferkuch W, Echternacht-Happle K, Happle R (1981) Effect of danazol on dysfunctional C1 inhibitor in a patient with angioedema. Arch Dermatol Res 270:119–122

Krause L, Shuster S (1983) Mode of action of H1 antihistamines in itch. Br J Dermatol 109 (Suppl 24): 30

Lagrue G, Moisy M, Intrator L, Belghiti D, Sobel A (1978) Traitement de l'oedème angio-neurotique héréditaire par les androgènes. Nouv Presse Méd 7:2927–2931

Landerman NS, Webster ME, Becker EL, Ratcliffe HE (1962) Hereditary angioneurotic edema: II. Deficiency of inhibitor for serum globulin permeability factor and/or plasma kallikrein. J Allergy 33:330–341

Leigh IM, Ramsay CA (1975) Localized heat urticaria treated by inducing tolerance to heat. Br J Dermatol 92:191–194

Leigh IM, Ramsay CA, Calnan CD (1974) Cold urticaria: Desensitization. Trans St Johns Hosp Dermatol Soc 60:40–42

Levine PH, Hardin JC, Scoon KL, Krinsky NI (1981) Effect of corticosteroids on the production of superoxide and hydrogen peroxide and the appearance of chemiluminescence by phagocytosing polymorphonuclear leukocytes. Inflammation 5:19–27

Lichtenstein LM, Valentine MD, Sobotka AK (1979) Insect allergy: The state of the art. J Allergy Clin Immunol 64: 5–12

Lieberman P, Taylor WW Jr (1979) Recurrent idiopathic anaphylaxis. Arch Intern Med 139:1032–1034

Liebeskind H, Schwarze G (1974) Zur Problematik der Penizillintherapie der Kältekontakturtikaria. Hautarzt 25:482–485

Lopez LR, Davis KC, Kohler PF, Schocket AL (1984) The hypocomplementemic urticarial vasculitis syndrome: Therapeutic response to hydroxychloroquine. J Allergy Clin Immunol 73:600–603

Lumry WR, Curd JG, Zeiger RS, Pleskow WW, Stevenson DD (1983) Aspirin-sensitive rhinosinusitis: the clinical syndrome and effects of aspirin administration. J Allergy Clin Immunol 71:580–587

Lundh B, Laurell AB, Wetterquist H, White T, Granerus G (1968) A case of hereditary angioneurotic edema, successfully treated with epsilon-aminocaproic acid. Studies on C1 esterase inhibitor, C1 activation, plasminogen level and histamine metabolism. Clin Exp Immunol 3:733–745

Madanes AE, Farber M (1982) Danazol. Ann Int Med 96:625–630

Mallorga J, Tallman JF, Henneberry DC, Hirata F, Strittmatter WJ, Axelrod J (1980) Mepacrine blocks β-adrenergic agonist-induced desensitization in astrocytoma cells. Proc Natl Acad Sci USA 77:1341–1345

Marcussen PV (1950) Dermographic prurigo: a syndrome with constitutional, psychic and mechanical etiology. Acta Dermatol Venerol 30:95–113

Matthews CNA, Boss JM, Warin RP, Storari F (1979) The effect of H1 and H2 histamine antagonists on symptomatic dermographism. Br J Dermatol 101:57–61

Matthews CNA, Kirby JD, James J, Warin RP (1973) Dermographism: reduction in weal size by chlorpheniramine and hydroxizine. Br J Dermatol 88: 279–282

Matthews CNA, Saihan EM, Warin RP (1978) Urticaria-like lesions associated with systemic lupus erythematosus: response to dapsone. Br J Dermatol 99:455–457

McDuffie FC, Sams WM, Maldonado JE, Andreini PH, Conn DL, Samayoa EA (1973) Hypocomplementemia with cutaneous vasculitis and arthritis. Possible immune complex syndrome. Mayo Clin Proc 48:340–348

Ménardo JL, Bousquet J, Delair L, Michel FB (1984) Treatment failures during maintenance therapy in honey bee venom allergy. J Allergy Clin Immunol 73:188

Michaelsson G, Ros AM (1971) Familial localized heat urticaria of delayed type. Acta Derm Venereol 51:279–283

Michell P, Hawk JLM, Shafrir A, Corbett MF, Magnus IA (1980) Assessing the treatment of solar urticaria: the dose-response as a quantifying approach. Dermatologica 160:198–207

Middleton C Jr, Drzewiecki G, Krishnarao D (1981) Quercitin: an inhibitor of antigen-induced human basophil histamine release. J Immunol 127:546–550

Millns JL, Randle HW, Solley GO, Dicken CH (1980) The therapeutic response of urticarial vasculitis to indomethacin. J Am Acad Dermatol 3:349–355

Monroe EW, Cohen SH, Kalbfleisch J, Schulz CI (1981) Combined H1 and H2 antihistamine therapy in chronic urticaria. Arch Dermatol 117:404–407

Moore PK, Hoult JRS (1980) Anti-inflammatory steroids reduce tissue PG synthetase activity and enhance PG breakdown. Nature 288:269–270

Moore-Robinson M, Warin RP (1968) Some clinical aspects of cholinergic urticaria. Br J Dermatol 80:794–799

Müller U (1981) Diagnose und Therapie der Insektenstichallergie heute. Allergologie 4:51–55

Myers G, Bloom F (1981) Cimetidine (Tagamet R) combined with steroids and H1 antihistamines for the prevention of serious radiographic contrast media reactions. Cathet Cardiovasc Diagn 7:65–71

Naclerio R, Mizrahi EA, Adkinson NF (1983) Immunologic observations during desensitization and maintenance of clinical tolerance to penicillin. J Allergy Clin Immunol 71:294–301

Neittaanmäki H, Myöhänen T, Fräki JE (1984) Comparison of cinnarizine, cyproheptadine, doxepin, and hydroxyzine in treatment of idiopathic cold urticaria: Usefulness of doxepin. J Am Acad Dermatol 11:483–489

Norman PS (1980) An overview of immunotherapy: Implications for the future. J Allergy Clin Immunol 65: 87–96

O'Loughlin S, Schroeter AL, Jordon RE (1978) Chronic urticaria-like lesions in systemic lupus erythematosus. A review of 12 cases. Arch Dermatol 114:879–883

Opferkuch W, Echternacht K, Gronemeyer W, Hammar CH, Jaeger U, Niemczyk H, Rieger C (1980) Klinische Ausprägung und Therapie des hereditären angioneurotischen Ödems (HANE). Immun Infekt 8:56–60

Orr TSC, Elliott EV, Altounyan REC, Stern MA (1980) Modulation of release of neutrophil chemotactic factor (NCF). Clinical Allergy 10 (Suppl):491–496

Parker CW (1975) Drug allergy (Third of three parts). N Engl J Med 292:957–960

Parrish JA, Jaenicke KF, Morison WL, Momtaz K, Shea C (1982) Solar urticaria: treatment with PUVA and mediator inhibitors. Br J Dermatol 106:575–580

Pence HL, Evans R, Guernsey LH, Gerhard RC (1974) Prophylactic use of epsilon aminocaproic acid for oral surgery in a patient with hereditary angioneurotic edema. J Allergy Clin Immunol 53:298–302

Peremans W, Mertens RLJ, Morias J, Campaert H (1981) Oxatomide in the treatment of chronic urticaria. A double-blind placebo-controlled trial. Dermatologica 162:42–50

Phanuphak P, Schocket Al, Kohler PF (1978) Treatment of chronic idiopathic urticaria with combined H1 and H2 blockers. Clin Allergy 8:429–433

Pickering RJ, Kelly JR, Good RA, Gewurz H (1969) Replacement therapy in hereditary angioedema. Successful treatment of two patients with fresh frozen plasma. Lancet I:326–330

Pitts JS, Donaldson VH, Firristal J, Wyatt RJ (1978) Remissions induced in hereditary angioneurotic edema with an attenuated androgen (danazol): correlation between concentrations of C1-inhibitor and the fourth and second components of complement. J Lab Clin Med 92:501–507

Pleskow WW, Stevenson DD, Mathison DA, Simon RA, Schatz M, Zeiger RS (1982) Aspirin desensitization in aspirin-sensitive asthmatic patients: clinical manifestations and characterization of the refractory period. J Allergy Clin Immunol 69:11–19

Pokropp A, Czarnetzki BM (1983) Untersuchungen zur Wirkung von intravenösem Kalzium auf experimentelle Quaddel- und Erythembildung. Allergologie 6:82–83

Ramsay CA (1977) Solar urticaria treatment by inducing tolerance to artificial radiation and natural light. Arch Dermatol 113:1222–1225

Ratanen T, Suhonen R (1980) Solar urticaria. A case with increased skin mast cells and good therapeutic response to an antihistamine. Acta Derm Venereol 60:363–365

Ravits M, Armstrong RB, Harber LC (1982) Solar urticaria. Clinical features and wavelength dependency. Arch Dermatol 118:228–231

Roberts LJ, Turk JW, Oates JA (1982) Shock syndrome associated with mastocytosis: pharmacologic reversal of the acute episode and therapeutic prevention of recurrent attacks. Adv Shock Res 8:145–152

Rosen FS, Austen KF (1976) Androgen therapy in hereditary angioneurotic edema. N Engl J Med 295:1476–1477

Rosse WF, Logue GL, Silberman HR, Frank MM (1976) The effect of synthetic androgens in hereditary angioneurotic edema: alteration of C1 inhibitor and C4 levels. Trans Ass Am Phys 89:122–132

Ruzicka T, Goerz G (1981) Systemic lupus erythematosus and vasculitic urticaria. Effect of dapsone and complement levels. Dermatologica 162:203–205

Saihan EM (1981) Ketotifen and terbutaline in urticaria. Br J Dermatol 104:205–206

Saihan EM, Littlewood SN (1983) Ketotifen and terbutaline in chronic urticaria. Br J Dermatol 109 (Suppl 24):31

Sauer RR, Steigleder GK (1983) The effect of ketotifen and oxatomide on histamine liberation following exposure in cold urticaria. Z Hautkr 58:1768–1772

Schleimer RP, MacGlashan DW Jr, Gillespie E, Lichtenstein LM (1982) Inhibition of basophil histamine release by antiinflammatory steroids. II. Studies on the mechanism of action. J Immunol 129:1632–1636

Schulz K-H (1974) Hereditäres Quincke-Ödem. Neuere Wege der Therapie. Der Hautarzt 25:12–16

Shea C, Morse ED (1978) Inhibition of human neutrophil chemotaxis by corticosteroids. Ann Clin Lab Sci 8:30–33

Sheffer AL, Craig JM, Willms-Kretschmer K, Austen KF, Rosen FS (1971) Histopathological and ultrastructural observations on tissues from patients with hereditary angioneurotic edema. J Allergy 47:292–297

Sheffer AL, Fearon DT, Austen KF (1979) Clinical and biochemical effects of impeded androgen (oxymetholone) therapy of hereditary angioedema. J Allergy Clin Immunol 64:275–280

Sigler RW, Evans R, Horakova Z, Ottesen E, Kaplan AP (1980) The role of cyproheptadine in the treatment of cold urticaria. J Allergy Clin Immunol 65:309–312

Sissons JGP, Williams DG, Peters DK (1974) Skin lesions, angioedema and hypocomplementemia. Lancet II:1350–1352

Smith JA, Mansfield LE, de Shazo RD, Nelson HS (1980) An evaluation of the pharmacologic inhibition of the immediate and late cutaneous reaction to allergen. J Allergy Clin Immunol 65:118–121

Soter NA (1977) Chronic urticaria as a manifestation of necrotizing venulitis. N Engl J Med 296:1440–1442

Soter NA, Austen KF, Wasserman SI (1979) Oral sodium cromoglycate in the treatment of systemic mastocytosis. N Engl J Med 301:465–469

Spangler DL, Vanderpool GE, Carroll MS, Tinkelman DG (1980) Terbutaline in the treatment of chronic urticaria. Ann Allergy 45:246–247

Spaulding WB (1960) Methyltestosterone therapy for hereditary episodic edema (hereditary angioneurotic edema). Ann Int Med 53:739–745

Starr JC, Brasher GW, Hammerschmidt DE (1980) Localized heat urticaria. Ann Allergy 44:164–165

Staub AM, Bovet D (1937) Action de la thymoxyéthyldiéthylamine (929 F) et des éthers phénoliques sur le choc anaphylactique du cobaye. CR Séanc Soc Biol 125:818–823

Stevenson DD, Pleskow WW, Simon RA, Mathison DA, Lumry WR, Schatz M, Zeiger RS (1984) Aspirin sensitive rhinosinusitis asthma: A double-blind crossover study of treatment with aspirin. J Allergy Clin Immunol 73:500–507

Sussman GL, Harvey RP, Schocket AL (1982) Delayed pressure urticaria. J Allergy Clin Immunol 70:337–342

Tappeiner G, Hintner H, Glatzl J, Wolff K (1979) Hereditary angio-oedema: Treatment with danazol. Report of a case. Br J Dermatol 100:207–212

Thormann J, Laurberg G, Zachariae H (1980) Oral sodium cromoglycate in chronic urticaria. Allergy 35:139–141

Urbanek R, Kuhn W, Forster J (1984) Prolonged venom immunotherapy: Specific IgE and IgG antibodies as criteria for discontinuation of treatment. J Allergy Clin Immunol 73:188

Valsecchi R, Cainelli T, Serra M (1977) Clinical use of cinnarizine in chronic urticaria. Chron Dermatol 8:883–887

Van der Horst J, Bronsveld W (1981) Urticarial vasculitis in a patient with systemic lupus erythematosus: a case report. Clin Exp Dermatol 6:489–494

Vaz GA, Tan LKT, Gerrard JW (1978) Oral cromoglycate in treatment of adverse reactions to foods. Lancet I:1066–1068

Vella Briffa D, Eady RAJ, James MP, Gatti S, Bleehen SS (1983) Photochemotherapy (PUVA) in the treatment of urticaria pigmentosa. Br J Dermatol 109:67–75

Verhaegen H, De Cree J (1980) Oxatomide in the treatment of idiopathic chronic urticaria. A placebo-controlled study. Allergologie 3:30–33

Verschave A, Stevens E, Degreef H (1983) Pseudo-allergen-free diet in chronic urticaria. Dermatologica 167:256–259

Wahn U, Müller J (1983) Mast cells and basophils: Models for studying the antianaphylactic potency of drugs. Ped Pharmacol 3:287–292

Wanderer AA, St Pierre JP, Ellis EF (1977) Primary acquired cold urticaria. Double-blind comparative study of treatment with cyproheptadine, chlorpheniramine, and placebo. Arch Dermatol 113:1375–1377

Wang SSM, Wang SR, Shieh WS (1984) The inhibitory effects of ketotifen on SRS activity and SRS production from human leukocytes. J Allergy Clin Immunol 73:193

Warin RP, Champion RH (1974) Urticaria. WB Saunders Co, London

Webster GF, Alexander JC, McArthur WP, Leyden JJ (1984) Inhibition of chemiluminescence in human neutrophils by dapsone. Br J Dermatol 110:657–663

Welch EA, Alper JC, Bogaars H, Farrell DS (1983) Treatment of bullous mastocytosis with disodium cromoglycate. J Am Acad Dermatol 9:349–353

Wells E, Mann J (1983) Phosphorylation of a mast cell protein in response to treatment with anti-allergic compounds. Biochem Pharmacol 32:837–842

Wennersten G (1980) Carotenoid treatment for light sensitivity: A reappraisal and six years' experience. Acta Derm Venereol 60:251–255

Werb Z (1978) Biochemical actions of glycocorticoids on macrophages in culture. Specific inhibition of elastase, collagenase, and plasminogen activator secretion and effects on other metabolic functions. J Exp Med 147:1695–1712

Werman BS, Rietschel RL (1981) Chronic urticaria from tantalum staples. Arch Dermatol 117:438–439

Willis I, Epstein JH (1974) Solar vs heat-induced urticaria. Arch Dermatol 110:389–392

Wise RD, Malkinson FD, Luskin A, Gewurs AT, Zeitz HJ (1978) Localized heat urticaria. Arch Dermatol 114:1079–1080

Wüthrich B (1979) Clinical and immunological studies on acquired heat contact urticaria. Dermatologica 159:371–376

Wüthrich B (1984) Allergie: Wer sollte hyposensibilisiert werden? Z Allg Med 60:67–75

Zachariae H, Laurberg G, Hjortshoj A (1975) Tranexamic acid in hereditary angioneurotic edema. Ugeskr Laeg 137:1106–1108

Zachariae H, Niordson AM, Henningsen SJ (1969) Indomethacin in urticaria and histamine induced wealing. A double-blind evaluation. Acta Derm Venereol 49:49–54

Index

MIX
Papier aus verantwortungsvollen Quellen
Paper from responsible sources
FSC® C105338

If you have any concerns about our products,
you can contact us on
ProductSafety@springernature.com

In case Publisher is established outside the EU,
the EU authorized representative is:
Springer Nature Customer Service Center GmbH
Europaplatz 3, 69115 Heidelberg, Germany

Printed by Libri Plureos GmbH
in Hamburg, Germany